A Clinician's Guide to Arteriogenesis

A Clinician's Guide to Arteriogenesis

Editor: Taryn Solomon

hayle medical
New York

Hayle Medical,
750 Third Avenue, 9th Floor,
New York, NY 10017, USA

Visit us on the World Wide Web at:
www.haylemedical.com

ISBN 978-1-64647-553-7 (Hardback)

Cataloging-in-Publication Data

A clinician's guide to arteriogenesis / edited by Taryn Solomon.
p. cm.
Includes bibliographical references and index.
ISBN 978-1-64647-553-7
1. Arteries--Growth. 2. Collateral circulation. 3. Neovascularization.
4. Blood-vessels--Growth. 5. Cardiology. I. Solomon, Taryn.
QP106.2 .C55 2023
612.133--dc23

Contents

Preface

The main aim of this book is to educate learners and enhance their research focus by presenting diverse topics covering this vast field. This is an advanced book which compiles significant studies by distinguished experts in the area of analysis. This book addresses successive solutions to the challenges arising in the area of application, along with it; the book provides scope for future developments.

Arteriogenesis is the increase in the diameter of arterial vessels. The process of development of arteries is supplemented by the migration of pericytes and smooth muscle cells (SMCs) from the epicardium. Majority of the SMCs of the coronary artery stem from the epicardium, however, SMCs of proximal coronary arteries originate from the neural chest. In terms of mechanical simulation, arteriogenesis is associated with elevated pressure which intensifies the stress on the radial wall, and elevates the flow which then intensifies the stress on endothelial surface. The diameter is increased by the vessel until the normalization of the stress. In terms of chemical simulation arteriogenesis is associated with upregulation of cell adhesion and cytokines receptors. The book aims to shed light on some of the unexplored aspects of arteriogenesis and the recent researches in this area of study. It will serve as a reference to a broad spectrum of readers.

It was a great honour to edit this book, though there were challenges, as it involved a lot of communication and networking between me and the editorial team. However, the end result was this all-inclusive book covering diverse themes in the field.

Finally, it is important to acknowledge the efforts of the contributors for their excellent chapters, through which a wide variety of issues have been addressed. I would also like to thank my colleagues for their valuable feedback during the making of this book.

Editor

1

Heterogeneity of Vascular Endothelial Cells, De Novo Arteriogenesis and Therapeutic Implications in Pancreatic Neuroendocrine Tumors

Bin Ren [1,2,3,4,5,6,*], J. Bart Rose [1,2], Yehe Liu [7], Renata Jaskular-Sztul [1,2,5], Carlo Contreras [1,2], Adam Beck [1] and Herbert Chen [1,2,5,6]

[1] Department of Surgery, University of Alabama at Birmingham, Birmingham, AL 35294, USA; jbrose@uabmc.edu (J.B.R.); rjsztul@uabmc.edu (R.J.-S.); ccontreras@uabmc.edu (C.C.); awbeck@uabmc.edu (A.B.); hchen@uabmc.edu (H.C.)

[2] O'Neal Comprehensive Cancer Center, University of Alabama at Birmingham, Birmingham, AL 35294, USA

[3] Nutrition & Obesity Research Center, University of Alabama at Birmingham, Birmingham, AL 35294, USA

[4] Diabetes Research Center, University of Alabama at Birmingham, Birmingham, AL 35294, USA

[5] Department of Biomedical Engineering, University of Alabama at Birmingham, Birmingham, AL 35294, USA

[6] Graduate Biomedical Science Program of the Graduate School, University of Alabama at Birmingham, Birmingham, AL 35294, USA

[7] Department of Biomedical Engineering, Case Western Reserve University, Cleveland, OH 44106, USA; yx1448@case.edu

* Correspondence: bren98@uab.edu

Abstract: Arteriogenesis supplies oxygen and nutrients in the tumor microenvironment (TME), which may play an important role in tumor growth and metastasis. Pancreatic neuroendocrine tumors (pNETs) are the second most common pancreatic malignancy and are frequently metastatic on presentation. Nearly a third of pNETs secrete bioactive substances causing debilitating symptoms. Current treatment options for metastatic pNETs are limited. Importantly, these tumors are highly vascularized and heterogeneous neoplasms, in which the heterogeneity of vascular endothelial cells (ECs) and de novo arteriogenesis may be critical for their progression. Current anti-angiogenetic targeted treatments have not shown substantial clinical benefits, and they are poorly tolerated. This review article describes EC heterogeneity and heterogeneous tumor-associated ECs (TAECs) in the TME and emphasizes the concept of de novo arteriogenesis in the TME. The authors also emphasize the challenges of current antiangiogenic therapy in pNETs and discuss the potential of tumor arteriogenesis as a novel therapeutic target. Finally, the authors prospect the clinical potential of targeting the FoxO1-CD36-Notch pathway that is associated with both pNET progression and arteriogenesis and provide insights into the clinical implications of targeting plasticity of cancer stem cells (CSCs) and vascular niche, particularly the arteriolar niche within the TME in pNETs, which will also provide insights into other types of cancer, including breast cancer, lung cancer, and malignant melanoma.

Keywords: angiogenesis; arteriogenesis; CD36; cancer stem cells; FoxO1; Notch; protein kinase D; neuroendocrine tumor; transdifferentiation

1. Introduction

Pancreatic neuroendocrine tumors (pNETs) represent a group of rare neoplasms that originate from pancreatic endocrine cells [1]. They are highly vascularized and heterogeneous neoplasms, which are characterized by high levels of vascular endothelial growth factor (VEGF) and its receptors [2], the potential driver in the metastatic process of pNETs [3], particularly in hepatic metastases [4]. PNETs also highly express platelet-derived growth factor receptors (PDGF-Rs), suggesting an increase in vascular maturation and arteriolar formation in the tumor microenvironment (TME). Sunitinib, a receptor tyrosine kinase (RTK) inhibitor and angiogenesis inhibitor targeting VEGFRs and PDGF-Rs, has been approved for the treatment of advanced pNETs. However, the therapeutic efficacy is limited, accompanied by high rates of progression. Therefore, tailoring antiangiogenic therapy to patients with pNETs requires novel insight into tumor angiogenesis. Recent advances in the understanding of the microenvironment biology of pNETs made VEGF and PDGF pathways interesting targets due to their associations with tumor angiogenesis [5,6], particularly their associations with the development of more mature tumor vessels and arterioles or "de novo arteriogenesis" in the TME.

Angiogenesis is considered one of the hallmarks in tumor growth and metastasis [7], in which the heterogeneity of vascular endothelial cells (ECs) and de novo arteriogenesis may play important roles and serve as new therapeutic targets, especially in highly angiogenic tumors such as pNETs. John Hunter, a British surgeon, was the first to coin the term angiogenesis by describing blood vessels that grow in reindeer antlers in 1787 [8]. Two centuries later, Dr. Judah Folkman, a surgeon at Harvard Medical School, further developed the concept of angiogenesis, which was defined as the development of new blood vessels from preexisting vessels via sprouting [9]. Mechanistically, angiogenesis is the growth and remodeling process of primitive networks into a complex network [10].

Broadly speaking, the growth of new blood vessels includes vasculogenesis, angiogenesis, arteriogenesis and venogenesis. Vasculogenesis is defined as the generation of blood vessels from hemangioblasts (endothelial precursors) during embryonic development of the cardiovascular system [11], including the initial formation of blood islands and tubes. This is followed by the development of vascular trees with the myriad of blood vessels to nourish all tissues and organs. Vasculogenesis can also occur during tumor progression, which may lead to the formation of immature and poorly functioning vascular networks [10].

Angiogenesis is a more generic concept referring to the formation of new microvessels [12]. This process is also known as neoangiogenesis under both ischemic and neoplastic conditions [13], where new capillaries are formed by sprouting or longitudinally splitting of preexisting blood vessels [14,15]. The capillary networks are fed by the arterioles, the terminal components of the arterial system via arteriogenesis.

Arteriogenesis refers to a process in which smooth muscle cells (SMCs) cover ECs during vascular myogenesis, accompanied by vascular stabilization. A typical change seen in arteriogenesis is the enlargement of preexisting arterioles [10]. However, an adult arteriogenesis can be a de novo process that occurs by blood vessel expansion and capillary arterialization [16–18]. Previous studies suggested that de novo arteriogenesis in adult organisms under ischemic and oncogenic conditions [19–21] could be associated with CD36 expression. CD36 is a key regulator in angiogenesis and fatty acid metabolism [22,23] and is a potential driver in metastatic cancer stem cells (CSCs) [24–26].

Venogenesis is used to define the formation of new venous vessels [27]. Similar to the ECs in the arteriogenesis, the venous ECs may generate different batches or concentrations of similar factors to complete the recruitment and differentiation of venous SMCs and the formation of new venules during angiogenic processes. The venule is the first ramification of the venous system that can drain blood and components in the microcirculation away from the capillary networks.

As for the tumor vasculature, it is highly heterogeneous with regard to their organization, function, and structure. Six distinct types of tumor-associated blood vessels have been identified in several types of human cancers and replicated in an animal model. These vessels develop into neoangiogenesis by three distinct but parallel interrelated processes: angiogenesis, arteriogenesis, and venogenesis [20,27,28], as well as vasculogenesis by the formation of capillaries via endothelial progenitor cells or cancer stem cells [29,30] (Figure 1).

These different angiogenic processes may be determined by heterogeneous groups of vascular ECs that constitute the linings of the entire vascular system within TMEs. Therefore, ECs that are heterogeneous in different microenvironments may determine the complexity and diversity of their functions by serving as versatile and multifunctional organs [31–33].

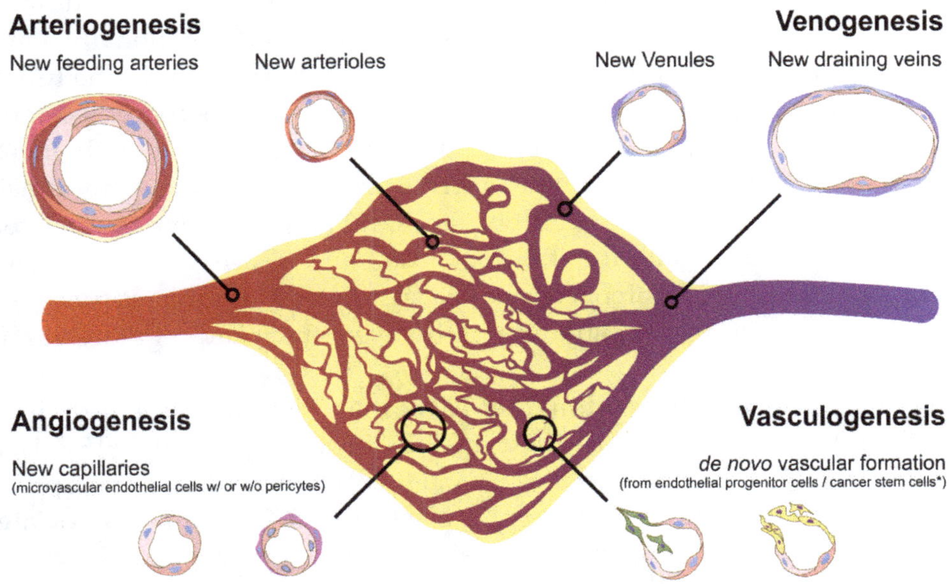

Figure 1. Heterogeneity of blood vessels in the tumor microenvironment. During tumor progression, new blood vascular networks will be developed to provide nutrients and oxygen and remove the metabolic wastes. They can also interact with other types of cells within the vascular niche. Shown is the formation of several types of blood vessels through processes, including de novo arteriogenesis, venogenesis, vascular remodeling, angiogenesis, and vasculogenesis.

2. Heterogeneity of Vascular Endothelial Cells

A variety of vascular ECs are the key cell type that constitutes different kinds of blood vessels, and capillary angiogenesis is primarily mediated by the assembly of ECs. However, ECs are extremely heterogeneous. This EC heterogeneity is responsible for the formation of heterogeneous blood vessels and is involved in normal tissue homeostasis and various pathologies. The local microenvironment likely causes phenotypic differences in vascular ECs via genetic, epigenetic, signaling, and cellular differentiation mechanisms [21,32,34]. The morphological, functional, and behavioral heterogeneity existing in the vascular ECs is accompanied by various differential gene expression profiles [19,21,34–37]. Additionally, ECs can sense and respond to various signals such as changes in local oxygenation, altered hemodynamic forces, and concentrations of signaling molecules from their microenvironment to maintain their functional heterogeneity. Paracrine signaling in the TME can regulate EC gene transcription, allowing for adaptive changes in a tissue-dependent manner. Therefore, the vascular endothelium should be considered as a consortium of distinct individual organs located within blood vessels, which are uniquely adapted to meet the demands of the specific microenvironments [32], such as TMEs.

EC heterogeneity actually occurs during angiogenic sprouting, where tip cells lead the way, followed by morphologically and functionally distinct stalk cells. During this process, Notch/VEGFR-signaling regulates the differential dynamics of VE-cadherin junctions and drives functional EC rearrangements [38]. Recent studies suggest that ECs such as microvascular ECs (MVECs) may undergo transdifferentiation and change into arteriolar ECs in response to specific environmental cues via stimulation of the protein kinase D (PKD-1) signaling pathway and epigenetic regulation of the activities of transcriptional factor FoxO1 [21,39]. Furthermore, forced expression of PKD-1, an important kinase in VEGF-mediated angiogenesis [40], can induce a tip cell phenotype [35]. These data suggested that certain ECs may inherently have genetic traits of tip cells, which can be induced epigenetically under specific temporal and spatial conditions, thereby coordinating with stalk cells to promote functional angiogenesis [41].

Phenotypic heterogeneity may also occur in tumor endothelium, including that of pNETs. Tumor-associated EC (TAEC) heterogeneity can be additive to the TME, tumor cell, and CSC heterogeneity. The ECs lining the tumor vessels are structurally and functionally abnormal, showing growth properties of cancer cells and projecting into the vessel lumen [42]. The tumor endothelium is covered by morphologically abnormal pericytes and demonstrates increased fenestrations with widened intercellular junctions or gaps. Therefore, the permeability is generally increased in certain tumor-associated vessels [43]. The TME where TAECs are exposed is unique, consisting of cancer and stromal cells such as tumor-associated fibroblasts (TAF) [44] and tumor-associated macrophages (TAM) [45]. Cancer cells may hijack the TAECs, TAFs, and TAMs for their own advantage via paracrine stromal interactions [46]. Moreover, hypoxia significantly stimulates tumor vessel growth by upregulating multiple pro-angiogenic signaling pathways, which can regulate vascular patterning, maturation, and function [47,48].

Intriguingly, the stromal cells within the TME may release cytokines, including soluble growth stimulators and inhibitors such as VEGF, FGF-2, thrombospondin-1 (TSP-1), and endostatin. These factors may regulate the behavior of TAECs via interaction with their receptors and influence the angiogenic status during tumor progression [20,39,40,49–53]. The tumor-associated vessels often appear to be more dilated and tortuous, show excessive branching morphogenesis, form arteriovenous shunts, and lack normal artery–capillary–vein hierarchy [54]. However, the vascular networks should have feeding arteriolar vessels, which can provide blood and nutrients in tumor tissues [55] and may also occur in pNETs. Therefore, TAECs may be critical in determining the angiogenic status and formation of the type of blood vessels within the TME. Unlike what researchers originally thought, TAECs are actually not genetically stable but unstable and show a different gene expression profile and respond differently to growth factors compared to normal ECs [56]. This may create complexity but also opportunities to discover new targeted therapy against tumor angiogenesis.

Added to the complexity of TAEC heterogeneity are the possibilities of CSC transformation into ECs. It has been shown that a sub-population of stem-like cells can generate ECs [30,57] due to the plasticity and transdifferentiation of cancer cells. These abnormal TAECs, in turn, release a variety of factors and cytokines to affect the tumor growth [58–60] and possibly to promote tumor metastasis. Moreover, tumors hijack physiological or developmental vascular endothelial processes, including angiogenic sprouting or vasculogenesis. They can develop vascular networks via vessel co-option or intussusception (splitting of pre-existing mother vessels to give rise to daughter vessels), and parasitize the host's vascular system to promote malignant progression [27,61,62], which may be involved in different TAECs and likely cooperates with stromal vascular cells, TAFs, TAMs, and other immune cells. Thus, TAEC heterogeneity may have a different impact on cancer behavior. Due to the heterogeneity of TAECs, it is a huge challenge to pinpoint a single overall function that defines the EC population. The arteriolar TAECs may express high levels of delta-like 4 (DLL4), a Notch ligand, which can interact with Notch receptors in CSCs to promote CSC maintenance and self-renewal. Therefore, arterial differentiation and arteriolar TAECs could be critical for the development of de novo arteriogenesis under ischemic conditions within the TME of well-vascularized tumors such as pNETs, thereby facilitating metastasis and leading to therapeutic resistance.

3. De Novo Arteriogenesis, an Emerging Concept of Formation of New Vascular Networks

Angiogenesis, as a hallmark of cancer, supplies oxygen and nutrients and disposes wastes, which is critical for tumor growth and metastatic spreading [9,63,64]. Tumor angiogenesis originally referred to new capillary growth by regeneration of a population of capillary ECs within a neoplasm [63]. Tumor cells cannot grow more than 2–3 mm in diameter without angiogenesis [65]. Tumor angiogenesis is regulated by VEGF prominently via VEGF receptor 2 (VEGFR-2) signaling in vascular ECs [53]. This signaling pathway is also required for angiogenic remodeling [66], an important process of vascular maturation and arteriogenesis. The anti-VEGF monoclonal antibody bevacizumab has shown certain clinical significance in multiple tumor types with limited efficacy, which probably results from its targeting mainly at the newly formed capillaries but not at matured tumor-associated vessels and newly formed tumor-associated arterioles [27] that we call de novo arteriogenesis.

There is a general belief that arteriogenesis refers to the remodeling process of pre-existing arteries or the increase in the lumen volume and size of the vessel wall, in which smooth muscle cell (SMC) proliferation may play an essential role [10,67,68]. However, de novo arteriogenesis represents the formation of new arteriolar networks via capillary arterialization, in which the proliferation and arteriolar differentiation of ECs, particularly MVECs, may be critical [17–19,21,69–72].

EphrinB2 represents the earliest specific marker for arterial ECs [73]. In Zebrafish, the gridlock gene, an HLH gene required for assembly of the aorta, specifies arterial fate [74,75] and regulates the Notch signaling pathway [76,77]. Inhibition of the Notch pathway in ECs by gridlock determines an arterial fate, while VEGF can upregulate the expression of ephrinB2 and stimulates the arterial fate of ECs [78–80]. Angiopoietins, a multifaceted cytokine that functions in angiogenesis, also regulates an arterial fate of ECs via modifying VEGF functions [80]. The small chemical molecule GS4898 can rescue the gridlock function in a Zebrafish model with a gridlock mutant phenotype [81,82]. This small chemical molecule promotes arterial differentiation via stimulating the MAPK/Erk pathway during postnatal angiogenesis in a mouse hindlimb ischemia model [19]. These studies suggest a role of de novo arteriogenesis during development and under ischemic conditions. The micro-CT imaging actually documented the occurrence of the newly formed arterioles under ischemic conditions [19].

Recent studies have shown that lysophosphatidic acid (LPA), a lipid signaling mediator, may facilitate the formation of functional arterioles in cooperation with VEGF in vivo [21]. This biological effect may be associated with FoxO-1 regulation of VEGF expression and crosstalk between VEGF signaling and the CD36 pathway [39]. Studies suggest that MVECs may be converted to arteriolar ECs. This process is likely to be involved in the CD36-mediated priming of VEGF signaling and capillary arterialization [22,35,40,41,83]. In fact, the crosstalk between angiogenic and antiangiogenic signaling could be critical to the specification of arterial ECs [39,40].

Venous ECs can be converted to arterial ECs by VEGF both in vitro and in vivo [79,80], further exemplifying the plasticity of vascular EC phenotypes. This phenomenon is supported by the fact that shear stress in circulation may determine the phenotypes of ECs [84], leading to the formation of either arterioles or venules through differentiation of two distinct types of ECs.

Vascular ECs are indeed critical for the regulation of arteriogenesis. In response to VEGF and other cytokines, ECs can be activated to increase the expression of FGF-2, platelet-derived growth factor PDGF-B and TGF-β1, thereby inducing the regrowth of SMCs and vessel enlargement [10,85]. Moreover, VEGF-mediated arteriogenic gene expression and Notch signaling may be essential for arterial differentiation and arteriolar remodeling in the TME [19,21,35,66], and may determine the arterial fate and stimulate de novo arteriogenesis via preferential activation of downstream MAPK/Erk rather than PI3Kinase/Akt signaling as shown in animal models [19,81]. We propose that during adult angiogenesis, arteriolar ECs can signal recruitment and appropriate differentiation of arteriolar SMCs, thus leading to the development of arterioles, particularly under ischemic and oncological conditions. Furthermore, arteriolar ECs will generate a variety of factors, including PDGF-B, TGF-β1, FGF-2, and thrombospondin 1 (TSP-1) to facilitate the recruitment and proliferation of arteriolar SMCs to form arterioles. This is accompanied by a corresponding formation of the extracellular matrix, leading to the development of a mature arteriolar network.

The arterioles that feed into a capillary network in the TME [55] represent a long-term structural adaptation to the altered metabolic demand [86], likely occurring via de novo arteriolar remodeling of capillaries into arterioles [17,19,21,70,87,88]. The significant increase in intratumoral capillaries during tumor progression [89,90] reasonably requires the concurrent expansion of upstream arterioles [20,55,89,91]. The analysis of tumor angiogenesis based on TAEC proliferation and pericyte recruitment demonstrated that there is active angiogenesis in several types of human tumors [92].

The results actually implicate the formation of feeding arterioles or de novo arteriogenesis [20,27,28] since the staining for the tumor vessels was not confirmed with other specific markers other than α-SMA, a key marker for SMCs [92]. Dr. Harold Dvorak's group elegantly documented the appearance of arteries and arterioles in the TME [27].

Most tumors continue to generate a significant amount of VEGF over long periods of time, thus, continually inducing the formation of new blood vessels [27]. In collaboration with LPA and/or FGF-2, the VEGF might concurrently lead to previously formed vessels to develop into more stable forms of arteriolar vasculature [21,85,93] within the TME. In response to VEGF overexpression, capillaries are enlarged and transformed toward an arterial phenotype in a process that is known as capillary arterialization [94] or arteriogenesis. Similarly, Dvorak's group showed that in the TME of VEGF-secreting tumors, Ad-VEGF-A164 stimulates abnormal arteriogenesis and venogenesis via remodeling of pre-existing arteries and veins to feed and drain the angiogenic vascular bed in animal models [27].

In fact, extensive studies show that arteriogenesis may likely occur within the TME in animal models and in patients with cancer [21,27,28,55,88,89,91,95–97], possibly within the TME of pNETs. NETs, including pNETs, classically, are most easily apparent in the early arterial phase of a computed tomography (CT) scan. For decades, it has been clinically appreciated that many primary gastrointestinal NETs and metastatic sites have a pattern of early arterial enhancement on cross-sectional imaging. Consequently, contrasted multiphase CT or magnetic resonance imaging is an important component in the evaluation of a patient with suspected primary or recurrent NETs [98,99]. Compared with normal pancreatic islets, pNETs have increased expression of nestin, probably contributing to vascular remodeling within the TME of pNETs [27,28,55,100]. Though the vessels in grade 3, NETs display the highest EC angiogenic activity, and they have regained pericyte coverage [101]. These studies suggest an increase in the formation of matured blood vessels and possibly the development into arterioles within the TME of pNETs. The development of arteriogenesis is supported by studies showing the high levels of pro-arteriogenic factors VEGF, VEGF receptors, and FGF-2 in NETs, but not in normal islet cells. Moreover, recent studies suggest that MVEC transdifferentiation into arteriolar ECs is likely an approach for facilitating the formation of arterioles under physiological or pathological conditions [20,21]. Intriguingly, during development, different types of blood vessels may be generated from different origins. Pulmonary capillaries are developed by angiogenesis, while pulmonary arteries are developed by vasculogenesis [102], which further supports the concept that de novo arteriogenesis exists under physiological and pathological conditions [19,20].

Maturation of the endothelial networks within the TME involves remodeling and 'pruning' capillary-like vessels with uniform size, and irregular organization into a structured network of branching vessels. Blood flow in tumor vessels is often chaotic, slow, and not efficient in meeting metabolic demands in some tumors [103]. However, blood vessels in tumor beds should be functional enough to allow oxygen and nutrients to be supplied and metabolic wastes to be removed. De novo arteriogenesis may be the case in highly angiogenic pNETs, in which the antiangiogenic drug sunitinib is partially effective as a targeted therapy against tumor vessels [104].

4. Tumor Arteriogenesis: Potential Target in pNETs

Tumor angiogenesis has been extensively studied since Folkman coined this concept more than three decades ago [63], whereas the role of de novo arteriogenesis within the TME is important but under-appreciated, and the mechanisms remain largely unknown. The arterioles to supply the vascular beds of tumors [55] might be generated by de novo arteriogenesis. The arteriolar differentiation of TAECs (a key component of the CSC niche [105]) and arteriolar remodeling within the TME might serve as a unique vascular niche for CSC maintenance and self-renewal in malignant progression of pNETs and other types of cancers, including breast and lung cancers, and malignant melanoma.

Actually, not only do ECs serve as gatekeepers of organ homeostasis [106], but they are also essential to maintain the function of arterioles in providing nutrients to cancer cells [19,20,107], including CSCs.

EC differentiation likely plays a key role in tumor arteriogenesis [20,27,55,91,108] in that arteriolar ECs may recruit SMCs to form arterioles and promote tumor progression by serving as an arteriolar niche for CSC maintenance and self-renewal. Prior studies have shown that the LPA/PKD-1-CD36 signaling axis switches MVECs to an "arteriolar phenotype" [21,71,109]. We postulated that TAECs also possess plasticity and may be reprogrammed for arteriolar differentiation toward arteriolar remodeling in response to microenvironmental factors within the TME for the progression of pNETs.

NETs are regarded as neoplasms originating in the hormone-producing cells of the endocrine system. PNETs represent 1–2% of all pancreatic tumors and 7% of NETs in general, second only to gastrointestinal carcinoid [110–112]. Current studies suggest that NETs may derive from mature neuroendocrine cells that undergo dedifferentiation due to genetic mutations or the progenitors of the neuroendocrine cells that undergo mutations, and even from the non-neuroendocrine cells that acquire neuroendocrine characteristics during carcinogenesis due to the loss of certain genes [113]. These studies indicate that the cellular plasticity contributes to the formation of NETs, including pNETs, and suggests the existence of CSC plasticity.

PNETs can be hormonal non-functioning or functioning. Up to 30% of tumors can secrete bioactive substances, including insulin, gastrin, glucagon, and somatostatin [114]. PNETs are often asymptomatic and grow slowly over several years before becoming symptomatic from mass effect, with a favorable five-year relative survival rate of 54% across all Surveillance, Epidemiology, and End Results (SEER) stages combined (www.cancer.org/cancer/pancreatic-neuroendocrine-tumor). However, a small, poorly differentiated subset is associated with a very aggressive phenotype [115]. More than 10% of pNETs present hepatic metastases upon diagnosis based on several multi-center studies [116], and approximately 85% of patients will develop hepatic metastases during a follow-up period of 20 years [117]. Current surgical and medical management have limited efficacy in the metastatic setting and show a poor prognosis compared to resected local-only disease [118,119]. Intriguingly, pNETs are highly vascularized and heterogeneous neoplasms [120], which are characterized by high levels of VEGF and its receptors [2]. Cytokine VEGF is a potential driver in the metastatic process of pNETs [3], particularly in hepatic metastases [4]. PNETs also highly express PDGFRs, which promote vascular maturation and arteriogenesis [121]. Both VEGFRs and PDGFRs are targets for the RTK sunitinib, which has shown limited antiangiogenic effects though the drug can increase progression-free survival by six months only in some patients with advanced pNETs [122,123].

Antiangiogenic therapy may show clinical benefits in patients with pNETs with a high intensity of neoangiogenesis [124]. The antiangiogenic drug bevacizumab was tested in phase II studies of advanced pNETs in combination with octreotide and chemotherapy with acceptable toxicity but showed limited improvement [125,126]. The limited response in these early studies may be a result of limited VEGF targeting that only inhibits the growth of the newly formed capillaries in the TME but has limited action against stable tumor vasculature [127].

Studies implicate that arteriolar formation or de novo arteriogenesis may play a critical role in tumor progression [20,55]. The concept that targeting arterioles improves prognosis is supported by the fact that the inhibition of the PDGF pathway enhances the efficacy of agents targeting VEGF [128] since PDGFs promote vascular maturation and arteriogenesis by mediating the recruitment of pericytes or SMCs to the newly formed blood vessels [10]. LPA likely promotes de novo arteriogenesis in the TME [20]. It is reasonable to speculate that in the early phases of cancer progression, the neoangiogenesis is dependent more on the VEGF pathway than PDGF and LPA signaling. However, this VEGF dependency may be reduced or lost in later phases when mature blood vessels are present [27]. It is during this later phase that arteriogenic drivers such as PDGF and LPA are likely more important because of their leading to angiogenic inhibitor-resistance [20,21,28,128,129]. Therefore, it is essential to establish appropriate animal cancer models that can mimic human cancer vasculature, including the formation of later stage and matured vascular networks, feeding arterioles, and drainage veins. Better understanding pathways that regulate tumor arteriogenesis may be a fundamental step to discovering an approach for controlling the progression of different types of cancer, including pNETs.

5. Antiangiogenic Therapy in pNETs: Challenges and Prospective

PNETs often present with metastases. Conventional therapies for advanced disease are rarely curative, and cytoreductive surgery showed limited results [130]. Targeting angiogenesis in pNETs results in therapeutic resistance. However, targeted antiangiogenic therapies like sunitinib are promising treatment options in the clinic. A phase III trial comparing sunitinib to placebo in well differentiated, unresectable pNETs showed a significant benefit in progression free survival (PFS) and suggested an improvement in overall survival [122]. Five-year follow-up of this study confirmed a benefit in PFS but failed to show an improvement in overall survival, possibly confounded by cross-over [104]. However, a phase IV trial supports the outcome of the phase III trial, further confirming that sunitinib is an efficacious and safe treatment option [131].

A recent study analyzed a small cohort of pNET patients with sunitinib treatment in a real-world clinical setting [132]. In this clinical scenario, over 98.8% had received three or more therapeutic regimens before initiating sunitinib therapy. Among those patients, 80% had been treated with everolimus, and 95% with somatostatin analogs. Additionally, it appears that there was a synergic effect between somatostatin analogs and sunitinib based on median PFS. This study demonstrated that sunitinib was safe and effective in the clinical setting even if the patients were undergone pre-treatment. However, the significance is limited due to a retrospective investigation of a low number of patients.

Everolimus (an mTOR inhibitor) as a target agent is also effective in advanced, well-differentiated progression pNETs [133]. The RADIANT-3 trial found that everolimus also significantly prolonged progression-free survival among patients with low or intermediate grade pNETs with progressive advanced disease [133]. However, everolimus may only show a limited effect in targeting tumor angiogenesis when compared with sunitinib. Furthermore, both sunitinib and everolimus are non-specific and may target many different types of cells and show severe side-effects.

Somatostatin analogs have shown antitumor effects via direct inhibition of cellular proliferation and tumor progression and indirect regulation of angiogenesis in gastroenteropancreatic neuroendocrine tumors [134]. In a randomized, double-blind study, lanreotide, the somatostatin analog, was used in patients with metastatic enteropancreatic NETs and showed prolonged progression-free survival through mechanisms that were not completely understood [135]. Early in 1991, somatostatin analogs were reported to inhibit angiogenesis of normal vascular development in vitro [136]. Their antiangiogenic activity in the TME was elegantly discussed in the literature about tumor angiogenesis [137,138], possibly via acting on the VEGF pathway in TAECs [139,140].

Current antiangiogenic therapy is based on the concept that the molecular phenotype of neoangiogenesis in the TME is active and immature, in which VEGF is a key player. Researchers try to target these immature vessels selectively, without affecting the quiescent organ vasculature [141–144]. Unfortunately, tumors often evade current single-agent antiangiogenic therapy via the induction of alternative proangiogenic pathways [3,145]. Moreover, some tumors even increase invasiveness and metastasis in response to current antiangiogenic therapy [48,146].

VEGF is considered as a key driver in the metastatic process of pNETs [3]. Targeting the VEGF pathway shows antitumor effects in mouse models of pNETs. However, human patients will potentially become resistant over time and develop metastases [147], which may be associated with FGF-associated intratumor hypoxia [3,146]. Moreover, hypoxia-induced hypoxia-inducible factor (HIF)-1α or HIF-2α stimulates the formation of normalized functioning vessels [48]. This also supports the existence of arteriogenesis within the TME [28,90,91] and suggests that the formation of functional arterioles within the TME in pNETs may play an important role in malignant progression and liver metastasis. Intriguingly, concomitant inhibition of c-Met and VEGF signaling has synergistic effects in pNETs [6], indicating that inhibition of multiple signaling pathways may increase the efficacy of anti-angiogenesis drugs. Recently, clinical trials are undergoing to investigate the combinations of immunotherapy with anti-angiogenesis treatment [148]. However, to maximize the efficacy of anti-angiogenesis, one widely adopted strategy is to combine drugs targeting multiple pathways in angiogenesis. We will focus on the Notch signaling pathway and vascular niche and CSC plasticity.

5.1. Notch Pathway: The Potential Target in pNETs

Expression of Notch receptors and ligands continue to be present in mature vessels to maintain vascular integrity and homeostasis [149], whereas inhibition of DLL4/Notch signaling enhances non-functional vessel growth and significantly limits tumor growth by reducing blood perfusion in lung malignancies [150]. DLL4-mediated Notch signaling is also critical during active vascularization, but less important for the maintenance of normal blood vessels [151]. Blocking DLL4 signaling inhibits tumor growth, which may be associated with defective maturation of the tumor vascular network and poor tissue perfusion [152]. These studies, thus, support the concept that functional angiogenesis and arteriolar networks in the TME may promote malignant progression.

Intriguingly, forced expression of DLL4 in tumor cells affects the morphogenesis of tumor vasculature, leading to the non-functional angiogenesis in the TME [150]. DLL4 expression in myotubes can activate Notch3 in adjacent myoblasts, thereby signaling those cells for quiescence [153]. This suggests that the DLL4/Notch axis restores the SC pool via SC self-renewal. Because arteriolar ECs express DLL4 and CSCs express Notch receptors, it is reasonable to hypothesize that this crosstalk exists between TAECs in the arterioles and CSCs within the TME. Moreover, this interaction may be critical for CSC maintenance and self-renewal in pNETs. Blocking DLL4 signaling may disrupt the crosstalk of arteriolar ECs with CSCs via targeting the Notch pathway. Therefore, the combination of sunitinib with anti-DLL4 can be a potential strategy to increase therapeutic efficacy. However, to develop an optimal therapeutic strategy, it is imperative to have a better understanding of the mechanisms of tumor arteriogenesis and the oncogenic signaling essential for pNET progression.

Currently, little is known about the degree of active angiogenesis and the functional status of the vasculature within human cancers, including pNETs. The optimal vascular network should be highly organized, including venules, capillaries, and arterioles, to supply all cells with sufficient nutrients. This may not be the case in the TME for different types of cancers, but a similar organization could exist in pNETs as the early arterial phase of a CT scan can easily show pNETs and targeting the arteriogenic pathway by sunitinib had certain therapeutic effects.

Additionally, the prognostic value of microvascular density (MVD) in NETs is controversial: some studies showed that low MVD and high endothelial proliferation index are unfavorable prognostic values [154], whereas other studies suggest that MVD was by no means a prognostic factor in pNETs [155]. In low-grade pNETs, the blood vessels are well branched, and the total surface area is expanded, whereas vessels in high-grade pNETs are plump, non-branched, and accompanied by a decreased vessel surface [156]. Increased blood vessel size or altered shape may be a marker of poor prognosis in other cancers such as squamous cell carcinoma of the vulva [157]. The observation, thus, suggests that the functional status and formation of arterioles or de novo arteriogenesis could be an important prognostic index and contribute to the progression of pNETs.

Moreover, the Notch pathway may be a key regulator of both tumor angiogenesis [150] and tumorigenesis, specifically in NETs [158,159]. Prior studies [160–164] have shown that Notch1 signaling is minimal or absent in pulmonary, thyroid, adrenal, and pNETs. Overexpression of Notch1 in a human pNET cell-line (BON cells) using an inducible construct demonstrated the suppression of tumor growth, an increase in the downstream target of the Notch1 Hes, a decrease in NET marker ASCL1 [161], and inhibition of neuroendocrine differentiation [164]. The inhibition of differentiation suggests that Notch1 signaling may promote the development of the stemness of CSCs in pNETs, which is supported by another study [165]. In contrast, a tissue microarray of 120 well-differentiated NETs arising from the pancreas ($n = 74$) reveals significant variability in Notch1 signaling across different tissue types, with an elevated Notch1 expression in 34% of human pNETs [166]. In patients with well-differentiated pNETs, 43.7% demonstrated positive Notch1 expression [167], suggesting heterogeneous expression of this pathway in pNETs. Moreover, Notch1 signaling shows significant variability in tumor status across different tissue types, which may promote or inhibit tumor progression [168,169]. Further studies are needed to elucidate the mechanisms of Notch1 in pNET progression.

Intriguingly, another Notch isoform, Notch3, has been shown to inhibit the progression of medullary thyroid carcinoma [170,171] and may be a therapeutic target [172]. Notch3 inhibits the progression of small cell lung cancer [173], likely as a result of deregulated Notch functions in cell fate decisions [174]. Functionally, Notch may serve as either an oncogene or a tumor suppressor, depending on cellular context. Targeting Notch/Notch-ligands interplay may be an effective strategy for pNETs. DLL3 inhibits Notch activation by interfering with DLL1/Notch interaction, leading to failure of cell membrane translocation. A DLL3 monoclonal antibody conjugated with a toxic chemotherapeutic agent appears to be an effective therapeutic strategy in preclinical models of small cell lung cancer [175]. The novel DLL3-targeting antibody-drug conjugate Rovalpituzumab is currently being utilized in clinical trials [176]. Antibody-drug conjugates targeting DLL3 are able to eliminate CSCs in xenograft models of pulmonary neuroendocrine cancers [177]. These studies indicate that significant genetic and epigenetic heterogeneity could exist among different types of NETs in terms of expression of Notch receptors and target genes. It is worthy of noting that the Notch pathway is known as the key regulator of tumor angiogenesis and arterial differentiation, a key process in de novo arteriogenesis [19,21,39,71,178]. Therefore, elucidating the mechanisms by which Notch signaling crosstalk between arteriolar ECs and CSCs of pNETs in the vascular niche may hold the key to successful therapeutic approaches to targeting this pathway in both cancer and vascular compartments at the same time.

5.2. Control of pNET Progression by Targeting Vascular Niche and CSC Plasticity

Emerging evidence supports that tumor recurrence and metastasis are driven by a subpopulation of CSCs that can undergo self-renewal and differentiation. Intact tumors harbor CSCs in dedicated niches (microenvironment) [179–184]. Intriguingly, the plasticity of this cell population allows them to alternate between CSC and non-CSCs, representing a substantial difference when compared to normal SCs. [185]. These phenotypic transitions can be driven by environmental stimuli [186–190]. A new and emerging concept indicates that CSCs may be much more plastic and abundant and can proliferate vigorously [191–193], rather than presenting as hierarchies as normal SCs. This plasticity in CSCs may be an important driver of drug resistance via change of its status into quiescence. Interestingly, pancreatic adenocarcinoma xenografts appear not to be driven by quiescent CSCs but rather by the successive activation of transiently active CSCs [193]. Both differentiated and transient amplifying cancer cells can be reprogrammed into CSCs if appropriate niche signals exist in the TME [185]. On the other hand, genetic mutations may occur to sustain the self-renewal of CSCs during tumor progression and render CSCs progressive independent of niche signals. An autonomous CSC phenotype can significantly increase numbers of CSCs within tumor tissue via blocking differentiation [185]. While CSCs have also been shown to be present in pNETs [165], it is not clear what degree of CSCs plasticity exists in this disease. Given the intratumor plasticity on top of the inherent mutability of cancer cells [194], it may be an attractive therapeutic strategy to modulate stem cell-niche functions such as vascular niche rather than to pursue therapies that are only based on intrinsic CSC features in order to keep CSC dormant or induce its differentiation into normal cells.

Moreover, mitochondrial respiration may play an important role in the maintenance and self-renewal of CSCs [195]. Like quiescent muscle SCs, which are dependent on oxidative phosphorylation mainly through mitochondrial fatty acid oxidation [196], quiescent CSCs might also rely on oxidative metabolism via fatty acid oxidation for their maintenance. Inhibition of oxidative phosphorylation and fatty acid metabolism could deplete this cell population, thereby improving responses to chemotherapeutics and targeted therapies. This was shown in mouse models of pancreatic cancer [197–199]. To achieve optimal therapeutic responses, targeting CD36, a fatty acid receptor and antiangiogenic receptor, could be beneficial because CD36 not only inhibits tumor angiogenesis and is associated with arteriolar differentiation and remodeling [20,21,108,200] but is also expressed in a subpopulation of highly aggressive disseminated CSCs to increase metastatic potential [25]. CD36 as a fatty acid receptor may facilitate the uptake and metabolism of fatty acids in CSCs, possibly representing an opportunity to treat the late stages of disease by controlling CD36-mediated metastasis [25,26,201,202] and by inhibiting arteriogenesis in TMEs.

Muscle SCs (satellite cells) are deeply quiescent, yet they localize to aerobic niches close to capillary vessels and use oxidative phosphorylation mainly through mitochondrial fatty acid oxidation [196]. Inhibition of fatty acid uptake and metabolism via CD36 indeed inhibits metastasis, though it does not affect the growth of primary oral squamous carcinomas [25]. The arterioles in the TME can provide free oxygen to tumor tissues and could serve as a unique vascular niche for the maintenance and self-renewal of CSCs in a variety of cancers, such as pNETs and breast cancer, that can rely on fatty acid as energy sources. However, the most aggressive forms of CSCs become independent of normal niche signals [190,203,204]. Therefore, it is worthy of studying the arteriolar differentiation and remodeling as a unique arteriolar niche in promoting CSC aggressiveness.

Furthermore, transcription factors may be involved in CSC stemness and plasticity via the regulation of CD36 transcription. The forkhead box O (FoxO) transcription factors are required for the maintenance of somatic and CSCs [205–207], whereas FoxO1 regulates CD36 transcription [21], which could play a key role in the development of metastatic CSCs. Moreover, FoxO1 may be an important player in the formation of a vascular niche by acting on ECs. In blood vessels, FoxO1 is highly expressed in vascular ECs, including MVECs, and is essential for the regulation of EC stability, vascular development, angiogenesis, and arteriolar differentiation [21,200,208,209]. FoxO1 also functions as a potent regulator of adult vascular homeostasis [208] and endothelial quiescence via a coordinated reduction in the proliferative and metabolic activity of vascular ECs [209]. In a Zebrafish model, FoxO1 is able to restore oxidative stress-compromised vascular regeneration via interaction with the Notch pathway [41]. In MVECs and TAECs, FoxO1 can regulate the transcriptional expression of CD36 in response to LPA/PKD-1 signaling [20,21]. These studies strongly suggest the role of FoxO1 in arteriolar differentiation and vascular maturation and implicate the involvement of FoxO1 in the formation of functional arterioles [20,21,39] via priming proangiogenic VEGF signaling [20–22,35,39,83]. Therefore, FoxO1 might not only play an important role in the maintenance of the CSC pool but also mediate the formation of a unique vascular niche for the maintenance and self-renewal of CSCs in cancers, including pNETs.

Therefore, future potential therapeutic strategies may include combinations of antiangiogenic therapy with anti-CSC strategy by targeting both the FoxO-1-CD36 signaling axis and Notch pathways (Figure 2). This combination might significantly limit the growth of cancers, including pNETs, and inhibit their metastasis by targeting both arteriolar niche and CSCs despite the caveats that CSC plasticity evokes toward the design of anti-CSC therapies. Additionally, venous components could be involved in the regulation of CSC behavior via venogenesis, the functional role of which needs to be further investigated in pNETs but is not discussed in this review. It will also be worthy of a better understanding of the mechanisms by which the vascular niche within the TME specifies the CSC state and plasticity in the setting of pNETs. Moreover, developing clinically relevant pNET models with robust angiogenesis, matured vasculature, and arteriogenesis in animals should facilitate the understanding of mechanisms and early diagnosis.

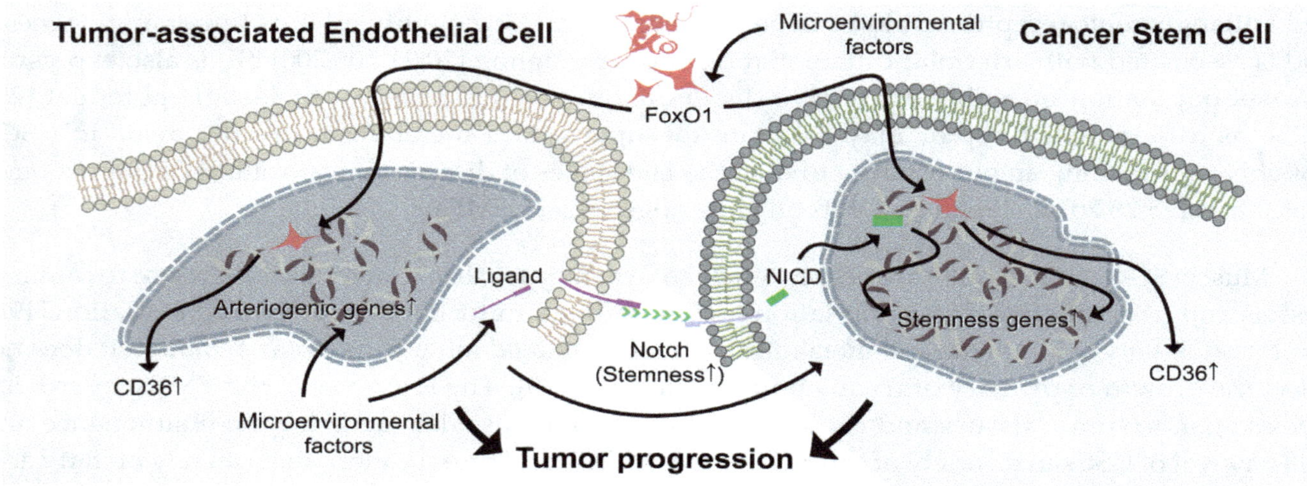

Figure 2. FoxO-1-CD36 and Notch signaling in tumor-associated endothelial cells (TAECs) and cancer stem cells (CSCs). Targeting both the FoxO1-CD36 signaling and Notch pathway may inhibit TAECs and attenuate maintenance and self-renewal of CSCs. Shown in this figure are the upregulated CD36 expression in both TAECs and CSCs via FoxO1. Whereas, the Notch pathway may upregulate arteriogenic genes or Notch ligands in TAECs, thus promoting interactions between TAECs and CSCs. Inhibition of CD36 may attenuate the generation of metastatic CSCs. Combined inhibition of the Notch pathway with CD36 signaling, both arteriogenic TAECs and CSCs will be targeted, subsequently leading to tumor regression and inhibition of tumor metastasis.

The transdifferentiation of TAECs and CSCs of pNETs may be explored and targeted since TAEC heterogeneity may respond to antiangiogenic drugs differently, and the CSC plasticity concept represents the capacity of CSCs undergoing both differentiation and transdifferentiation. Because targeting vascular niche may reactivate and sensitize quiescent CSCs to anti-cancer therapy, an approach to targeting both vascular niche and CSC compartment may present an attractive strategy via the identification of key regulators of arteriolar differentiation and CSC metabolism and differentiation in cancers, including pNETs. In this regard, the PKD-1/CD36-FoxO1 signaling axis is likely to be a promising and potential candidate target. Dissecting this pathway will facilitate the identification of key and targetable regulators because of its close association with both tumor neoangiogenesis (de novo arteriogenesis) and stemness and plasticity of CSCs.

In summary, pNETs exhibit a wide range of biologic behaviors ranging from long dormancy to rapid progression. Currently, only limited therapeutic options are available to patients with advanced pNETs. The efficacy of systemic therapy is poor, with high progression rates. It is well-known that pNETs are highly angiogenic and heterogeneous, with variable prognosis. Sunitinib is the only targeted therapy approved for pNETs, and relapse after an initial response. Carrasco et al., recently reviewed classical antiangiogenic therapies, and discussed some new angiogenic targets in NETs [210]. Here, we summarize some novel antiangiogenic "drug" molecules/agents, which may be promising and potential therapeutic targets in pNETs (Table 1).

Table 1. Drugs/molecules/agents for potential antiangiogenic treatment in pNETs.

Name	Mechanisms & Functions	Reference(s)
CVM-1118	Phase II clinical trial for patients with advanced NETs, including pNETs; de novo development of vascular networks via vascular mimicry, which is associated with a malignant phenotype and a poor clinical outcome. Vascular mimicry was presented in pNET animal models.	https://clinicaltrials.gov/ct2/show/NCT03600233; Chu et al., *Am J Pathol 2013*; Wagenblast, et al., *Nature* 2015; Hendrix, et al., *Pharmacol Ther* 2016 [211–213]
Cabozantinib	Phase III clinical trial of in patients with advanced neuroendocrine tumors after progression on everolimus (CABINET) A VEGFR, c-MET and AXL inhibitor; attenuate sunitinib therapy-mediated pro-metastasis in xenograft mouse tumor models of renal cell carcinoma.	https://clinicaltrials.gov/ct2/show/NCT03375320; Zhou et al., *Oncogene*, 2015 [214]
Lenvatinib	A multi-kinase inhibitor with a preferential antiangiogenic activity.	Capdevila, et al. *J Clin Oncol*, 2019; Capozzi, et al., *Cancer Manag Res* 2019 [215,216]
TH-302 (evofosfamide)	A hypoxia-activated prodrug, which is metabolized to its active form, bromo-isophosphoramide mustard (Br-IPM), under hypoxic conditions. Used in combination with sunitinib.	Grande, et al., abstract. *J Clin Oncol*, 2019 [217]
Doublecortin-like kinase 1 (DCLK1)	A potential marker for pNET CSCs; induce epithelial-mesenchymal transition (EMT).	Ikezono, et al., *Mol Cancer Res*, 2017 [218]
MEDI3617	A monoclonal antibody targeting angiopoietin-2; in combination with VEGF-targeted therapies.	Rigamonti, et al., *Cell Rep* 2014; Biel, et al., *Cancer Letters*, 2016 [219,220]
Sema3A (Semaphorin 3A)	Overcome cancer hypoxia and metastatic dissemination induced by sunitinib treatment in mice. In combination with sunitinib, Sema3A synergistically enhanced RIP-Tag2 mouse survival.	Maione, F, et al., *J Clin Invest*, 2012 [221]
Brivanib	A dual FGF/VEGF inhibitor; vascular inhibition and tumor stability.	Allen, et al., *Clin Cancer Res*, 2011 [222]
PIGF signaling inhibitor?	High PIGF expression in pNET patients with poor outcome; overcome resistance to antiangiogenic factors.	Fischer et al., *Cell*, 2007; Hilfenhaus, et al., *Endocr Relat Cancer*, 2013 [223,224]
EZH2 inhibitor?	Sensitize tumor to sunitinib in cell lines and PDX models.	Marconcini, et al., 2016 [225]
Autotaxin (ATX) inhibitors? LPA receptor-specific antagonists?	High ATX expression in pNET tissues, which was associated with higher tumor grade, TNM staging and lymph node metastasis; ATX drives LPA expression, which is also linked to tumor angiogenesis and arteriolar differentiation and malignancy of tumor cells.	*Liu* et al., *Cancer Cell*, 2009; Chen, et al., *Front Biosci (Landmark Ed)* 2013; Ren, et al., *Arterioscler Thromb Vasc Biol*, 2016; Liu et al., *Cancer Lett* 2016; Dong et al., *Oncotarget*, 2017 [20]; Yang et al., *Endocr. Connect*, 2018 [21,226–229]

Many alternative pathways are involved in the formation of tumor vasculature, which may be independent of VEGF signaling, such as vascular mimicry formation and vascular intussusception. We need to identify the key regulator of heterogeneous tumor vascular networks in the development of pNETs. We also urgently need to elucidate mechanisms by which pNETs progress, relapse, and discover key signaling molecules in de novo arteriogenesis in order to identify new targets for effective therapy. Due to the complexity and dynamic properties of heterogeneous TAECs, we may consider personalized antiangiogenic therapies, likely in combination with checkpoint-inhibitor immunotherapy, based on a patient's specific profile of tumor tissues and TAECs in order to achieve optimal therapeutic responses in the clinic [230]. Furthermore, the feeding arterioles that are derived from de novo arteriogenesis or the mature, SMC-coated daughter blood vessels could be potentially valuable targets because they supply the smaller, angiogenic vessels enclosed within the tumor mass [19,20,27]. A better mechanistic understanding of angiogenesis and de novo arteriogenesis within the TME, and the role of CSCs in pNET progression may provide insight into novel and effective treatment strategies not only in pNETs but also other highly angiogenic and arteriogenic cancers.

Author Contributions: B.R. wrote the manuscript; J.B.R., R.J.-S., C.C., A.B., and H.C. edited the manuscript and Y.L. edited the manuscript and made figures.

Acknowledgments: Ren's work has been supported by the American Cancer Society (86-004-26; Institution Fund to BR, Medical College of Wisconsin), the American Heart Association (13SDG14800019; BR), the Ann's Hope Foundation (FP00011709; BR), Bioengineering Surgery Collaborative Award, University of Alabama at Birmingham (BR & AP), and the National Institute of Health (HL136423; BR).

References

1. Halfdanarson, T.R.; Rabe, K.G.; Rubin, J.; Petersen, G.M. Pancreatic neuroendocrine tumors (PNETs): Incidence, prognosis and recent trend toward improved survival. *Ann. Oncol.* **2008**, *19*, 1727–1733. [CrossRef] [PubMed]
2. Terris, B.; Scoazec, J.Y.; Rubbia, L.; Bregeaud, L.; Pepper, M.S.; Ruszniewski, P.; Belghiti, J.; Flejou, J.; Degott, C. Expression of vascular endothelial growth factor in digestive neuroendocrine tumours. *Histopathology* **1998**, *32*, 133–138. [CrossRef] [PubMed]
3. Casanovas, O.; Hicklin, D.J.; Bergers, G.; Hanahan, D. Drug resistance by evasion of antiangiogenic targeting of VEGF signaling in late-stage pancreatic islet tumors. *Cancer Cell* **2005**, *8*, 299–309. [CrossRef] [PubMed]
4. Gomez, D.; Malik, H.Z.; Al-Mukthar, A.; Menon, K.V.; Toogood, G.J.; Lodge, J.P.; Prasad, K.R. Hepatic resection for metastatic gastrointestinal and pancreatic neuroendocrine tumours: Outcome and prognostic predictors. *HPB (Oxford)* **2007**, *9*, 345–351. [CrossRef]
5. De Dosso, S.; Grande, E.; Barriuso, J.; Castellano, D.; Tabernero, J.; Capdevila, J. The targeted therapy revolution in neuroendocrine tumors: In search of biomarkers for patient selection and response evaluation. *Cancer Metastasis Rev.* **2013**, *32*, 465–477. [CrossRef]
6. Sennino, B.; Ishiguro-Oonuma, T.; Wei, Y.; Naylor, R.M.; Williamson, C.W.; Bhagwandin, V.; Tabruyn, S.P.; You, W.K.; Chapman, H.A.; Christensen, J.G.; et al. Suppression of tumor invasion and metastasis by concurrent inhibition of c-Met and VEGF signaling in pancreatic neuroendocrine tumors. *Cancer Discov.* **2012**, *2*, 270–287. [CrossRef]
7. Hanahan, D.; Weinberg, R.A. Hallmarks of cancer: The next generation. *Cell* **2011**, *144*, 646–674. [CrossRef]
8. Lenzi, P.; Bocci, G.; Natale, G. John Hunter and the origin of the term "angiogenesis". *Angiogenesis* **2016**, *19*, 255–256. [CrossRef]
9. Folkman, J. Angiogenesis in cancer, vascular, rheumatoid and other disease. *Nat. Med.* **1995**, *1*, 27–31. [CrossRef]
10. Carmeliet, P. Mechanisms of angiogenesis and arteriogenesis. *Nat. Med.* **2000**, *6*, 389–395. [CrossRef]

11. Shalaby, F.; Rossant, J.; Yamaguchi, T.P.; Gertsenstein, M.; Wu, X.F.; Breitman, M.L.; Schuh, A.C. Failure of blood-island formation and vasculogenesis in Flk-1-deficient mice. *Nature* **1995**, *376*, 62–66. [CrossRef] [PubMed]
12. Dvorak, H.F.; Brown, L.F.; Detmar, M.; Dvorak, A.M. Vascular permeability factor/vascular endothelial growth factor, microvascular hyperpermeability, and angiogenesis. *Am. J. Pathol.* **1995**, *146*, 1029–1039. [PubMed]
13. Bernardi, R.; Guernah, I.; Jin, D.; Grisendi, S.; Alimonti, A.; Teruya-Feldstein, J.; Cordon-Cardo, C.; Simon, M.C.; Rafii, S.; Pandolfi, P.P. PML inhibits HIF-1alpha translation and neoangiogenesis through repression of mTOR. *Nature* **2006**, *442*, 779–785. [CrossRef] [PubMed]
14. Potente, M.; Gerhardt, H.; Carmeliet, P. Basic and therapeutic aspects of angiogenesis. *Cell* **2011**, *146*, 873–887. [CrossRef]
15. Carmeliet, P.; Jain, R.K. Molecular mechanisms and clinical applications of angiogenesis. *Nature* **2011**, *473*, 298–307. [CrossRef]
16. Simons, M.; Ware, J.A. Therapeutic angiogenesis in cardiovascular disease. *Nat. Rev. Drug Discov.* **2003**, *2*, 863–871. [CrossRef]
17. Mac Gabhann, F.; Peirce, S.M. Collateral capillary arterialization following arteriolar ligation in murine skeletal muscle. *Microcirculation* **2010**, *17*, 333–347. [CrossRef]
18. Ren, B.; Best, B.; Weihrauch, D.; Jones, D.W.; Dong, L.; Opansky, C.; Yuan, R.; Pritchard, K.A.; Silverstein, R. Abstract 15673: LPA/PKD-1-FoxO1-CD36 Signaling Axis Regulates Capillary Arterialization in Ischemic Conditions. *Circulation* **2016**, *134*, A15673. [CrossRef]
19. Ren, B.; Deng, Y.; Mukhopadhyay, A.; Lanahan, A.A.; Zhuang, Z.W.; Moodie, K.L.; Mulligan-Kehoe, M.J.; Byzova, T.V.; Peterson, R.T.; Simons, M. ERK1/2-Akt1 crosstalk regulates arteriogenesis in mice and zebrafish. *J. Clin. Invest.* **2010**, *120*, 1217–1228. [CrossRef]
20. Dong, L.; Yuan, Y.; Opansky, C.; Chen, Y.; Aguilera-Barrantes, I.; Wu, S.; Yuan, R.; Cao, Q.; Cheng, Y.C.; Sahoo, D.; et al. Diet-induced obesity links to ER positive breast cancer progression via LPA/PKD-1-CD36 signaling-mediated microvascular remodeling. *Oncotarget* **2017**, *8*, 22550–22562. [CrossRef]
21. Ren, B.; Best, B.; Ramakrishnan, D.P.; Walcott, B.P.; Storz, P.; Silverstein, R.L. LPA/PKD-1-FoxO1 Signaling Axis Mediates Endothelial Cell CD36 Transcriptional Repression and Proangiogenic and Proarteriogenic Reprogramming. *Arter. Thromb. Vasc. Biol.* **2016**, *36*, 1197–1208. [CrossRef] [PubMed]
22. Ren, B.; Hale, J.; Srikanthan, S.; Silverstein, R.L. Lysophosphatidic acid suppresses endothelial cell CD36 expression and promotes angiogenesis via a PKD-1-dependent signaling pathway. *Blood* **2011**, *117*, 6036–6045. [CrossRef] [PubMed]
23. Aitman, T.J.; Glazier, A.M.; Wallace, C.A.; Cooper, L.D.; Norsworthy, P.J.; Wahid, F.N.; Al-Majali, K.M.; Trembling, P.M.; Mann, C.J.; Shoulders, C.C.; et al. Identification of Cd36 (Fat) as an insulin-resistance gene causing defective fatty acid and glucose metabolism in hypertensive rats. *Nat. Genet.* **1999**, *21*, 76–83. [CrossRef] [PubMed]
24. Yuan, Y.; Kohlenberg, J.D.; Chen, Y.; Komas, S.; Xin, G.; Yuan, G.; Cui, W.; Wu, S.; Ren, B. Abstract A09: Diet-induced obesity promotes breast cancer progression by LPA-signaling-mediated functional changes of mitochondria and angiogenesis. *Cancer Res.* **2015**, *75*, A09. [CrossRef]
25. Pascual, G.; Avgustinova, A.; Mejetta, S.; Martin, M.; Castellanos, A.; Attolini, C.S.; Berenguer, A.; Prats, N.; Toll, A.; Hueto, J.A.; et al. Targeting metastasis-initiating cells through the fatty acid receptor CD36. *Nature* **2017**, *541*, 41–45. [CrossRef]
26. Hale, J.S.; Otvos, B.; Sinyuk, M.; Alvarado, A.G.; Hitomi, M.; Stoltz, K.; Wu, Q.; Flavahan, W.; Levison, B.; Johansen, M.L.; et al. Cancer stem cell-specific scavenger receptor CD36 drives glioblastoma progression. *Stem Cells* **2014**, *32*, 1746–1758. [CrossRef]
27. Nagy, J.A.; Dvorak, H.F. Heterogeneity of the tumor vasculature: The need for new tumor blood vessel type-specific targets. *Clin. Exp. Metastasis* **2012**, *29*, 657–662. [CrossRef]
28. Sitohy, B.; Nagy, J.A.; Jaminet, S.C.; Dvorak, H.F. Tumor-surrogate blood vessel subtypes exhibit differential susceptibility to anti-VEGF therapy. *Cancer Res.* **2011**, *71*, 7021–7028. [CrossRef]
29. Ribatti, D. The involvement of endothelial progenitor cells in tumor angiogenesis. *J. Cell Mol. Med.* **2004**, *8*, 294–300. [CrossRef]

30. Wang, R.; Chadalavada, K.; Wilshire, J.; Kowalik, U.; Hovinga, K.E.; Geber, A.; Fligelman, B.; Leversha, M.; Brennan, C.; Tabar, V. Glioblastoma stem-like cells give rise to tumour endothelium. *Nature* **2010**, *468*, 829–833. [CrossRef]
31. Yuan, L.; Chan, G.C.; Beeler, D.; Janes, L.; Spokes, K.C.; Dharaneeswaran, H.; Mojiri, A.; Adams, W.J.; Sciuto, T.; Garcia-Cardena, G.; et al. A role of stochastic phenotype switching in generating mosaic endothelial cell heterogeneity. *Nat. Commun.* **2016**, *7*, 10160. [CrossRef] [PubMed]
32. Regan, E.R.; Aird, W.C. Dynamical systems approach to endothelial heterogeneity. *Circ. Res.* **2012**, *111*, 110–130. [CrossRef] [PubMed]
33. Ren, B. Endothelial Cells: A Key Player in Angiogenesis and Lymphangiogenesis. *MOJ Cell Sci. Rep.* **2015**, *2*. [CrossRef]
34. Chi, J.T.; Chang, H.Y.; Haraldsen, G.; Jahnsen, F.L.; Troyanskaya, O.G.; Chang, D.S.; Wang, Z.; Rockson, S.G.; van de Rijn, M.; Botstein, D.; et al. Endothelial cell diversity revealed by global expression profiling. *Proc. Natl. Acad. Sci. USA* **2003**, *100*, 10623–10628. [CrossRef] [PubMed]
35. Best, B.; Moran, P.; Ren, B. VEGF/PKD-1 signaling mediates arteriogenic gene expression and angiogenic responses in reversible human microvascular endothelial cells with extended lifespan. *Mol. Cell Biochem.* **2018**, *446*, 199–207. [CrossRef] [PubMed]
36. Nolan, D.J.; Ginsberg, M.; Israely, E.; Palikuqi, B.; Poulos, M.G.; James, D.; Ding, B.S.; Schachterle, W.; Liu, Y.; Rosenwaks, Z.; et al. Molecular signatures of tissue-specific microvascular endothelial cell heterogeneity in organ maintenance and regeneration. *Dev. Cell* **2013**, *26*, 204–219. [CrossRef] [PubMed]
37. Marcu, R.; Choi, Y.J.; Xue, J.; Fortin, C.L.; Wang, Y.; Nagao, R.J.; Xu, J.; MacDonald, J.W.; Bammler, T.K.; Murry, C.E.; et al. Human Organ-Specific Endothelial Cell Heterogeneity. *iScience* **2018**, *4*, 20–35. [CrossRef]
38. Bentley, K.; Franco, C.A.; Philippides, A.; Blanco, R.; Dierkes, M.; Gebala, V.; Stanchi, F.; Jones, M.; Aspalter, I.M.; Cagna, G.; et al. The role of differential VE-cadherin dynamics in cell rearrangement during angiogenesis. *Nat. Cell Biol.* **2014**, *16*, 309–321. [CrossRef]
39. Ren, B. FoxO1 transcriptional activities in VEGF expression and beyond: A key regulator in functional angiogenesis? *J. Pathol.* **2018**, *245*, 255–257. [CrossRef]
40. Ren, B. Protein Kinase D1 Signaling in Angiogenic Gene Expression and VEGF-Mediated Angiogenesis. *Front. Cell Dev. Biol.* **2016**, *4*, 37. [CrossRef]
41. Baek, K.I.; Packard, R.R.S.; Hsu, J.J.; Saffari, A.; Ma, Z.; Luu, A.P.; Pietersen, A.; Yen, H.; Ren, B.; Ding, Y.; et al. Ultrafine Particle Exposure Reveals the Importance of FOXO1/Notch Activation Complex for Vascular Regeneration. *Antioxid. Redox Signal.* **2018**, *28*, 1209–1223. [CrossRef]
42. Denekamp, J. Endothelial cell proliferation as a novel approach to targeting tumour therapy. *Br. J. Cancer* **1982**, *45*, 136–139. [CrossRef] [PubMed]
43. Morikawa, S.; Baluk, P.; Kaidoh, T.; Haskell, A.; Jain, R.K.; McDonald, D.M. Abnormalities in pericytes on blood vessels and endothelial sprouts in tumors. *Am. J. Pathol.* **2002**, *160*, 985–1000. [CrossRef]
44. Orimo, A.; Weinberg, R.A. Stromal fibroblasts in cancer: A novel tumor-promoting cell type. *Cell Cycle* **2006**, *5*, 1597–1601. [CrossRef] [PubMed]
45. Franklin, R.A.; Liao, W.; Sarkar, A.; Kim, M.V.; Bivona, M.R.; Liu, K.; Pamer, E.G.; Li, M.O. The cellular and molecular origin of tumor-associated macrophages. *Science* **2014**, *344*, 921–925. [CrossRef] [PubMed]
46. Ronca, R.; Van Ginderachter, J.A.; Turtoi, A. Paracrine interactions of cancer-associated fibroblasts, macrophages and endothelial cells: Tumor allies and foes. *Curr. Opin. Oncol.* **2018**, *30*, 45–53. [CrossRef]
47. Wilson, W.R.; Hay, M.P. Targeting hypoxia in cancer therapy. *Nat. Rev. Cancer* **2011**, *11*, 393–410. [CrossRef]
48. Krock, B.L.; Skuli, N.; Simon, M.C. Hypoxia-induced angiogenesis: Good and evil. *Genes Cancer* **2011**, *2*, 1117–1133. [CrossRef]
49. Senger, D.R.; Galli, S.J.; Dvorak, A.M.; Perruzzi, C.A.; Harvey, V.S.; Dvorak, H.F. Tumor cells secrete a vascular permeability factor that promotes accumulation of ascites fluid. *Science* **1983**, *219*, 983–985. [CrossRef]
50. Ren, B.; Hoti, N.; Rabasseda, X.; Wang, Y.Z.; Wu, M. The antiangiogenic and therapeutic implications of endostatin. *Methods Find. Exp. Clin. Pharm.* **2003**, *25*, 215–224. [CrossRef]
51. Ren, B.; Yee, K.O.; Lawler, J.; Khosravi-Far, R. Regulation of tumor angiogenesis by thrombospondin-1. *Biochim. Biophys. Acta* **2006**, *1765*, 178–188. [CrossRef] [PubMed]
52. Ren, B.; Song, K.; Parangi, S.; Jin, T.; Ye, M.; Humphreys, R.; Duquette, M.; Zhang, X.; Benhaga, N.; Lawler, J.; et al. A double hit to kill tumor and endothelial cells by TRAIL and antiangiogenic 3TSR. *Cancer Res.* **2009**, *69*, 3856–3865. [CrossRef] [PubMed]

53. Simons, M.; Gordon, E.; Claesson-Welsh, L. Mechanisms and regulation of endothelial VEGF receptor signalling. *Nat. Rev. Mol. Cell Biol.* **2016**, *17*, 611–625. [CrossRef] [PubMed]
54. Nagy, J.A.; Chang, S.H.; Shih, S.C.; Dvorak, A.M.; Dvorak, H.F. Heterogeneity of the tumor vasculature. *Semin. Thromb. Hemost.* **2010**, *36*, 321–331. [CrossRef]
55. Dvorak, H.F. Tumor Stroma, Tumor Blood Vessels, and Antiangiogenesis Therapy. *Cancer J.* **2015**, *21*, 237–243. [CrossRef]
56. Hida, K.; Hida, Y.; Amin, D.N.; Flint, A.F.; Panigrahy, D.; Morton, C.C.; Klagsbrun, M. Tumor-associated endothelial cells with cytogenetic abnormalities. *Cancer Res.* **2004**, *64*, 8249–8255. [CrossRef]
57. Ricci-Vitiani, L.; Pallini, R.; Biffoni, M.; Todaro, M.; Invernici, G.; Cenci, T.; Maira, G.; Parati, E.A.; Stassi, G.; Larocca, L.M.; et al. Tumour vascularization via endothelial differentiation of glioblastoma stem-like cells. *Nature* **2010**, *468*, 824–828. [CrossRef]
58. Samson, T.; Welch, C.; Monaghan-Benson, E.; Hahn, K.M.; Burridge, K. Endogenous RhoG is rapidly activated after epidermal growth factor stimulation through multiple guanine-nucleotide exchange factors. *Mol. Biol. Cell* **2010**, *21*, 1629–1642. [CrossRef]
59. Franses, J.W.; Edelman, E.R. The evolution of endothelial regulatory paradigms in cancer biology and vascular repair. *Cancer Res.* **2011**, *71*, 7339–7344. [CrossRef]
60. Franses, J.W.; Baker, A.B.; Chitalia, V.C.; Edelman, E.R. Stromal endothelial cells directly influence cancer progression. *Sci. Transl. Med.* **2011**, *3*, 66ra65. [CrossRef]
61. Jain, R.K.; Carmeliet, P. SnapShot: Tumor angiogenesis. *Cell* **2012**, *149*, 1408. [CrossRef] [PubMed]
62. Jain, R.K. Antiangiogenesis strategies revisited: From starving tumors to alleviating hypoxia. *Cancer Cell* **2014**, *26*, 605–622. [CrossRef] [PubMed]
63. Folkman, J. Tumor angiogenesis: Therapeutic implications. *N. Engl. J. Med.* **1971**, *285*, 1182–1186. [CrossRef] [PubMed]
64. Pluda, J.M. Tumor-associated angiogenesis: Mechanisms, clinical implications, and therapeutic strategies. *Semin. Oncol.* **1997**, *24*, 203–218.
65. Brem, H.; Folkman, J. Inhibition of tumor angiogenesis mediated by cartilage. *J. Exp. Med.* **1975**, *141*, 427–439. [CrossRef]
66. Hainaud, P.; Contreres, J.O.; Villemain, A.; Liu, L.X.; Plouet, J.; Tobelem, G.; Dupuy, E. The role of the vascular endothelial growth factor-Delta-like 4 ligand/Notch4-ephrin B2 cascade in tumor vessel remodeling and endothelial cell functions. *Cancer Res.* **2006**, *66*, 8501–8510. [CrossRef]
67. Heil, M.; Eitenmuller, I.; Schmitz-Rixen, T.; Schaper, W. Arteriogenesis versus angiogenesis: Similarities and differences. *J. Cell Mol. Med.* **2006**, *10*, 45–55. [CrossRef]
68. Cai, W.J.; Koltai, S.; Kocsis, E.; Scholz, D.; Kostin, S.; Luo, X.; Schaper, W.; Schaper, J. Remodeling of the adventitia during coronary arteriogenesis. *Am. J. Physiol.-Heart Circ. Physiol.* **2003**, *284*, H31–H40. [CrossRef]
69. Lanahan, A.; Zhang, X.; Fantin, A.; Zhuang, Z.; Rivera-Molina, F.; Speichinger, K.; Prahst, C.; Zhang, J.; Wang, Y.; Davis, G.; et al. The neuropilin 1 cytoplasmic domain is required for VEGF-A-dependent arteriogenesis. *Dev. Cell* **2013**, *25*, 156–168. [CrossRef]
70. Moraes, F.; Paye, J.; Mac Gabhann, F.; Zhuang, Z.W.; Zhang, J.; Lanahan, A.A.; Simons, M. Endothelial cell-dependent regulation of arteriogenesis. *Circ. Res.* **2013**, *113*, 1076–1086. [CrossRef]
71. Moran, P.; Guo, Y.; Yuan, R.; Barnekow, N.; Palmer, J.; Beck, A.; Ren, B. Translating Ribosome Affinity Purification (TRAP) for RNA Isolation from Endothelial Cells In vivo. *J. Vis. Exp.* **2019**, e59624. [CrossRef] [PubMed]
72. Moran, P.; Opansky, C.; Weihrauch, D.; Yuan, R.; Jones, D.W.; Ramchandran, R.; Ren, B. Abstract 14944: Transcriptional Reprogramming of Endothelial Cells for Arteriolar Differentiation by Small Chemical Molecule via Protein Kinase D1 Signaling Pathway. *Circulation* **2017**, *136*, A14944. [CrossRef]
73. Wang, H.U.; Chen, Z.F.; Anderson, D.J. Molecular distinction and angiogenic interaction between embryonic arteries and veins revealed by ephrin-B2 and its receptor Eph-B4. *Cell* **1998**, *93*, 741–753. [CrossRef]
74. Weinstein, B.M.; Stemple, D.L.; Driever, W.; Fishman, M.C. Gridlock, a localized heritable vascular patterning defect in the zebrafish. *Nat. Med.* **1995**, *1*, 1143–1147. [CrossRef]
75. Zhong, T.P.; Rosenberg, M.; Mohideen, M.A.; Weinstein, B.; Fishman, M.C. gridlock, an HLH gene required for assembly of the aorta in zebrafish. *Science* **2000**, *287*, 1820–1824. [CrossRef]
76. Zhong, T.P.; Childs, S.; Leu, J.P.; Fishman, M.C. Gridlock signalling pathway fashions the first embryonic artery. *Nature* **2001**, *414*, 216–220. [CrossRef]

77. Lawson, N.D.; Scheer, N.; Pham, V.N.; Kim, C.H.; Chitnis, A.B.; Campos-Ortega, J.A.; Weinstein, B.M. Notch signaling is required for arterial-venous differentiation during embryonic vascular development. *Development* **2001**, *128*, 3675–3683.
78. Weinstein, B.M.; Lawson, N.D. Arteries, veins, Notch, and VEGF. *Cold Spring Harb. Symp. Quant. Biol.* **2002**, *67*, 155–162. [CrossRef]
79. Mukouyama, Y.S.; Shin, D.; Britsch, S.; Taniguchi, M.; Anderson, D.J. Sensory nerves determine the pattern of arterial differentiation and blood vessel branching in the skin. *Cell* **2002**, *109*, 693–705. [CrossRef]
80. Visconti, R.P.; Richardson, C.D.; Sato, T.N. Orchestration of angiogenesis and arteriovenous contribution by angiopoietins and vascular endothelial growth factor (VEGF). *Proc. Natl. Acad. Sci. USA* **2002**, *99*, 8219–8224. [CrossRef]
81. Hong, C.C.; Peterson, Q.P.; Hong, J.Y.; Peterson, R.T. Artery/vein specification is governed by opposing phosphatidylinositol-3 kinase and MAP kinase/ERK signaling. *Curr. Biol.* **2006**, *16*, 1366–1372. [CrossRef] [PubMed]
82. Peterson, R.T.; Shaw, S.Y.; Peterson, T.A.; Milan, D.J.; Zhong, T.P.; Schreiber, S.L.; MacRae, C.A.; Fishman, M.C. Chemical suppression of a genetic mutation in a zebrafish model of aortic coarctation. *Nat. Biotechnol.* **2004**, *22*, 595–599. [CrossRef] [PubMed]
83. Kazerounian, S.; Duquette, M.; Reyes, M.A.; Lawler, J.T.; Song, K.; Perruzzi, C.; Primo, L.; Khosravi-Far, R.; Bussolino, F.; Rabinovitz, I.; et al. Priming of the vascular endothelial growth factor signaling pathway by thrombospondin-1, CD36, and spleen tyrosine kinase. *Blood* **2011**, *117*, 4658–4666. [CrossRef] [PubMed]
84. Dewey, J.F. Regional tectonics. *Science* **1981**, *214*, 550–551. [CrossRef] [PubMed]
85. Deindl, E.; Hoefer, I.E.; Fernandez, B.; Barancik, M.; Heil, M.; Strniskova, M.; Schaper, W. Involvement of the fibroblast growth factor system in adaptive and chemokine-induced arteriogenesis. *Circ. Res.* **2003**, *92*, 561–568. [CrossRef] [PubMed]
86. Aragones, J.; Fraisl, P.; Baes, M.; Carmeliet, P. Oxygen sensors at the crossroad of metabolism. *Cell Metab.* **2009**, *9*, 11–22. [CrossRef] [PubMed]
87. Helisch, A.; Schaper, W. Arteriogenesis: The development and growth of collateral arteries. *Microcirculation* **2003**, *10*, 83–97. [CrossRef]
88. Dong, L.; Yuan, Y.; Aguilera-Barrantes, I.; Chen, Y.; Sturich, A.; Yuan, R.; Wu, S.; Silverstein, R.; Ren, B. Abstract 482: Signaling Lipid Lysophosphatidic Acid Is a Critical Link to Diet-induced Obesity, Cellular Bioenergetics and Breast Cancer Angiogenesis. *Arterioscler. Thromb. Vasc. Biol.* **2015**, *35*, A482.
89. Yu, J.L.; Rak, J.W. Host microenvironment in breast cancer development: Inflammatory and immune cells in tumour angiogenesis and arteriogenesis. *Breast Cancer Res.* **2003**, *5*, 83–88. [CrossRef]
90. Skuli, N.; Majmundar, A.J.; Krock, B.L.; Mesquita, R.C.; Mathew, L.K.; Quinn, Z.L.; Runge, A.; Liu, L.; Kim, M.N.; Liang, J.; et al. Endothelial HIF-2alpha regulates murine pathological angiogenesis and revascularization processes. *J. Clin. Invest.* **2012**, *122*, 1427–1443. [CrossRef]
91. Skuli, N.; Liu, L.; Runge, A.; Wang, T.; Yuan, L.; Patel, S.; Iruela-Arispe, L.; Simon, M.C.; Keith, B. Endothelial deletion of hypoxia-inducible factor-2alpha (HIF-2alpha) alters vascular function and tumor angiogenesis. *Blood* **2009**, *114*, 469–477. [CrossRef] [PubMed]
92. Eberhard, A.; Kahlert, S.; Goede, V.; Hemmerlein, B.; Plate, K.H.; Augustin, H.G. Heterogeneity of angiogenesis and blood vessel maturation in human tumors: Implications for antiangiogenic tumor therapies. *Cancer Res.* **2000**, *60*, 1388–1393. [PubMed]
93. Buschmann, I.; Heil, M.; Jost, M.; Schaper, W. Influence of inflammatory cytokines on arteriogenesis. *Microcirculation* **2003**, *10*, 371–379. [CrossRef] [PubMed]
94. Rissanen, T.T.; Korpisalo, P.; Markkanen, J.E.; Liimatainen, T.; Orden, M.R.; Kholova, I.; de Goede, A.; Heikura, T.; Grohn, O.H.; Yla-Herttuala, S. Blood flow remodels growing vasculature during vascular endothelial growth factor gene therapy and determines between capillary arterialization and sprouting angiogenesis. *Circulation* **2005**, *112*, 3937–3946. [CrossRef] [PubMed]
95. Schechter, J.; Goldsmith, P.; Wilson, C.; Weiner, R. Morphological evidence for the presence of arteries in human prolactinomas. *J. Clin. Endocrinol. Metab.* **1988**, *67*, 713–719. [CrossRef] [PubMed]
96. Tinsley, J.H.; Teasdale, N.R.; Yuan, S.Y. Involvement of PKCdelta and PKD in pulmonary microvascular endothelial cell hyperpermeability. *Am. J. Physiol. Cell Physiol.* **2004**, *286*, C105–C111. [CrossRef]

97. Shin, D.; Garcia-Cardena, G.; Hayashi, S.; Gerety, S.; Asahara, T.; Stavrakis, G.; Isner, J.; Folkman, J.; Gimbrone, M.A., Jr.; Anderson, D.J. Expression of ephrinB2 identifies a stable genetic difference between arterial and venous vascular smooth muscle as well as endothelial cells, and marks subsets of microvessels at sites of adult neovascularization. *Dev. Biol.* **2001**, *230*, 139–150. [CrossRef]
98. Elias, D.; Lasser, P.; Ducreux, M.; Duvillard, P.; Ouellet, J.F.; Dromain, C.; Schlumberger, M.; Pocard, M.; Boige, V.; Miquel, C.; et al. Liver resection (and associated extrahepatic resections) for metastatic well-differentiated endocrine tumors: A 15-year single center prospective study. *Surgery* **2003**, *133*, 375–382. [CrossRef]
99. Dromain, C.; de Baere, T.; Baudin, E.; Galline, J.; Ducreux, M.; Boige, V.; Duvillard, P.; Laplanche, A.; Caillet, H.; Lasser, P.; et al. MR imaging of hepatic metastases caused by neuroendocrine tumors: Comparing four techniques. *Am. J. Roentgenol.* **2003**, *180*, 121–128. [CrossRef]
100. Calderone, A. The Biological Role of Nestin((+))-Cells in Physiological and Pathological Cardiovascular Remodeling. *Front. Cell Dev. Biol.* **2018**, *6*, 15. [CrossRef]
101. Yazdani, S.; Kasajima, A.; Tamaki, K.; Nakamura, Y.; Fujishima, F.; Ohtsuka, H.; Motoi, F.; Unno, M.; Watanabe, M.; Sato, Y.; et al. Angiogenesis and vascular maturation in neuroendocrine tumors. *Hum. Pathol.* **2014**, *45*, 866–874. [CrossRef] [PubMed]
102. Hall, S.M.; Hislop, A.A.; Pierce, C.M.; Haworth, S.G. Prenatal origins of human intrapulmonary arteries: Formation and smooth muscle maturation. *Am. J. Respir. Cell Mol. Biol.* **2000**, *23*, 194–203. [CrossRef] [PubMed]
103. Helmlinger, G.; Netti, P.A.; Lichtenbeld, H.C.; Melder, R.J.; Jain, R.K. Solid stress inhibits the growth of multicellular tumor spheroids. *Nat. Biotechnol.* **1997**, *15*, 778–783. [CrossRef] [PubMed]
104. Faivre, S.; Niccoli, P.; Castellano, D.; Valle, J.W.; Hammel, P.; Raoul, J.L.; Vinik, A.; Van Cutsem, E.; Bang, Y.J.; Lee, S.H.; et al. Sunitinib in pancreatic neuroendocrine tumors: Updated progression-free survival and final overall survival from a phase III randomized study. *Ann. Oncol.* **2017**, *28*, 339–343. [CrossRef] [PubMed]
105. Gu, J.W.; Rizzo, P.; Pannuti, A.; Golde, T.; Osborne, B.; Miele, L. Notch signals in the endothelium and cancer "stem-like" cells: Opportunities for cancer therapy. *Vasc. Cell* **2012**, *4*, 7. [CrossRef]
106. Rafii, S.; Butler, J.M.; Ding, B.S. Angiocrine functions of organ-specific endothelial cells. *Nature* **2016**, *529*, 316–325. [CrossRef]
107. Awgulewitsch, C.P.; Trinh, L.T.; Hatzopoulos, A.K. The Vascular Wall: A Plastic Hub of Activity in Cardiovascular Homeostasis and Disease. *Curr. Cardiol. Rep.* **2017**, *19*, 51. [CrossRef]
108. Kohlenberg, J.D.; Chen, Y.; Best, B.; Storz, P.; Peterson, R.T.; Silverstein, R.; Ren, B. Abstract LB-338: A novel LPA-PKD1-FoxO1 pathway in endothelial cells provides an angiogenic switch via down-regulation of CD36 transcription and induction of arteriogenic responses. *Cancer Res.* **2013**, *73*. [CrossRef]
109. Opansky, C.; Best, B.; Yuan, R.; Cao, Q.; Ren, B. Protein Kinase D1 Signaling is the Key to Arterial Differentiation of Vascular Endothelial Cells. *Circulation* **2016**, *134*, A14437.
110. Yao, J.C.; Eisner, M.P.; Leary, C.; Dagohoy, C.; Phan, A.; Rashid, A.; Hassan, M.; Evans, D.B. Population-based study of islet cell carcinoma. *Ann. Surg. Oncol.* **2007**, *14*, 3492–3500. [CrossRef]
111. Metz, D.C.; Jensen, R.T. Gastrointestinal neuroendocrine tumors: Pancreatic endocrine tumors. *Gastroenterology* **2008**, *135*, 1469–1492. [CrossRef] [PubMed]
112. Lawrence, B.; Gustafsson, B.I.; Chan, A.; Svejda, B.; Kidd, M.; Modlin, I.M. The epidemiology of gastroenteropancreatic neuroendocrine tumors. *Endocrinol. Metab. Clin. N. Am.* **2011**, *40*, 1–18. [CrossRef] [PubMed]
113. Cueto, A.; Burigana, F.; Nicolini, A.; Lugnani, F. Neuroendocrine tumors of the lung: Hystological classification, diagnosis, traditional and new therapeutic approaches. *Curr. Med. Chem.* **2014**, *21*, 1107–1116. [CrossRef] [PubMed]
114. Liakakos, T.; Roukos, D.H. Everolimus and sunitinib: From mouse models to treatment of pancreatic neuroendocrine tumors. *Future Oncol.* **2011**, *7*, 1025–1029. [CrossRef]
115. Hori, T.; Takaori, K.; Uemoto, S. Pancreatic neuroendocrine tumor accompanied with multiple liver metastases. *World J. Hepatol.* **2014**, *6*, 596–600. [CrossRef]
116. Rindi, G.; Klersy, C.; Albarello, L.; Baudin, E.; Bianchi, A.; Buchler, M.W.; Caplin, M.; Couvelard, A.; Cros, J.; de Herder, W.W.; et al. Competitive Testing of the WHO 2010 versus the WHO 2017 Grading of Pancreatic Neuroendocrine Neoplasms: Data from a Large International Cohort Study. *Neuroendocrinology* **2018**, *107*, 375–386. [CrossRef]

117. Proye, C. Natural history of liver metastasis of gastroenteropancreatic neuroendocrine tumors: Place for chemoembolization. *World J. Surg.* **2001**, *25*, 685–688. [CrossRef]
118. Fendrich, V.; Waldmann, J.; Bartsch, D.K.; Langer, P. Surgical management of pancreatic endocrine tumors. *Nat. Rev. Clin. Oncol.* **2009**, *6*, 419–428. [CrossRef]
119. Nguyen, S.Q.; Angel, L.P.; Divino, C.M.; Schluender, S.; Warner, R.R. Surgery in malignant pancreatic neuroendocrine tumors. *J. Surg. Oncol.* **2007**, *96*, 397–403. [CrossRef]
120. Villaume, K.; Blanc, M.; Gouysse, G.; Walter, T.; Couderc, C.; Nejjari, M.; Vercherat, C.; Cordier-Bussat, M.; Roche, C.; Scoazec, J.Y. VEGF secretion by neuroendocrine tumor cells is inhibited by octreotide and by inhibitors of the PI3K/AKT/mTOR pathway. *Neuroendocrinology* **2010**, *91*, 268–278. [CrossRef]
121. Zhang, J.; Cao, R.; Zhang, Y.; Jia, T.; Cao, Y.; Wahlberg, E. Differential roles of PDGFR-alpha and PDGFR-beta in angiogenesis and vessel stability. *FASEB J.* **2009**, *23*, 153–163. [CrossRef] [PubMed]
122. Raymond, E.; Dahan, L.; Raoul, J.L.; Bang, Y.J.; Borbath, I.; Lombard-Bohas, C.; Valle, J.; Metrakos, P.; Smith, D.; Vinik, A.; et al. Sunitinib malate for the treatment of pancreatic neuroendocrine tumors. *N. Engl. J. Med.* **2011**, *364*, 501–513. [CrossRef] [PubMed]
123. Valle, J.W.; Borbath, I.; Rosbrook, B.; Fernandez, K.; Raymond, E. Sunitinib in patients with pancreatic neuroendocrine tumors: Update of safety data. *Future Oncol.* **2019**, *15*. [CrossRef] [PubMed]
124. Capozzi, M.; VON Arx, C.; DE Divitiis, C.; Ottaiano, A.; Tatangelo, F.; Romano, G.M.; Tafuto, S. Antiangiogenic Therapy in Pancreatic Neuroendocrine Tumors. *Anticancer Res.* **2016**, *36*, 5025–5030. [CrossRef] [PubMed]
125. Berruti, A.; Fazio, N.; Ferrero, A.; Brizzi, M.P.; Volante, M.; Nobili, E.; Tozzi, L.; Bodei, L.; Torta, M.; D'Avolio, A.; et al. Bevacizumab plus octreotide and metronomic capecitabine in patients with metastatic well-to-moderately differentiated neuroendocrine tumors: The XELBEVOCT study. *BMC Cancer* **2014**, *14*, 184. [CrossRef] [PubMed]
126. Chan, J.A.; Stuart, K.; Earle, C.C.; Clark, J.W.; Bhargava, P.; Miksad, R.; Blaszkowsky, L.; Enzinger, P.C.; Meyerhardt, J.A.; Zheng, H.; et al. Prospective study of bevacizumab plus temozolomide in patients with advanced neuroendocrine tumors. *J. Clin. Oncol.* **2012**, *30*, 2963–2968. [CrossRef] [PubMed]
127. Helfrich, I.; Scheffrahn, I.; Bartling, S.; Weis, J.; von Felbert, V.; Middleton, M.; Kato, M.; Ergun, S.; Augustin, H.G.; Schadendorf, D. Resistance to antiangiogenic therapy is directed by vascular phenotype, vessel stabilization, and maturation in malignant melanoma. *J. Exp. Med.* **2010**, *207*, 491–503. [CrossRef]
128. Erber, R.; Thurnher, A.; Katsen, A.D.; Groth, G.; Kerger, H.; Hammes, H.P.; Menger, M.D.; Ullrich, A.; Vajkoczy, P. Combined inhibition of VEGF and PDGF signaling enforces tumor vessel regression by interfering with pericyte-mediated endothelial cell survival mechanisms. *FASEB J.* **2004**, *18*, 338–340. [CrossRef]
129. Sitohy, B.; Nagy, J.A.; Dvorak, H.F. Anti-VEGF/VEGFR therapy for cancer: Reassessing the target. *Cancer Res.* **2012**, *72*, 1909–1914. [CrossRef]
130. Uri, I.; Grozinsky-Glasberg, S. Current treatment strategies for patients with advanced gastroenteropancreatic neuroendocrine tumors (GEP-NETs). *Clin. Diabetes Endocrinol.* **2018**, *4*, 16. [CrossRef]
131. Raymond, E.; Kulke, M.H.; Qin, S.; Yu, X.; Schenker, M.; Cubillo, A.; Lou, W.; Tomasek, J.; Thiis-Evensen, E.; Xu, J.M.; et al. Efficacy and Safety of Sunitinib in Patients with Well-Differentiated Pancreatic Neuroendocrine Tumours. *Neuroendocrinology* **2018**, *107*, 237–245. [CrossRef] [PubMed]
132. Rinzivillo, M.; Fazio, N.; Pusceddu, S.; Spallanzani, A.; Ibrahim, T.; Campana, D.; Marconcini, R.; Partelli, S.; Badalamenti, G.; Brizzi, M.P.; et al. Sunitinib in patients with pre-treated pancreatic neuroendocrine tumors: A real-world study. *Pancreatology* **2018**, *18*, 198–203. [CrossRef] [PubMed]
133. Yao, J.C.; Shah, M.H.; Ito, T.; Bohas, C.L.; Wolin, E.M.; Van Cutsem, E.; Hobday, T.J.; Okusaka, T.; Capdevila, J.; de Vries, E.G.; et al. Everolimus for advanced pancreatic neuroendocrine tumors. *N. Engl. J. Med.* **2011**, *364*, 514–523. [CrossRef] [PubMed]
134. Baldelli, R.; Barnabei, A.; Rizza, L.; Isidori, A.M.; Rota, F.; Di Giacinto, P.; Paoloni, A.; Torino, F.; Corsello, S.M.; Lenzi, A.; et al. Somatostatin analogs therapy in gastroenteropancreatic neuroendocrine tumors: Current aspects and new perspectives. *Front. Endocrinol.* **2014**, *5*, 7. [CrossRef] [PubMed]
135. Caplin, M.E.; Pavel, M.; Cwikla, J.B.; Phan, A.T.; Raderer, M.; Sedlackova, E.; Cadiot, G.; Wolin, E.M.; Capdevila, J.; Wall, L.; et al. Lanreotide in metastatic enteropancreatic neuroendocrine tumors. *N. Engl. J. Med.* **2014**, *371*, 224–233. [CrossRef]

136. Woltering, E.A.; Barrie, R.; O'Dorisio, T.M.; Arce, D.; Ure, T.; Cramer, A.; Holmes, D.; Robertson, J.; Fassler, J. Somatostatin analogues inhibit angiogenesis in the chick chorioallantoic membrane. *J. Surg. Res.* **1991**, *50*, 245–251. [CrossRef]
137. Grozinsky-Glasberg, S.; Shimon, I.; Korbonits, M.; Grossman, A.B. Somatostatin analogues in the control of neuroendocrine tumours: Efficacy and mechanisms. *Endocr. Relat. Cancer* **2008**, *15*, 701–720. [CrossRef]
138. Dasgupta, P. Somatostatin analogues: Multiple roles in cellular proliferation, neoplasia, and angiogenesis. *Pharmacol. Ther.* **2004**, *102*, 61–85. [CrossRef]
139. Albini, A.; Florio, T.; Giunciuglio, D.; Masiello, L.; Carlone, S.; Corsaro, A.; Thellung, S.; Cai, T.; Noonan, D.M.; Schettini, G. Somatostatin controls Kaposi's sarcoma tumor growth through inhibition of angiogenesis. *FASEB J.* **1999**, *13*, 647–655. [CrossRef]
140. Mentlein, R.; Eichler, O.; Forstreuter, F.; Held-Feindt, J. Somatostatin inhibits the production of vascular endothelial growth factor in human glioma cells. *Int. J. Cancer* **2001**, *92*, 545–550. [CrossRef]
141. Boehm, T.; Folkman, J.; Browder, T.; O'Reilly, M.S. Antiangiogenic therapy of experimental cancer does not induce acquired drug resistance. *Nature* **1997**, *390*, 404–407. [CrossRef] [PubMed]
142. Mauceri, H.J.; Hanna, N.N.; Beckett, M.A.; Gorski, D.H.; Staba, M.J.; Stellato, K.A.; Bigelow, K.; Heimann, R.; Gately, S.; Dhanabal, M.; et al. Combined effects of angiostatin and ionizing radiation in antitumour therapy. *Nature* **1998**, *394*, 287–291. [CrossRef] [PubMed]
143. Friedlander, M.; Brooks, P.C.; Shaffer, R.W.; Kincaid, C.M.; Varner, J.A.; Cheresh, D.A. Definition of two angiogenic pathways by distinct alpha v integrins. *Science* **1995**, *270*, 1500–1502. [CrossRef] [PubMed]
144. Ferrara, N.; Chen, H.; Davis-Smyth, T.; Gerber, H.P.; Nguyen, T.N.; Peers, D.; Chisholm, V.; Hillan, K.J.; Schwall, R.H. Vascular endothelial growth factor is essential for corpus luteum angiogenesis. *Nat. Med.* **1998**, *4*, 336–340. [CrossRef] [PubMed]
145. Han, Z.B.; Ren, H.; Zhao, H.; Chi, Y.; Chen, K.; Zhou, B.; Liu, Y.J.; Zhang, L.; Xu, B.; Liu, B.; et al. Hypoxia-inducible factor (HIF)-1 alpha directly enhances the transcriptional activity of stem cell factor (SCF) in response to hypoxia and epidermal growth factor (EGF). *Carcinogenesis* **2008**, *29*, 1853–1861. [CrossRef] [PubMed]
146. Cooke, V.G.; LeBleu, V.S.; Keskin, D.; Khan, Z.; O'Connell, J.T.; Teng, Y.; Duncan, M.B.; Xie, L.; Maeda, G.; Vong, S.; et al. Pericyte depletion results in hypoxia-associated epithelial-to-mesenchymal transition and metastasis mediated by met signaling pathway. *Cancer Cell* **2012**, *21*, 66–81. [CrossRef]
147. Paez-Ribes, M.; Allen, E.; Hudock, J.; Takeda, T.; Okuyama, H.; Vinals, F.; Inoue, M.; Bergers, G.; Hanahan, D.; Casanovas, O. Antiangiogenic therapy elicits malignant progression of tumors to increased local invasion and distant metastasis. *Cancer Cell* **2009**, *15*, 220–231. [CrossRef]
148. Manegold, C.; Dingemans, A.C.; Gray, J.E.; Nakagawa, K.; Nicolson, M.; Peters, S.; Reck, M.; Wu, Y.L.; Brustugun, O.T.; Crino, L.; et al. The Potential of Combined Immunotherapy and Antiangiogenesis for the Synergistic Treatment of Advanced NSCLC. *J. Thorac. Oncol.* **2017**, *12*, 194–207. [CrossRef]
149. Mack, J.J.; Iruela-Arispe, M.L. NOTCH regulation of the endothelial cell phenotype. *Curr. Opin. Hematol.* **2018**, *25*, 212–218. [CrossRef]
150. Noguera-Troise, I.; Daly, C.; Papadopoulos, N.J.; Coetzee, S.; Boland, P.; Gale, N.W.; Lin, H.C.; Yancopoulos, G.D.; Thurston, G. Blockade of Dll4 inhibits tumour growth by promoting non-productive angiogenesis. *Nature* **2006**, *444*, 1032–1037. [CrossRef]
151. Ridgway, J.; Zhang, G.; Wu, Y.; Stawicki, S.; Liang, W.C.; Chanthery, Y.; Kowalski, J.; Watts, R.J.; Callahan, C.; Kasman, I.; et al. Inhibition of Dll4 signalling inhibits tumour growth by deregulating angiogenesis. *Nature* **2006**, *444*, 1083–1087. [CrossRef] [PubMed]
152. Scehnet, J.S.; Jiang, W.; Kumar, S.R.; Krasnoperov, V.; Trindade, A.; Benedito, R.; Djokovic, D.; Borges, C.; Ley, E.J.; Duarte, A.; et al. Inhibition of Dll4-mediated signaling induces proliferation of immature vessels and results in poor tissue perfusion. *Blood* **2007**, *109*, 4753–4760. [CrossRef] [PubMed]
153. Low, S.; Barnes, J.L.; Zammit, P.S.; Beauchamp, J.R. Delta-Like 4 Activates Notch 3 to Regulate Self-Renewal in Skeletal Muscle Stem Cells. *Stem Cells* **2018**, *36*, 458–466. [CrossRef] [PubMed]
154. Takahashi, Y.; Akishima-Fukasawa, Y.; Kobayashi, N.; Sano, T.; Kosuge, T.; Nimura, Y.; Kanai, Y.; Hiraoka, N. Prognostic value of tumor architecture, tumor-associated vascular characteristics, and expression of angiogenic molecules in pancreatic endocrine tumors. *Clin. Cancer Res. Off. J. Am. Assoc. Cancer Res.* **2007**, *13*, 187–196. [CrossRef]

155. Tan, G.; Cioc, A.M.; Perez-Montiel, D.; Ellison, E.C.; Frankel, W.L. Microvascular density does not correlate with histopathology and outcome in neuroendocrine tumors of the pancreas. *Appl. Immunohistochem. Mol. Morphol.* **2004**, *12*, 31–35. [CrossRef]
156. Laitakari, J.; Nayha, V.; Stenback, F. Size, shape, structure, and direction of angiogenesis in laryngeal tumour development. *J. Clin. Pathol.* **2004**, *57*, 394–401. [CrossRef]
157. Nayha, V.V.; Stenback, F.G. Increased angiogenesis is associated with poor prognosis of squamous cell carcinoma of the vulva. *Acta Obstet. Gynecol. Scand.* **2007**, *86*, 1392–1397. [CrossRef]
158. Crabtree, J.S.; Singleton, C.S.; Miele, L. Notch Signaling in Neuroendocrine Tumors. *Front. Oncol.* **2016**, *6*, 94. [CrossRef]
159. Radtke, F.; Raj, K. The role of Notch in tumorigenesis: Oncogene or tumour suppressor? *Nat. Rev. Cancer* **2003**, *3*, 756–767. [CrossRef]
160. Kunnimalaiyaan, M.; Chen, H. Tumor suppressor role of Notch-1 signaling in neuroendocrine tumors. *Oncologist* **2007**, *12*, 535–542. [CrossRef]
161. Kunnimalaiyaan, M.; Yan, S.; Wong, F.; Zhang, Y.W.; Chen, H. Hairy Enhancer of Split-1 (HES-1), a Notch1 effector, inhibits the growth of carcinoid tumor cells. *Surgery* **2005**, *138*, 1137–1142. [CrossRef] [PubMed]
162. Kunnimalaiyaan, M.; Traeger, K.; Chen, H. Conservation of the Notch1 signaling pathway in gastrointestinal carcinoid cells. *Am. J. Physiol. Gastrointest. Liver Physiol.* **2005**, *289*, G636–G642. [CrossRef] [PubMed]
163. Kunnimalaiyaan, M.; Vaccaro, A.M.; Ndiaye, M.A.; Chen, H. Overexpression of the NOTCH1 intracellular domain inhibits cell proliferation and alters the neuroendocrine phenotype of medullary thyroid cancer cells. *J. Biol. Chem.* **2006**, *281*, 39819–39830. [CrossRef] [PubMed]
164. Nakakura, E.K.; Sriuranpong, V.R.; Kunnimalaiyaan, M.; Hsiao, E.C.; Schuebel, K.E.; Borges, M.W.; Jin, N.; Collins, B.J.; Nelkin, B.D.; Chen, H.; et al. Regulation of neuroendocrine differentiation in gastrointestinal carcinoid tumor cells by notch signaling. *J. Clin. Endocrinol. Metab.* **2005**, *90*, 4350–4356. [CrossRef]
165. Krampitz, G.W.; George, B.M.; Willingham, S.B.; Volkmer, J.P.; Weiskopf, K.; Jahchan, N.; Newman, A.M.; Sahoo, D.; Zemek, A.J.; Yanovsky, R.L.; et al. Identification of tumorigenic cells and therapeutic targets in pancreatic neuroendocrine tumors. *Proc. Natl. Acad. Sci. USA* **2016**, *113*, 4464–4469. [CrossRef]
166. Wang, H.; Chen, Y.; Fernandez-Del Castillo, C.; Yilmaz, O.; Deshpande, V. Heterogeneity in signaling pathways of gastroenteropancreatic neuroendocrine tumors: A critical look at notch signaling pathway. *Mod. Pathol.* **2013**, *26*, 139–147. [CrossRef]
167. Krausch, M.; Kroepil, F.; Lehwald, N.; Lachenmayer, A.; Schott, M.; Anlauf, M.; Cupisti, K.; Knoefel, W.T.; Raffel, A. Notch 1 tumor expression is lacking in highly proliferative pancreatic neuroendocrine tumors. *Endocrine* **2013**, *44*, 182–186. [CrossRef]
168. Eliasz, S.; Liang, S.; Chen, Y.; De Marco, M.A.; Machek, O.; Skucha, S.; Miele, L.; Bocchetta, M. Notch-1 stimulates survival of lung adenocarcinoma cells during hypoxia by activating the IGF-1R pathway. *Oncogene* **2010**, *29*, 2488–2498. [CrossRef]
169. Sriuranpong, V.; Borges, M.W.; Strock, C.L.; Nakakura, E.K.; Watkins, D.N.; Blaumueller, C.M.; Nelkin, B.D.; Ball, D.W. Notch signaling induces rapid degradation of achaete-scute homolog 1. *Mol. Cell Biol.* **2002**, *22*, 3129–3139. [CrossRef]
170. Jaskula-Sztul, R.; Eide, J.; Tesfazghi, S.; Dammalapati, A.; Harrison, A.D.; Yu, X.M.; Scheinebeck, C.; Winston-McPherson, G.; Kupcho, K.R.; Robers, M.B.; et al. Tumor-suppressor role of Notch3 in medullary thyroid carcinoma revealed by genetic and pharmacological induction. *Mol. Cancer Ther.* **2015**, *14*, 499–512. [CrossRef]
171. Somnay, Y.R.; Yu, X.M.; Lloyd, R.V.; Leverson, G.; Aburjania, Z.; Jang, S.; Jaskula-Sztul, R.; Chen, H. Notch3 expression correlates with thyroid cancer differentiation, induces apoptosis, and predicts disease prognosis. *Cancer* **2017**, *123*, 769–782. [CrossRef] [PubMed]
172. Lou, I.; Odorico, S.; Yu, X.M.; Harrison, A.; Jaskula-Sztul, R.; Chen, H. Notch3 as a novel therapeutic target in metastatic medullary thyroid cancer. *Surgery* **2018**, *163*, 104–111. [CrossRef] [PubMed]
173. Zhou, M.; Jin, W.Y.; Fan, Z.W.; Han, R.C. Analysis of the expression of the Notch3 receptor protein in adult lung cancer. *Oncol. Lett.* **2013**, *5*, 499–504. [CrossRef] [PubMed]
174. Ito, T.; Udaka, N.; Yazawa, T.; Okudela, K.; Hayashi, H.; Sudo, T.; Guillemot, F.; Kageyama, R.; Kitamura, H. Basic helix-loop-helix transcription factors regulate the neuroendocrine differentiation of fetal mouse pulmonary epithelium. *Development* **2000**, *127*, 3913–3921. [PubMed]

175. Marcucci, F.; Caserta, C.A.; Romeo, E.; Rumio, C. Antibody-Drug Conjugates (ADC) Against Cancer Stem-Like Cells (CSC)-Is There Still Room for Optimism? *Front. Oncol.* **2019**, *9*, 167. [CrossRef]
176. Lashari, B.H.; Vallatharasu, Y.; Kolandra, L.; Hamid, M.; Uprety, D. Rovalpituzumab Tesirine: A Novel DLL3-Targeting Antibody-Drug Conjugate. *Drugs R D* **2018**, *18*, 255–258. [CrossRef]
177. Saunders, L.R.; Bankovich, A.J.; Anderson, W.C.; Aujay, M.A.; Bheddah, S.; Black, K.; Desai, R.; Escarpe, P.A.; Hampl, J.; Laysang, A.; et al. A DLL3-targeted antibody-drug conjugate eradicates high-grade pulmonary neuroendocrine tumor-initiating cells in vivo. *Sci. Transl. Med.* **2015**, *7*, 302ra136. [CrossRef]
178. Kuhnert, F.; Kirshner, J.R.; Thurston, G. Dll4-Notch signaling as a therapeutic target in tumor angiogenesis. *Vasc. Cell* **2011**, *3*, 20. [CrossRef]
179. Driessens, G.; Beck, B.; Caauwe, A.; Simons, B.D.; Blanpain, C. Defining the mode of tumour growth by clonal analysis. *Nature* **2012**, *488*, 527–530. [CrossRef]
180. Schepers, A.G.; Snippert, H.J.; Stange, D.E.; van den Born, M.; van Es, J.H.; van de Wetering, M.; Clevers, H. Lineage tracing reveals Lgr5+ stem cell activity in mouse intestinal adenomas. *Science* **2012**, *337*, 730–735. [CrossRef]
181. Kozar, S.; Morrissey, E.; Nicholson, A.M.; van der Heijden, M.; Zecchini, H.I.; Kemp, R.; Tavare, S.; Vermeulen, L.; Winton, D.J. Continuous clonal labeling reveals small numbers of functional stem cells in intestinal crypts and adenomas. *Cell Stem Cell* **2013**, *13*, 626–633. [CrossRef] [PubMed]
182. Zomer, A.; Ellenbroek, S.I.; Ritsma, L.; Beerling, E.; Vrisekoop, N.; Van Rheenen, J. Intravital imaging of cancer stem cell plasticity in mammary tumors. *Stem Cells* **2013**, *31*, 602–606. [CrossRef] [PubMed]
183. Chen, J.; Li, Y.; Yu, T.S.; McKay, R.M.; Burns, D.K.; Kernie, S.G.; Parada, L.F. A restricted cell population propagates glioblastoma growth after chemotherapy. *Nature* **2012**, *488*, 522–526. [CrossRef] [PubMed]
184. Oshimori, N.; Oristian, D.; Fuchs, E. TGF-beta promotes heterogeneity and drug resistance in squamous cell carcinoma. *Cell* **2015**, *160*, 963–976. [CrossRef] [PubMed]
185. Batlle, E.; Clevers, H. Cancer stem cells revisited. *Nat. Med.* **2017**, *23*, 1124–1134. [CrossRef] [PubMed]
186. Mathis, R.A.; Sokol, E.S.; Gupta, P.B. Cancer cells exhibit clonal diversity in phenotypic plasticity. *Open Biol.* **2017**, *7*. [CrossRef]
187. Gupta, P.B.; Fillmore, C.M.; Jiang, G.; Shapira, S.D.; Tao, K.; Kuperwasser, C.; Lander, E.S. Stochastic state transitions give rise to phenotypic equilibrium in populations of cancer cells. *Cell* **2011**, *146*, 633–644. [CrossRef]
188. Hoeck, J.D.; Biehs, B.; Kurtova, A.V.; Kljavin, N.M.; de Sousa, E.M.F.; Alicke, B.; Koeppen, H.; Modrusan, Z.; Piskol, R.; de Sauvage, F.J. Stem cell plasticity enables hair regeneration following Lgr5(+) cell loss. *Nat. Cell Biol.* **2017**, *19*, 666–676. [CrossRef]
189. Lenos, K.J.; Miedema, D.M.; Lodestijn, S.C.; Nijman, L.E.; van den Bosch, T.; Romero Ros, X.; Lourenco, F.C.; Lecca, M.C.; van der Heijden, M.; van Neerven, S.M.; et al. Stem cell functionality is microenvironmentally defined during tumour expansion and therapy response in colon cancer. *Nat. Cell Biol.* **2018**, *20*, 1193–1202. [CrossRef]
190. de Sousa e Melo, F.; Kurtova, A.V.; Harnoss, J.M.; Kljavin, N.; Hoeck, J.D.; Hung, J.; Anderson, J.E.; Storm, E.E.; Modrusan, Z.; Koeppen, H.; et al. A distinct role for Lgr5(+) stem cells in primary and metastatic colon cancer. *Nature* **2017**, *543*, 676–680. [CrossRef]
191. Drost, J.; van Boxtel, R.; Blokzijl, F.; Mizutani, T.; Sasaki, N.; Sasselli, V.; de Ligt, J.; Behjati, S.; Grolleman, J.E.; van Wezel, T.; et al. Use of CRISPR-modified human stem cell organoids to study the origin of mutational signatures in cancer. *Science* **2017**, *358*, 234–238. [CrossRef]
192. Clevers, H. STEM CELLS. What is an adult stem cell? *Science* **2015**, *350*, 1319–1320. [CrossRef]
193. Ball, C.R.; Oppel, F.; Ehrenberg, K.R.; Dubash, T.D.; Dieter, S.M.; Hoffmann, C.M.; Abel, U.; Herbst, F.; Koch, M.; Werner, J.; et al. Succession of transiently active tumor-initiating cell clones in human pancreatic cancer xenografts. *EMBO Mol. Med.* **2017**, *9*, 918–932. [CrossRef]
194. McGranahan, N.; Swanton, C. Clonal Heterogeneity and Tumor Evolution: Past, Present, and the Future. *Cell* **2017**, *168*, 613–628. [CrossRef]
195. Jagust, P.; de Luxan-Delgado, B.; Parejo-Alonso, B.; Sancho, P. Metabolism-Based Therapeutic Strategies Targeting Cancer Stem Cells. *Front. Pharmacol.* **2019**, *10*, 203. [CrossRef]
196. Ryall, J.G.; Dell'Orso, S.; Derfoul, A.; Juan, A.; Zare, H.; Feng, X.; Clermont, D.; Koulnis, M.; Gutierrez-Cruz, G.; Fulco, M.; et al. The NAD(+)-dependent SIRT1 deacetylase translates a metabolic switch into regulatory epigenetics in skeletal muscle stem cells. *Cell Stem Cell* **2015**, *16*, 171–183. [CrossRef]

197. Buffie, C.G.; Bucci, V.; Stein, R.R.; McKenney, P.T.; Ling, L.; Gobourne, A.; No, D.; Liu, H.; Kinnebrew, M.; Viale, A.; et al. Precision microbiome reconstitution restores bile acid mediated resistance to Clostridium difficile. *Nature* **2015**, *517*, 205–208. [CrossRef]
198. Viale, A.; Pettazzoni, P.; Lyssiotis, C.A.; Ying, H.; Sanchez, N.; Marchesini, M.; Carugo, A.; Green, T.; Seth, S.; Giuliani, V.; et al. Oncogene ablation-resistant pancreatic cancer cells depend on mitochondrial function. *Nature* **2014**, *514*, 628–632. [CrossRef]
199. Sancho, P.; Burgos-Ramos, E.; Tavera, A.; Bou Kheir, T.; Jagust, P.; Schoenhals, M.; Barneda, D.; Sellers, K.; Campos-Olivas, R.; Grana, O.; et al. MYC/PGC-1alpha Balance Determines the Metabolic Phenotype and Plasticity of Pancreatic Cancer Stem Cells. *Cell Metab.* **2015**, *22*, 590–605. [CrossRef]
200. Barnekow, N.; Yuan, R.; Moran, P.; Ren, B. Abstract 16740: Foxo1-Activated Cd36 Transcription Switches Arteriolar Differentiation of Endothelial Cells. *Circulation* **2018**, *138*, A16740. [CrossRef]
201. Ladanyi, A.; Mukherjee, A.; Kenny, H.A.; Johnson, A.; Mitra, A.K.; Sundaresan, S.; Nieman, K.M.; Pascual, G.; Benitah, S.A.; Montag, A.; et al. Adipocyte-induced CD36 expression drives ovarian cancer progression and metastasis. *Oncogene* **2018**, *37*, 2285–2301. [CrossRef]
202. Ye, H.; Adane, B.; Khan, N.; Sullivan, T.; Minhajuddin, M.; Gasparetto, M.; Stevens, B.; Pei, S.; Balys, M.; Ashton, J.M.; et al. Leukemic Stem Cells Evade Chemotherapy by Metabolic Adaptation to an Adipose Tissue Niche. *Cell Stem Cell* **2016**, *19*, 23–37. [CrossRef]
203. Fumagalli, A.; Drost, J.; Suijkerbuijk, S.J.; van Boxtel, R.; de Ligt, J.; Offerhaus, G.J.; Begthel, H.; Beerling, E.; Tan, E.H.; Sansom, O.J.; et al. Genetic dissection of colorectal cancer progression by orthotopic transplantation of engineered cancer organoids. *Proc. Natl. Acad. Sci. USA* **2017**, *114*, E2357–E2364. [CrossRef]
204. Fujii, M.; Shimokawa, M.; Date, S.; Takano, A.; Matano, M.; Nanki, K.; Ohta, Y.; Toshimitsu, K.; Nakazato, Y.; Kawasaki, K.; et al. A Colorectal Tumor Organoid Library Demonstrates Progressive Loss of Niche Factor Requirements during Tumorigenesis. *Cell Stem Cell* **2016**, *18*, 827–838. [CrossRef]
205. Zhang, X.; Yalcin, S.; Lee, D.F.; Yeh, T.Y.; Lee, S.M.; Su, J.; Mungamuri, S.K.; Rimmele, P.; Kennedy, M.; Sellers, R.; et al. FOXO1 is an essential regulator of pluripotency in human embryonic stem cells. *Nat. Cell Biol.* **2011**, *13*, 1092–1099. [CrossRef]
206. Tothova, Z.; Gilliland, D.G. FoxO transcription factors and stem cell homeostasis: Insights from the hematopoietic system. *Cell Stem Cell* **2007**, *1*, 140–152. [CrossRef]
207. Sykes, S.M.; Lane, S.W.; Bullinger, L.; Kalaitzidis, D.; Yusuf, R.; Saez, B.; Ferraro, F.; Mercier, F.; Singh, H.; Brumme, K.M.; et al. AKT/FOXO signaling enforces reversible differentiation blockade in myeloid leukemias. *Cell* **2011**, *146*, 697–708. [CrossRef]
208. Paik, J.H.; Kollipara, R.; Chu, G.; Ji, H.; Xiao, Y.; Ding, Z.; Miao, L.; Tothova, Z.; Horner, J.W.; Carrasco, D.R.; et al. FoxOs are lineage-restricted redundant tumor suppressors and regulate endothelial cell homeostasis. *Cell* **2007**, *128*, 309–323. [CrossRef]
209. Wilhelm, K.; Happel, K.; Eelen, G.; Schoors, S.; Oellerich, M.F.; Lim, R.; Zimmermann, B.; Aspalter, I.M.; Franco, C.A.; Boettger, T.; et al. FOXO1 couples metabolic activity and growth state in the vascular endothelium. *Nature* **2016**, *529*, 216–220. [CrossRef]
210. Carrasco, P.; Zuazo-Gaztelu, I.; Casanovas, O. Sprouting strategies and dead ends in anti-angiogenic targeting of NETs. *J. Mol. Endocrinol.* **2017**, *59*, R77–R91. [CrossRef]
211. Chu, X.; Gao, X.; Jansson, L.; Quach, M.; Skogseid, B.; Barbu, A. Multiple microvascular alterations in pancreatic islets and neuroendocrine tumors of a Men1 mouse model. *Am. J. Pathol.* **2013**, *182*, 2355–2367. [CrossRef]
212. Wagenblast, E.; Soto, M.; Gutierrez-Angel, S.; Hartl, C.A.; Gable, A.L.; Maceli, A.R.; Erard, N.; Williams, A.M.; Kim, S.Y.; Dickopf, S.; et al. A model of breast cancer heterogeneity reveals vascular mimicry as a driver of metastasis. *Nature* **2015**, *520*, 358–362. [CrossRef]
213. Hendrix, M.J.; Seftor, E.A.; Seftor, R.E.; Chao, J.T.; Chien, D.S.; Chu, Y.W. Tumor cell vascular mimicry: Novel targeting opportunity in melanoma. *Pharmacol. Ther.* **2016**, *159*, 83–92. [CrossRef]
214. Zhou, L.; Liu, X.D.; Sun, M.; Zhang, X.; German, P.; Bai, S.; Ding, Z.; Tannir, N.; Wood, C.G.; Matin, S.F.; et al. Targeting MET and AXL overcomes resistance to sunitinib therapy in renal cell carcinoma. *Oncogene* **2016**, *35*, 2687–2697. [CrossRef]

215. Capdevila, J.; Fazio, N.; López-López, C.; Teule, A.; Valle, J.W.; Tafuto, S.; Custodio, A.B.; Reed, N.; Raderer, M.; Grande, E.; et al. Progression-free survival (PFS) and subgroups analyses of lenvatinib in patients (pts) with G1/G2 advanced pancreatic (panNETs) and gastrointestinal (giNETs) neuroendocrine tumors (NETs): Updated results from the phase II TALENT trial (GETNE 1509). *J. Clin. Oncol.* **2019**, *37*, 332. [CrossRef]

216. Capozzi, M.; De Divitiis, C.; Ottaiano, A.; von Arx, C.; Scala, S.; Tatangelo, F.; Delrio, P.; Tafuto, S. Lenvatinib, a molecule with versatile application: From preclinical evidence to future development in anti-cancer treatment. *Cancer Manag. Res.* **2019**, *11*, 3847–3860. [CrossRef]

217. Grande, E.; Lopez, C.; Alonso-Gordoa, T.; Benavent, M.; Capdevila, J.; Teule, A.; Custodio, A.; Sevilla, I.; Gajate, P.; Molina-Cerrillo, J.; et al. The SUNEVO (GETNE-1408) trial to evaluate the activity and safety of thecombination of sunitinib with evofosfamide (TH-302) in patients with G1/G2 metastatic pancreatic neuroendocrine tumours (pNETs) naïve forsystemic treatment: A phase II study of the Spanish Task Force Group for Neuroendocrine and Endocrine Tumors (GETNE). *J. Clin. Oncol.* **2019**, *37*, 4105. [CrossRef]

218. Ikezono, Y.; Koga, H.; Akiba, J.; Abe, M.; Yoshida, T.; Wada, F.; Nakamura, T.; Iwamoto, H.; Masuda, A.; Sakaue, T.; et al. Pancreatic Neuroendocrine Tumors and EMT Behavior Are Driven by the CSC Marker DCLK1. *Mol. Cancer Res.* **2017**, *15*, 744–752. [CrossRef]

219. Rigamonti, N.; Kadioglu, E.; Keklikoglou, I.; Wyser Rmili, C.; Leow, C.C.; De Palma, M. Role of angiopoietin-2 in adaptive tumor resistance to VEGF signaling blockade. *Cell Rep.* **2014**, *8*, 696–706. [CrossRef]

220. Biel, N.M.; Siemann, D.W. Targeting the Angiopoietin-2/Tie-2 axis in conjunction with VEGF signal interference. *Cancer Lett.* **2016**, *380*, 525–533. [CrossRef]

221. Maione, F.; Capano, S.; Regano, D.; Zentilin, L.; Giacca, M.; Casanovas, O.; Bussolino, F.; Serini, G.; Giraudo, E. Semaphorin 3A overcomes cancer hypoxia and metastatic dissemination induced by antiangiogenic treatment in mice. *J. Clin. Invest.* **2012**, *122*, 1832–1848. [CrossRef]

222. Allen, E.; Walters, I.B.; Hanahan, D. Brivanib, a dual FGF/VEGF inhibitor, is active both first and second line against mouse pancreatic neuroendocrine tumors developing adaptive/evasive resistance to VEGF inhibition. *Clin. Cancer Res. Off. J. Am. Assoc. Cancer Res.* **2011**, *17*, 5299–5310. [CrossRef]

223. Hilfenhaus, G.; Gohrig, A.; Pape, U.F.; Neumann, T.; Jann, H.; Zdunek, D.; Hess, G.; Stassen, J.M.; Wiedenmann, B.; Detjen, K.; et al. Placental growth factor supports neuroendocrine tumor growth and predicts disease prognosis in patients. *Endocr. Relat. Cancer* **2013**, *20*, 305–319. [CrossRef]

224. Fischer, C.; Jonckx, B.; Mazzone, M.; Zacchigna, S.; Loges, S.; Pattarini, L.; Chorianopoulos, E.; Liesenborghs, L.; Koch, M.; De Mol, M.; et al. Anti-PlGF inhibits growth of VEGF(R)-inhibitor-resistant tumors without affecting healthy vessels. *Cell* **2007**, *131*, 463–475. [CrossRef]

225. Marconcini, R.; Faviana, P.; Campani, D.; Galli, L.; Antonuzzo, A.; Orlandini, C.; Falcone, A.; Ricci, S. Enhancer of zest homolog 2 (EZH2) expression in well and moderately differentiated pancreatic neuroendocrine tumor (pNET). *Ann. Oncol.* **2016**, *27*. [CrossRef]

226. Yang, L.; Yu, X.; Yang, Y. Autotaxin upregulated by STAT3 activation contributes to invasion in pancreatic neuroendocrine neoplasms. *Endocr. Connect.* **2018**, *7*, 1299–1307. [CrossRef]

227. Chen, Y.; Ramakrishnan, D.P.; Ren, B. Regulation of angiogenesis by phospholipid lysophosphatidic acid. *Front. Biosci. (Landmark Ed)* **2013**, *18*, 852–861.

228. Liu, S.; Umezu-Goto, M.; Murph, M.; Lu, Y.; Liu, W.; Zhang, F.; Yu, S.; Stephens, L.C.; Cui, X.; Murrow, G.; et al. Expression of autotaxin and lysophosphatidic acid receptors increases mammary tumorigenesis, invasion, and metastases. *Cancer Cell* **2009**, *15*, 539–550. [CrossRef]

229. Liu, Y.; An, S.; Ward, R.; Yang, Y.; Guo, X.X.; Li, W.; Xu, T.R. G protein-coupled receptors as promising cancer targets. *Cancer Lett.* **2016**, *376*, 226–239. [CrossRef]

230. Zecchin, A.; Kalucka, J.; Dubois, C.; Carmeliet, P. How Endothelial Cells Adapt Their Metabolism to Form Vessels in Tumors. *Front. Immunol.* **2017**, *8*, 1750. [CrossRef]

2

Is there a Chance to Promote Arteriogenesis by DPP4 Inhibitors Even in Type 2 Diabetes?

Srinivasan Vedantham [1,2], Anna-Kristina Kluever [3] and Elisabeth Deindl [3,*]

1 MedGenome Labs Ltd., Bangalore, Karnataka 560099, India; srinivasan.vedantham@gmail.com
2 School of Chemical Biotechnology, SASTRA University, Thanjavur 613401, India
3 Walter-Brendel-Centre of Experimental Medicine, University Hospital, LMU Munich, 80336 Munich, Germany; annakluever97@gmail.com
* Correspondence: elisabeth.deindl@med.uni-muenchen.de

Abstract: Cardiovascular diseases (CVD) are still the prevailing cause of death not only in industrialized countries, but even worldwide. Type 2 diabetes mellitus (type 2 DM) and hyperlipidemia, a metabolic disorder that is often associated with diabetes, are major risk factors for developing CVD. Recently, clinical trials proved the safety of gliptins in treating patients with type 2 DM. Gliptins are dipeptidyl-peptidase 4 (DPP4/CD26) inhibitors, which stabilize glucagon-like peptide-1 (GLP-1), thereby increasing the bioavailability of insulin. Moreover, blocking DPP4 results in increased levels of stromal cell derived factor 1 (SDF-1). SDF-1 has been shown in pre-clinical animal studies to improve heart function and survival after myocardial infarction, and to promote arteriogenesis, the growth of natural bypasses, compensating for the function of an occluded artery. Clinical trials, however, failed to demonstrate a superiority of gliptins compared to placebo treated type 2 DM patients in terms of cardiovascular (CV) outcomes. This review highlights the function of DPP4 inhibitors in type 2 DM, and in treating cardiovascular diseases, with special emphasis on arteriogenesis. It critically addresses the potency of currently available gliptins and gives rise to hope by pointing out the most relevant questions that need to be resolved.

Keywords: cardiovascular disease (CVD); arteriogenesis; diabetes mellitus; dipeptidyl-peptidase-4 (DPP4) inhibitors; stromal-cell-derived factor-1 (SDF-1); gliptins

---

1. Introduction

Cardiovascular diseases (CVD), such as coronary heart disease, cerebrovascular disease, and peripheral artery disease, are still the major cause of morbidity and death worldwide. For 2030, the World Health Organization (WHO) projected around 23 million deaths due to CVD [1]. Hyperlipidemia and diabetes mellitus are major risk factors for CVD by increasing atherosclerosis [2]. Moreover, collateral artery growth (arteriogenesis), which compensates for the functional loss of an artery due to atherosclerosis, is compromised in diabetes [3,4], a disease which is often associated with hyperlipidemia (see below). Accordingly, there is a pressing need for effective drugs to treat CVD, which also show positive effects in patients with diabetes, even with insulin resistance. In particular, these drugs should have the capacity to promote arteriogenesis, which is a tissue-, and even life-saving, process. Dipeptidyl-peptidase 4 (DPP4/CD26) inhibitors might present such drugs.

2. Arteriogenesis

The detrimental consequences of arterial stenosis, such as stroke, myocardial infarction, or peripheral artery disease, are a huge burden for affected patients worldwide. Occlusion of main blood conducting arteries results in severe ischemic damage of distal tissue, which might not be only associated with tissue damage, but even death. However, in the clinic, it is repeatedly observed that patients with occluded arteries show only minimal symptoms. These patients profited from arteriogenesis as a response to slow progressive stenosis [5]. Our whole body, not only the brain and the heart, but also the periphery, is pervaded with a collateral artery network. Upon slow progression of stenosis formation, blood flow is redirected into pre-existing collateral arteries bypassing the stenosing artery. Due to the increased blood flow, the endothelial cells of detouring arterioles experience elevated mechanical load, i.e. fluid shear stress [6], leading to their activation [7]. In contrast to angiogenesis, which is defined as the sprouting of capillaries, collateral artery growth not only involves the proliferation of endothelial cells, but also of smooth muscle cells. Recently, a mechanosensory complex consisting of vascular endothelial growth factor receptor 2 (VEGFR2), platelet endothelial cell adhesion molecule (PECAM)-1, and the adaptor protein vascular endothelial cell cadherin (VE-cadherin) has been identified [8]. It has been discussed for a long time whether the VEGFR2 ligand, vascular endothelial growth factor-A (VEGF-A), plays a role in arteriogenesis [9]. Whereas blocking of VEGFR2 significantly interfered with the process of arteriogenesis, administration of VEGF-A showed only little or no effect. We were recently able to show that the process of collateral artery growth is associated with elevated levels of VEGF-A [10], and that these levels of VEGF-A are not only necessary, but also sufficient to drive arteriogenesis. Accordingly, application of VEGF-A will not further promote the growth of collaterals, whereas blocking its cognate receptor, VEGFR2, dramatically interferes with vessel growth. As endothelial cells do not produce VEGF-A [11], the question arises, what is the source of VEGF-A. The endothelial glycocalyx consists of hyaluronic acid, glycoproteins, and proteoglycans, conferring it a negative charge. In the extended endothelial cell surface layer, plasma proteins and growth factors, among them VEGF-A, are stored [12]. Due to locally increased fluid shear stress, VEGF-A binds to VEGFR2, which involves Neuropilin-1 amplifying VEGFR2 signaling [13]. Thereupon, probably several cascades become activated in endothelial cells. Amongst them, the phosphatidylinositide 3-kinases (PI3K)/Akt pathway is relevant for increased expression levels of endothelial nitric oxide synthase (eNOS) and neuronal nitric oxide synthase (nNOS). Both isoforms are relevant for endothelial cell proliferation and are likely able to substitute for each other [10]. Moreover, VEGFR2/Neuropilin-1 signaling has been engaged in releasing the major ligand of the platelet receptor glycoprotein 1bα (GPIbα), the van Willebrand factor (vWF), from endothelial cells [14]. In recent investigations, we have demonstrated that GPIbα is essential for transient interaction of platelets with the endothelium [15], which is likely to trigger surface expression of P-selectin on platelets [16]. Upon binding of P-selectin to P-selectin glycoprotein ligand 1 (PSGL-1) on neutrophils, platelet-neutrophil aggregates (PNAs) are formed, resulting in neutrophil-NADPH oxidase 2 (Nox2) activation and translocation of urokinase plasminogen activator (uPA) on the surface of neutrophils [17]. Neutrophil uPA, together with endothelial cell uPA, whose expression is increased during the process of arteriogenesis [18], are relevant for paracellular transmigration and extravasation of neutrophils [19]. In the perivascular space, reactive oxygen species (ROS)- derived from neutrophil Nox-2 activate mast cells [17]. Mast cells, in turn, recruit further neutrophils by increasing the bioavailability of tumor necrosis factor α (TNF α). Neutrophils are a rich source of VEGF-A, the expression and release of which is mediated by midkine [10], enforcing VEGF-A signal transduction cascades resulting in endothelial cell proliferation and mast cell activation. In addition to neutrophils, activated mast cells also recruit T cells [17]. Moreover, by increasing the bioavailability of monocyte chemoattractant protein-1 (MCP-1), they recruit monocytes to the perivascular space [17]. Upon maturation to macrophages, these cells supply a variety of cytokines and growth factors—among them VEGF-A—to the growing vessel [20,21]. Altogether, arteriogenesis is a local inflammatory process, in which mast cells play an essential role by recruiting growth promoting leukocytes.

Angiogenesis is also a local inflammatory process [22]. Whereas capillaries have the function to provide oxygen and metabolites for tissues locally, arteries transport oxygenated blood through the body. Accordingly, only arteriogenesis, the growth of pre-existing arteriolar connections to functional arteries, is capable to compensate for the loss an artery (Figure 1).

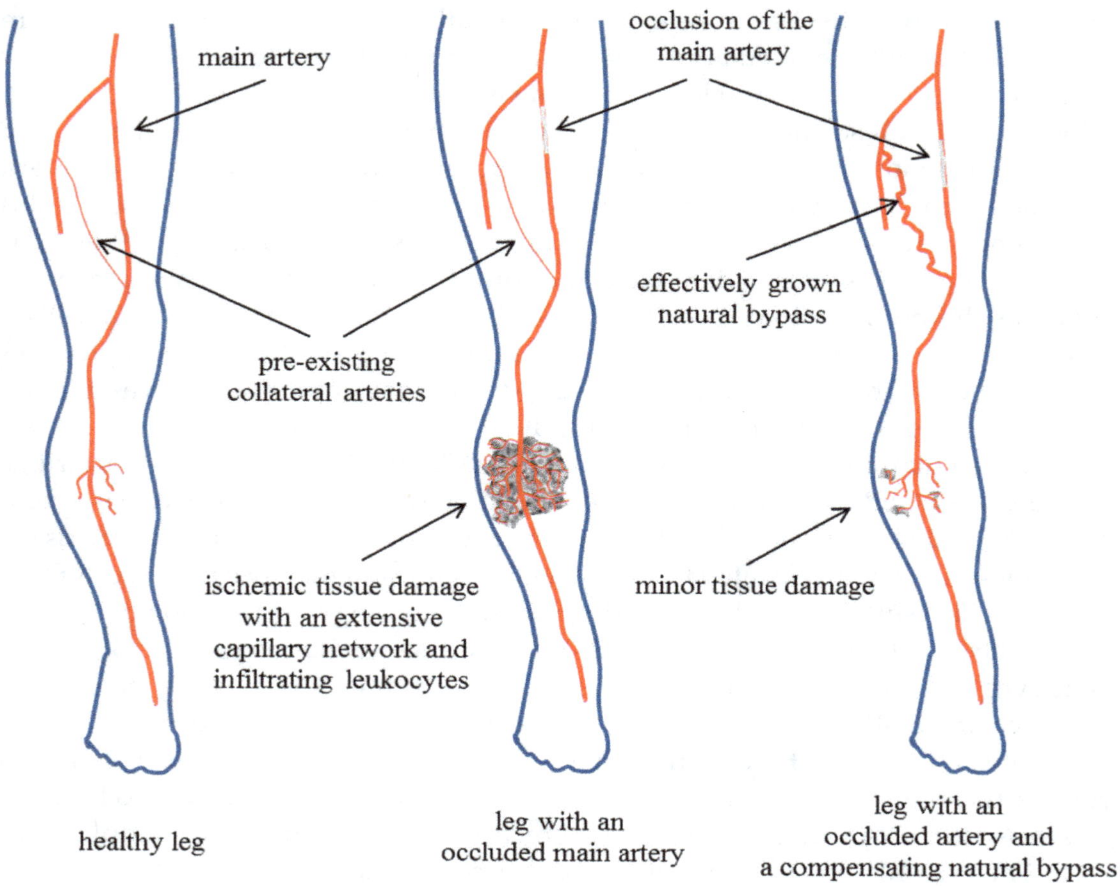

Figure 1. Arteriogenesis versus angiogenesis. The left picture displays a healthy human leg. In the left and the middle picture, a pre-existing collateral artery is shown. As arteries have the function to transport oxygenated blood to distal parts of the body—in the case of the femoral artery to the lower leg—occlusion of the femoral artery results in severe ischemic damage in the lower leg (middle picture). This is associated with extensive angiogenesis. However, the reason for capillary sprouting in this case is not to locally provide oxygen and metabolites—this is simply not possible as long as the feeding artery is occluded, or the bypassing pre-existing collateral has not yet been enlarged by growth—but to remove cell debris from tissue damaged by ischemia. The right picture shows a human leg with a completely occluded artery, which is bypassed by an effectively grown collateral artery compensating for the function of the occluded artery. Accordingly, there is minor ischemic damage in the lower leg with only little capillary sprouting. This picture reflects the tissue saving property of the process of arteriogenesis. Adapted from Chillo et al., 2016 [17] with the permission of Cell Reports.

Patients with diabetes show a high prevalence of high-grade coronary atherosclerosis [23]. Unfortunately, in these patients, the growth of compensating coronary collateral arteries is severely impaired [24]. Peripheral artery disease is also a common complication in type 2 diabetes mellitus (type 2 DM) [25]. It is associated with lower extremity function, critical limb ischemia, and foot ulceration [26,27], and, due to impaired arteriogenesis [28], with limb amputation [29]. The long-term prognosis of patients with DM and peripheral artery disease is extremely poor, with a high mortality rate [30].

3. Glucose Uptake and the Metabolic Disorder Diabetes Mellitus

3.1. Incretins, Insulin, and the Adrenergic System

Glucose in chyme stimulates the release of the metabolic hormones, gastric inhibitory polypeptide (GIP) and glucose-dependent insulinotropic peptide-1 (GLP-1), from intestinal mucosa. Thereupon, these incretins augment the secretion of insulin, a polypeptide hormone, which is produced by beta cells of the pancreatic islets. This endocrine pancreatic activity is reciprocally regulated by the adrenergic system. While activation of the β_2-adrenoreceptor (β_2-AR) promotes insulin release [31], it is repressed when the α_2-AR becomes activated [32]. In the blood, insulin reduces the blood glucose levels by stimulating cells to absorb glucose from the blood. Again, this process is potentiated through activation of β_2-AR by adrenaline [33] and antagonized by noradrenergic α_1-AR stimulation [34,35]. Moreover, insulin is a functional opponent of glucagon. Glucagon is a peptide hormone, which is released from the pancreas to the bloodstream upon stimulation of β-adrenergic receptors mainly due to hypoglycemia, protein rich food, and stress. In the liver, glucagon stimulates gluconeogenesis and glycogenolysis, resulting in increased blood glucose levels. Insulin and GLP-1 inhibit glucagon secretion, resulting in reduction of blood glucose levels. Binding of insulin to its receptor results in cross-talk with β_2-AR, and β_2-AR gene deletion results in hepatic insulin resistance [36]. Increased prevalence of insulin resistance in elderly patients with type 2 diabetes mellitus has been related to reduced expression of β_2-AR [31,37,38]. Resistance to insulin is characterized by defects in muscle glucose uptake and hepatic glucose overproduction.

The adrenergic system has also been implicated in angiogenesis. While stimulation of α_1-AR interfered with endothelial cell proliferation, migration, and tube formation, antagonizing the receptor showed the opposite effect. Moreover, blocking the receptor resulted in enhanced extracellular signal regulated kinase (ERK) activation and retinoblastoma phosphorylation, relevant for cell proliferation [39]. Deficiency of the β_2-AR on endothelial cells, in contrast, impaired nuclear factor 'kappa-light-chain-enhancer' (NF-κB) activation and tube formation in vitro and angiogenesis in vivo [40]. However, further investigations are necessary to define the exact molecular mechanisms and signal transduction cascades associated with adrenoreceptor signaling in endothelial cells.

3.2. *Diabetes Mellitus and Glucose-Dependent Insulinotropic* Peptide-1 *(GLP-1)*

Diabetes mellitus refers to a metabolic disorder resulting in high blood glucose levels due to either reduced insulin levels caused by destruction of insulin-producing beta-cells (type 1 DM), or insulin resistance (type 2 DM). Out of the two, type 2 DM is the prevailing form, with 95% of all DM cases being type 2 [41]. Moreover, about 85% of type 2 DM exhibit insulin resistance [42]. Besides hyperlipidemia, DM is a major risk factor for coronary and peripheral artery diseases [2].

Increasing insulin resistance elicits increased levels of free fatty acids in the blood. Accordingly, hyperglycemia in type 2 DM is often associated with hyperlipidemia, a metabolic disorder, which is characterized by high concentrations of triglycerides and low-density lipoprotein (LDL) cholesterol in the blood. Besides its action on insulin release, GLP-1 also regulates cholesterol and triglycerides. It reduces VLDL triglyceride production in the liver and regulates reverse cholesterol transport [43–48]. GLP-1 as well as GIP are rapidly inactivated by the enzyme, DPP4 [49], whose activity correlates with insulin resistance in type 2 DM [50,51].

Whether GLP-1 acts on hepatocytes, thereby directly exerting a function in the liver, is controversially discussed. Although there are data available showing the expression of the GLP-1 receptor (GLP-1R) on hepatocytes [52], these results were not confirmed by others [53]. As insulin resistance is a common problem in patients with type 2 DM, it is of major importance to clarify whether GLP-1 and, accordingly, GLP-1-based drugs (GLP-1 analogues, see below) have the capacity to exert their beneficial effects not only indirectly via insulin and glucagon, but also directly by binding the GLP-1R on hepatocytes. When treating healthy subjects with GLP-1 (45 pmol/kg per h), D'Alessio et al. found that GLP-1 improves glucose tolerance, and suggested that this is due to stimulation of insulin release and of insulin-independent glucose disposal [54]. In contrast, by infusing physiological postprandial levels of GLP-1 (0.4 pmol/kg per min), Seghieri et al. found a reduction in hepatic glucose production, but no effect on glucose disposal, and concluded that GLP-1 either directly inhibits hepatic gluconeogenesis or has a neutral effect [55]. Since GLP-1 is rapidly degraded by DPP4, it is not suitable as a drug to treat patients. Accordingly, DPP4–resistant mimetics of GLP-1 have been developed. These include exenatide [56], which is the synthetic form of the naturally occurring peptide, exendin-4 [57]. Interestingly, exendin-4 has been described to increase glucokinase enzyme activity in the liver independent of insulin (probably by acting on the hepatic GLP-1R) [58] and to improve insulin sensitivity [59]. For the latter, several mechanisms are discussed [60–64]. Since GLP-1 analogues are not applicable orally, non-peptide agonists would be desirable, which do not require self-injection by patients.

Recently, it has been shown that GLP-1 also stimulates nitric oxide (NO) production, thereby reducing blood pressure and the risk of atherosclerosis [65]. Indeed, it has been described that endothelial NO synthase (eNOS) is uncoupled in type 2 DM, thereby resulting in decreased levels of NO [66–68]. Interestingly, it has been demonstrated that blocking DPP4 activity gives rise to increased NO production, even independent of GLP-1, by promoting phosphorylation of endothelial NO synthase (eNOS) [69]. Orally applicable DPP4 inhibitors are currently used to treat type 2 DM (see below).

4. Molecular Functions of Dipeptidyl-Peptidase-4 (DPP4)

Proteases are involved in all kinds of physiological and pathophysiological processes, such as inflammation, fertilization, cell proliferation and death, tumor growth, and tissue remodeling [70]. DPP4 belongs to a class of specialized proteases, which cleave proline adjacent bonds. These proteases consist of (1) metallopeptidases, such as aminopeptidase P, carboxypeptidase P, and prolidase; and (2) three serine proteases, i.e. prolyloligopeptidase, DPP2, and DPP4 [70]. DPP4 belongs to prolyloliogopeptidases, which have evolved by independent convergent evolution [71,72]. A number of DPP4-like proteins are identified, which show either similarity to DPP4 activity, or are structurally related to DPP4, but enzymatically inactive. These proteins are called DPP4 activity and/or structure homologues (DASH) [73] and, for example, include fibroblast activation protein (FAP) [74], DPP4b [75], DPP6 [76], DPP7 [77], and DPP8 [78].

DPP4 is an intrinsic membrane glycoprotein that cleaves X-proline dipeptides from the N-terminus of polypeptides, however, it also exists in a soluble form [79]. Thus, DPP4 plays a major role in the regulation and activation of paracrine and autocrine as well as of extracellular endocrine peptides [80]. The protein is expressed in a variety of cells, although mainly in adipocytes [51], macrophages [81], T cells [82], endothelial cells [83], epithelial cells [84], and hepatocytes [85].

Beyond glucose control, DPP4 has a variety of functions, and not all of them are mediated by the enzymatic activity of the protein. The extracellular domain, which is involved in adenosine deaminase (ADA)/extracellular matrix binding, is exclusively responsible for the enzymatic activity of the enzyme [86]. Besides cleaving GLP-1 and GIP, both of which stimulate insulin secretion (see above), DPP4 also cleaves the regulatory peptides, glucagon-like peptide-2 (GLP-2), which plays a part in intestinal growth and function [87]; gastrin-releasing peptide (GRP) [88], which is involved in gastric acid secretion; and growth-hormone-releasing factor (GHRF), which stimulates growth hormone production [89]. However, DPP4 also modifies neuropeptides enzymatically. Among them are B-type natriuretic peptide (BNP), playing a role in vasodilation [90]; substance P, a neurotransmitter [91]; peptide YY, which is involved in electrolyte absorption in the colon [92]; and neuropeptide Y (NPY), which is linked to learning and memory [93]. Moreover, DPP4 cleaves a variety of chemokines, which are all involved in chemotaxis and leukocyte recruitment, including interferon-inducible T cell α chemoattractant (ITAC) [94], interferon-γ-induced protein-10 (IP-10) [94], Eotaxin [95], monokine induced by interferon γ (MIG) [96], macrophage derived chemokine (MDC) [97], regulated on activation normal T cell expressed and presumably secreted (RANTES) [98], granulocyte colony stimulating factor (G-CSF) [99], granulocyte monocyte colony stimulating factor (GM-CSF) [99], and stromal-cell-derived factor-1 (SDF-1) [94]. For an overview of the DPP4 mediated effects see Table 1.

Table 1. DPP4 activity.

Function	Protein	Result of DPP4 Cleavage
Regulatory peptides	GLP-1	Inactivation
	GLP-2	Inactivation
	GIP	Inactivation
	GRP	Inactivation
	GHRF	Inactivation
Neuropeptides	BNP	Activity reduced
	Substance P	Inactivation
	Peptide YY	Receptor specificity
	NPY	Receptor specificity
Chemokines	ITAC	Inactivation
	IP-10	Inactivation
	Eotaxin	Inactivation
	MIG	Altered cell type specificity
	MDC	Inactivation
	RANTES	Inactivation
	G-CSF	Inactivation
	GM-CSF	Inactivation

Abbreviations: Glucagon-like peptide 1 (GLP-1); glucose-dependent insulinotropic peptide (GIP); glucagon-like peptide-2 (GLP-2); gastrin-releasing peptide (GRP); growth-hormone-releasing factor (GHRF); B-type natriuretic peptide (BNP); neuropeptide Y (NPY); interferon-inducible T cell α chemoattractant (ITAC); interferon-γ-induced protein-10 (IP-10); monokine induced by interferon γ (MIG); macrophage derived chemokine (MDC); regulated on activation normal T cell expressed and presumably secreted (RANTES); granulocyte colony stimulating factor (G-CSF); granulocyte monocyte colony stimulating factor (GM-CSF); stromal-cell-derived factor-1 (SDF-1).

Besides its enzymatic activity, DPP4 can interact with several other ligands. By binding to adenosine deaminase (ADA) [100], caveolin-1 [101], insulin growth factor receptor 2 (IGFR2) [102], and protein tyrosine phosphatase receptor type C (PTPRC, D45) [103], DPP4 positively regulates T cell co-activation. Moreover, it triggers T cell proliferation by binding to caveolin-1 and caspase recruitment domain-containing protein 11 (CARD11) [101]. It also promotes the proteolysis of the extracellular matrix and the migration of endothelial cells by interacting with separase [104]. Furthermore, DPP4 induces CD68 upregulation on monocytes by binding to caveolin-1 [105]. By associating with the Na^+-H^+ ion exchanger isoform sodium–hydrogen exchanger 3 (NHE3), DPP4 has been suggested to regulate NH3 activity and surface expression [106], and it is postulated that DPP4 also interacts with the thromboxane A2 receptor [107].

5. Cardiovascular Functions of Stromal-Cell-Derived Factor-1

The substrate of DPP4 SDF-1/CXCL12 plays a particularly important role in the cardiovascular system (see below). By interacting with its receptor, CXC-motive-chemokine receptor 4 (CXCR4), SDF-1 recruits leukocytes, such as neutrophils, monocytes, T-, and B cells, as well as other bone marrow derived CXCR4$^+$ cells, such as stem cells and mast cells [17]. Askari et al. described SDF-1 as a key regulator involved in the homing of stem cells to ischemic myocardium, and showed that SDF-1 levels are already upregulated one hour after myocardial infarction, but return to baseline levels seven days later [108]. In rodent models, it was shown that overexpression of SDF-1 improved myocardial function after infarction and promoted revascularization [109,110]. Zhang et al. have shown that stem cells are not involved in the regeneration of cardiac myocytes after myocardial infarction, but that they play a beneficial paracrine role in cardiac myocyte survival and vascularization by supplying SDF-1 [111].

As SDF-1 is cleaved and hence inactivated by DPP4 [112], it was suggested that inhibition of DPP4 activity and thus stabilization of SDF-1 might be a promising approach to treat cardiovascular and peripheral artery diseases (for an example see Figure 2).

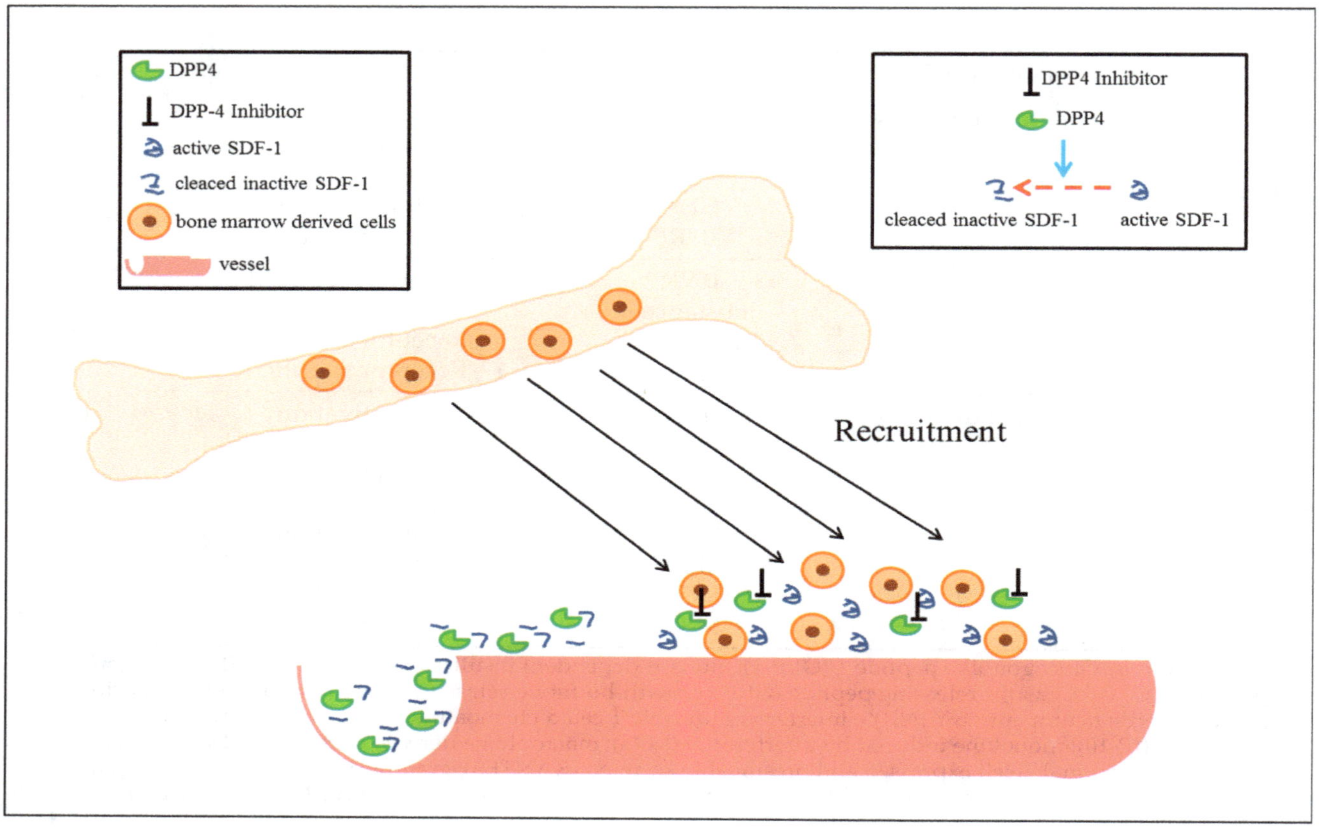

Figure 2. Recruitment of bone marrow derived cells by inhibition of dipeptidyl-peptidase 4 (DPP4). Stromal-cell-derived factor-1 (SDF-1) is cleaved by DPP4 (blue arrow) resulting in inactivation of the chemokine (red arrow). Blocking the enzymatic activity of DPP4 by specific (pharmacological) inhibitors preserves SDF-1. By binding to the receptor, CXC-motive-chemokine receptor 4 (CXCR-4), which is expressed on stem cells, leukocytes, and mast cells, SDF-1 locally recruits bone marrow derived cells, which in turn promote e.g. vessel growth (see Section 6.1).

6. DPP4 Inhibitors and Cardiovascular Diseases

6.1. DPP4 Inhibitors in Pre-Clinical Studies

Particularly due to the function of SDF-1 to recruit bone marrow derived cells, DPP4 inhibitors have been used to increase SDF-1 levels, aiming to improve CVD in pre-clinical animal studies. In several studies, the DPP4 inhibitor, Diprotin A, which is administered intraperitoneally (i.p.), has been applied. Referring to the studies of Christopherson et al. [112], who showed that Diprotin A increased the transmigration of progenitor cells towards an SDF-1 gradient, Zaruba et al. [113] performed studies in a murine model of myocardial infarction. This investigation showed that Diprotin A treatment decreased DPP4 activity in the myocardium (but not in the serum), which was associated with increased levels of SDF-1 and homing of CXCR-4^{+} stem cells, finally resulting in reduced cardiac remodeling, increased neovascularization, and improved myocardial function and survival. Similar results were obtained by Dingenouts et al. [114], who moreover showed that Diprotin A treatment results in a shift towards regenerative M2 macrophages in infarcted myocardium. We performed studies on a murine hindlimb model of arteriogenesis, a shear stress triggered process that relies on local recruitment of leukocytes, which promote the proliferation of endothelial- and smooth muscle cells of pre-existing collateral arterioles, finally resulting in natural bypass growth [5]. Our studies demonstrated that Diprotin A treatment increased SDF-1 levels in collaterals (but not an improved perfusion recovery in atherosclerosis prone ApoE-/- mice [115]. Interestingly, their results in serum), which resulted in increased mast cell recruitment. In turn, mast cell recruited leukocytes (neutrophils, T cells, and macrophages) significantly enhanced arteriogenesis [17]. Using the same model of arteriogenesis, although with sitagliptin as a DPP4 inhibitor, Haverslag et al. also found suggested that DPP4 inhibition showed no adverse side effects on atherogenesis and might even contribute to plaque stability. In accordance with our study, Haverslag et al. observed an increased accumulation of macrophages in the perivascular space of growing collaterals. Moreover, their results demonstrated an increased expression of the monocyte activation marker, CD11b, and of the SDF-1 receptor, CXCR-4, relevant for leukocyte activation and transmigration through activation of lymphocyte function-associated antigen-1 (LFA-1), and of very late antigen-4 and -5 (VLA-4, VLA-5) [116] on circulating monocytes. However, enhanced SDF-1 mediated CXCR-4 activation is also likely to induce NF-κB signaling in leukocytes [117] as well as phosphatidylinositol 3-kinase (PI3K), p44/42 mitogen-activated protein kinase (Erk 1 and Erk 2) [117], transforming growth factor-β (TGF-β), and tumor necrosis factor-α (TNF-α) [118] signaling in vascular cells, which are all relevant for effective collateral artery growth [10,119–122]. In a parallel study, it was shown by Krieger et al. that hydrogels locally releasing SDF-1 supported sustained natural bypass growth by recruiting M2 polarized macrophages [123], which have been shown to enhance arteriogenesis by promoting vascular remodeling [124]. This is an interesting finding, since Brenner et al. showed that sitagliptin treatment of mice (see below) mitigated atherosclerosis by priming monocytes into M2 macrophages [125]. Accordingly, these results strengthen the findings of Haverslag on atherogenesis in the mouse model of arteriogenesis in ApoE-/- mice.

In recent investigations, we were able to show that insulin treatment rescued arteriogenesis in streptozotocin-induced type 2 DM in mice by restoring leukocyte recruitment (unpublished own data). These data give rise to hope for treatment of type 2 DM patients with vascular occlusive diseases. Since the stabilization of GLP-1 through DPP4 inhibitors resulted in increased bioavailability of and sensitivity to insulin [126], and since DPP4 inhibitors have a positive effect on hypercholesterolemia, which also interferes with arteriogenesis [127], DPP4 inhibitors might not only restore arteriogenesis in type 2 DM patients, but even enhance it due to the local increase of SDF-1 levels. Moreover, DPP4 inhibitors evoked increased bioavailability of NO, relevant for proper arteriogenesis [10], which might also contribute to beneficial effects. Since G-CSF and GM-CSF are also substrates of DPP4, blocking its activity might additionally promote arteriogenesis since both factors were shown to enhance collateral artery growth when administered exogenously [128,129]. The importance of arteriogenesis has recently been demonstrated in a meta-analysis showing that high collateralization in patients with coronary artery disease (CAD) is associated with a 36% reduction of mortality risk [130]. Promoting natural bypass growth by drugs presents an elegant and non-invasive alternative to current clinical interventions, such as percutaneous transluminal angioplasty (PTA), percutaneous transluminal coronary angioplasty (PTCA), and bypass transplantation.

6.2. DPP4 Inhibitors in Clinical Studies

As DDP4 inhibitors represent a promising tool to treat patients with type 2 DM, several clinical studies were performed (for a short overview see Table 2). As diprotin A cannot be used for treating patients [131], other orally applicable DPP4 inhibitors, so-called gliptins, were applied. First results of meta-analyses of randomized controlled trials (RCTs), such as TECOS (Trial Evaluating Cardiovascular outcomes with Sitagliptin) [132], SAVOR-TIMI (Saxagliptin Assessment of Vascular Outcomes Recorded in Patients with Type 2 Diabetes Mellitus) [133], or EXAMINE (Examination of Cardiovascular Outcomes: Alogliptin vs. Standard Care in Patients With Type 2 Diabetes Mellitus and Acute Coronary Syndrome) [134], displayed a trend toward a lower incidence of major cardiovascular events (MACE), paving the way for further studies (recently reviewed in [135]).

Table 2. Meta-analyses of clinical trials using DPP4 inhibitors.

Study	Endpoint
SAVOR-TIMI, Saxagliptin Assessment of Vascular Outcomes Recorded in Patients with Type 2 Diabetes Mellitus [133]	cardiovascular death, nonfatal myocardial infarction, nonfatal stroke
TECOS, Trial Evaluating Cardiovascular Outcomes with Sitagliptin [132]	cardiovascular death, nonfatal myocardial infarction, nonfatal stroke
EXAMINE, Examination of Cardiovascular Outcomes: Alogliptin vs. Standard Care in Patients with Type 2 Diabetes Mellitus and Acute Coronary Syndrome [134]	cardiovascular death, nonfatal myocardial infarction, nonfatal stroke
CAROLINA, Cardiovascular Outcome Study of Linagliptin v.s. Glimepride in Patients with Type 2 Diabetes Mellitus [136]	cardiovascular death, nonfatal myocardial infarction, nonfatal stroke, unstable angina pectoris

Reviewed 2018 by S. J. Scheen, see [135].

All the subsequent trials showed that DPP4 inhibitors have a good safety profile. Due to the positive effects of DPP4 inhibitors on angiogenesis and arteriogenesis shown in pre-clinical studies, one would expect detrimental effects on retinopathy and nephropathy, which are caused by excessive vascularization [137] and are highly prevalent in patients with type 2 DM [137–139]. Yet the opposite was the case. Several clinical studies reported retino- as well as renoprotective effects of DPP4 inhibitors [140–143]. However, in terms of CVD, DPP4 inhibitors were not superior compared to placebo. This may be explained by several facts: (1) The trials were primarily designed to prove the safety of DPP4 inhibitors and not their superiority in terms of CVD outcomes; (2) the duration of these studies was probably too short (two to three years) to show any differences in CV (cardiovascular) outcomes; (3) that the positive effect in some patient subgroups may be compensated by zero (or even negative) outcomes in other subgroups. At this point, it is relevant to mention that the first trials only included patients with a rather low risk of CVD. Accordingly, the number of patients with surgical interventions, such as PTCA or intensive pharmacological treatment, was very low. This is an important point in terms of arteriogenesis. When the process of stenosis occurs (very slowly), the blood flow is redirected into pre-existing collateral arteries, triggering them to grow. However, if the stenotic artery is re-vascularized by PTA or PTCA, growing or grown collaterals are degraded as they are not needed anymore. Moreover, drugs, such as, for example, angiotensin-converting enzyme inhibitors, which degrade SDF-1 [144], might interfere with the positive effect of DPP4 inhibitors in arteriogenesis. Accordingly, new analyses are necessary, which take surgical and pharmacological treatment of patients into account; furthermore (4) the dose as well as the administration route might play a role. Recent studies on animal models using sitagliptin, which has been shown to be safe in the TECOS study, addressed this point (see Section 6.3).

6.3. DPP4 Inhibitors Revisited in Pre-Clinical Studies

Sitagliptin is administered orally in patients at a dose of 100 mg/d. The bioavailability is 87%, but 79% of the drug is excreted unchanged in the urine. Theiss et al. [145] performed a study on outcomes of myocardial infarction in mice using different dosages of orally administered sitagliptin ranging from 5 mg/kg/d to 500 mg/kg/d, and showed that only the treatment with 500 mg/kg significantly reduced DPP4 activity in the blood, whereby significantly increased numbers of bone marrow derived cells homing in the myocardium after infarction were already observed at a dose of 50 mg/kg. Treatment regimens with 500 mg/kg/d resulted in significantly reduced cardiac remodeling, increased capillary density, and improved myocardial function and survival of mice. The same results were obtained when the DPP4 inhibitor, vildagliptin, was used at an equal dosage. Brenner and co-workers, who also used 500 mg/kg/d of sitagliptin for oral treatment of mice, reported ameliorated atherosclerosis based on priming monocytes into M2 macrophages [125]. Moreover, they demonstrated that SDF-1, independent of GLP-1 action, shows a direct proliferative effect on endothelial cells [146], a process that is decisive for arteriogenesis [147].

Ghorpade et al. [148], recently published a study showing that oral administration of 35–40 mg/kg/d of sitagliptin significantly decreased plasma DPP4 activity in diet-induced obese (DIO) mice. The same result was obtained when mice were treated intravenously (i.v.) with a short hairpin RNA (shRNA) that specifically silenced DPP4 in the liver. However, in contrast to orally administered sitagliptin, only liver specific silencing of DPP4 decreased liver DPP4 protein levels and hepatocyte DPP4 activity.

Moreover, liver specific silencing of DPP4 lowered plasma insulin, improved glucose uptake, and suppressed insulin resistance in DIO mice. These data are in accordance with studies reporting that oral DPP4 inhibitors do not lower plasma insulin in insulin-resistant, hyperinsulinemic patients [149–154]. These facts throw a completely new light on orally administered DPP4 inhibitors in patients with type 2 DM in terms of rescuing or even enhancing the process of arteriogenesis. Several questions thus need to be addressed in pre-clinical studies.

6.4. Questions

As oral DPP4 inhibitors do not suppress insulin resistance, the first question is whether this is due to the oral application form or due to the dosage. GLP-1 receptor agonists, such as exenatide or semaglutide, used to increase insulin sensitivity in patients, are administered subcutaneously [155,156]. DPP4 increases insulin resistance by enzymatically cleaving GLP-1. However, it still remains to be elucidated whether insulin sensitivity is additionally promoted by a non-enzymatic function of DPP4. Therefore, the question arises of whether gliptins really are the best choice to treat insulin resistance. Another question is whether gliptins work equally well in rodents and humans concerning the specific recognition of DPP4 or whether differences in efficacy are due to differences in species. The next question is whether currently available DPP4 inhibitors reach all desired target organs (including the liver). Accordingly, the final question arises: Do we have to develop a new class of DPP4 inhibitors? Last, but not least, the data on patients in terms of improvements of CVD need to be (re-)addressed, considering whether the overall surgical and pharmacological treatment of each subject might interfere with the process of arteriogenesis.

7. Conclusions

DPP4 inhibitors have been shown to be safe in clinical trials and might efficiently promote arteriogenesis even in patients with type 2 DM. However, several problems need to be resolved before we will be able to efficiently promote arteriogenesis even in patients with type 2 DM.

Author Contributions: S.V., A.-K.K. and E.D. wrote the article.

References

1. World-Health-Organisation. *Cardiovascular Diseases (cvds)*; World-Health-Organisation: Geneva, Switzerland, 2013.
2. Kannel, W.B.; McGee, D.L. Diabetes and cardiovascular disease. The Framingham study. *JAMA* **1979**, *241*, 2035–2038. [CrossRef] [PubMed]
3. Abaci, A.; Oguzhan, A.; Kahraman, S.; Eryol, N.K.; Unal, S.; Arinc, H.; Ergin, A. Effect of diabetes mellitus on formation of coronary collateral vessels. *Circulation* **1999**, *99*, 2239–2242. [CrossRef] [PubMed]
4. Rivard, A.; Silver, M.; Chen, D.; Kearney, M.; Magner, M.; Annex, B.; Peters, K.; Isner, J.M. Rescue of diabetes-related impairment of angiogenesis by intramuscular gene therapy with adeno-VEGF. *Am. J. Pathol.* **1999**, *154*, 355–363. [CrossRef]
5. Deindl, E.; Schaper, W. The art of arteriogenesis. *Cell Biochem. Biophys.* **2005**, *43*, 1–15. [CrossRef]

6. Lasch, M.; Nekolla, K.; Klemm, A.H.; Buchheim, J.I.; Pohl, U.; Dietzel, S.; Deindl, E. Estimating hemodynamic shear stress in murine peripheral collateral arteries by two-photon line scanning. *Mol. Cell. Biochem.* **2018**. [CrossRef] [PubMed]
7. Pipp, F.; Boehm, S.; Cai, W.J.; Adili, F.; Ziegler, B.; Karanovic, G.; Ritter, R.; Balzer, J.; Scheler, C.; Schaper, W.T.S.-R. Elevated fluid shear stress enhances postocclusive collateral artery growth and gene expression in the pig hind limb. *Arterioscler. Thromb. Vasc. Biol.* **2004**, *24*, 1664–1668. [CrossRef] [PubMed]
8. Tzima, E.; Irani-Tehrani, M.; Kiosses, W.B.; Dejana, E.; Schultz, D.A.; Engelhardt, B.; Cao, G.; DeLisser, H.; Schwartz, M.A. A mechanosensory complex that mediates the endothelial cell response to fluid shear stress. *Nature* **2005**, *437*, 426–431. [CrossRef] [PubMed]
9. Jazwa, A.; Florczyk, U.; Grochot-Przeczek, A.; Krist, B.; Loboda, A.; Jozkowicz, A.; Dulak, J. Limb ischemia and vessel regeneration: Is there a role for VEGF? *Vasc. Pharmacol.* **2016**, *86*, 18–30. [CrossRef] [PubMed]
10. Lautz, T.; Lasch, M.; Borgolte, J.; Troidl, K.; Pagel, J.I.; Caballero-Martinez, A.; Kleinert, E.C.; Walzog, B.; Deindl, E. Midkine Controls Arteriogenesis by Regulating the Bioavailability of Vascular Endothelial Growth Factor A and the Expression of Nitric Oxide Synthase 1 and 3. *EBioMedicine* **2018**, *27*, 237–246. [CrossRef] [PubMed]
11. Deindl, E.; Buschmann, I.; Hoefer, I.E.; Podzuweit, T.; Boengler, K.; Vogel, S.; van Royen, N.; Fernandez, B.; Schaper, W. Role of ischemia and hypoxia-inducible genes in arteriogenesis after femoral artery occlusion in the rabbit. *Circ. Res.* **2001**, *89*, 779–786. [CrossRef] [PubMed]
12. Givens, C.; Tzima, E. Endothelial Mechanosignaling: Does One Sensor Fit All? *Antioxid. Redox Signal.* **2016**, *25*, 373–388. [CrossRef] [PubMed]
13. Kofler, N.M.; Simons, M. Angiogenesis versus arteriogenesis: Neuropilin 1 modulation of VEGF signaling. *F1000Prime Rep.* **2015**, *7*, 26. [CrossRef] [PubMed]
14. Fischer, S.; Nishio, M.; Peters, S.C.; Tschernatsch, M.; Walberer, M.; Weidemann, S.; Heidenreich, R.; Couraud, P.O.; Weksler, B.B.; Romero, I.A.; et al. Signaling mechanism of extracellular RNA in endothelial cells. *FASEB J.* **2009**, *23*, 2100–2109. [CrossRef] [PubMed]
15. Chandraratne, S.; von Bruehl, M.L.; Pagel, J.I.; Stark, K.; Kleinert, E.; Konrad, I.; Farschtschi, S.; Coletti, R.; Gartner, F.; Chillo, O.; et al. Critical role of platelet glycoprotein ibalpha in arterial remodeling. *Arterioscler. Thromb. Vasc. Biol.* **2015**, *35*, 589–597. [CrossRef] [PubMed]
16. Goto, S.; Ichikawa, N.; Lee, M.; Goto, M.; Sakai, H.; Kim, J.J.; Yoshida, M.; Handa, M.; Ikeda, Y.; Handa, S. Platelet surface P-selectin molecules increased after exposing platelet to a high shear flow. *Int. Angiol.* **2000**, *19*, 147–151. [PubMed]
17. Chillo, O.; Kleinert, E.C.; Lautz, T.; Lasch, M.; Pagel, J.I.; Heun, Y.; Troidl, K.; Fischer, S.; Caballero-Martinez, A.; Mauer, A.; et al. Perivascular Mast Cells Govern Shear Stress-Induced Arteriogenesis by Orchestrating Leukocyte Function. *Cell Rep.* **2016**, *16*, 2197–2207. [CrossRef] [PubMed]
18. Deindl, E.; Ziegelhoffer, T.; Kanse, S.M.; Fernandez, B.; Neubauer, E.; Carmeliet, P.; Preissner, K.T.; Schaper, W. Receptor-independent role of the urokinase-type plasminogen activator during arteriogenesis. *FASEB J.* **2003**, *17*, 1174–1176. [CrossRef] [PubMed]
19. Reichel, C.A.; Uhl, B.; Lerchenberger, M.; Puhr-Westerheide, D.; Rehberg, M.; Liebl, J.; Khandoga, A.; Schmalix, W.; Zahler, S.; Deindl, E.; et al. Urokinase-type plasminogen activator promotes paracellular transmigration of neutrophils via Mac-1, but independently of urokinase-type plasminogen activator receptor. *Circulation* **2011**, *124*, 1848–1859. [CrossRef] [PubMed]
20. Arras, M.; Ito, W.D.; Scholz, D.; Winkler, B.; Schaper, J.; Schaper, W. Monocyte activation in angiogenesis and collateral growth in the rabbit hindlimb. *J. Clin. Investig.* **1998**, *101*, 41–50. [CrossRef] [PubMed]
21. Morrison, A.R.; Yarovinsky, T.O.; Young, B.D.; Moraes, F.; Ross, T.D.; Ceneri, N.; Zhang, J.; Zhuang, Z.W.; Sinusas, A.J.; Pardi, R.; et al. Chemokine-coupled beta2 integrin-induced macrophage Rac2-Myosin IIA interaction regulates VEGF-A mRNA stability and arteriogenesis. *J. Exp. Med.* **2014**, *211*, 1957–1968. [CrossRef] [PubMed]
22. Szade, A.; Grochot-Przeczek, A.; Florczyk, U.; Jozkowicz, A.; Dulak, J. Cellular and molecular mechanisms of inflammation-induced angiogenesis. *IUBMB Life* **2015**, *67*, 145–159. [CrossRef] [PubMed]
23. Goraya, T.Y.; Leibson, C.L.; Palumbo, P.J.; Weston, S.A.; Killian, J.M.; Pfeifer, E.A.; Jacobsen, S.J.; Frye, R.L.; Roger, V.L. Coronary atherosclerosis in diabetes mellitus: A population-based autopsy study. *J. Am. Coll. Cardiol.* **2002**, *40*, 946–953. [CrossRef]

24. Weihrauch, D.; Lohr, N.L.; Mraovic, B.; Ludwig, L.M.; Chilian, W.M.; Pagel, P.S.; Warltier, D.C.; Kersten, J.R. Chronic hyperglycemia attenuates coronary collateral development and impairs proliferative properties of myocardial interstitial fluid by production of angiostatin. *Circulation* **2004**, *109*, 2343–2348. [CrossRef] [PubMed]
25. American Diabetes Association. Peripheral Artery Disease in People with Diabetes. *Diabetes Care* **2003**, *26*, 3333–3341.
26. Dolan, N.C.; Liu, K.; Criqui, M.H.; Greenland, P.; Guralnik, J.M.; Chan, C.; Schneider, J.R.; Mandapat, A.L.; Martin, G.; McDermott, M.M. Peripheral artery disease, diabetes, and reduced lower extremity functioning. *Diabetes Care* **2002**, *25*, 113–120. [CrossRef] [PubMed]
27. Prompers, L.; Schaper, N.; Apelqvist, J.; Edmonds, M.; Jude, E.; Mauricio, D.; Uccioli, L.; Urbancic, V.; Bakker, K.; Holstein, P.; et al. Prediction of outcome in individuals with diabetic foot ulcers: Focus on the differences between individuals with and without peripheral arterial disease. The EURODIALE Study. *Diabetologia* **2008**, *51*, 747–755. [CrossRef] [PubMed]
28. Ruiter, M.S.; van Golde, J.M.; Schaper, N.C.; Stehouwer, C.D.; Huijberts, M.S. Diabetes impairs arteriogenesis in the peripheral circulation: Review of molecular mechanisms. *Clin. Sci. (Lond.)* **2010**, *119*, 225–238. [CrossRef] [PubMed]
29. Ziegler-Graham, K.; MacKenzie, E.J.; Ephraim, P.L.; Travison, T.G.; Brookmeyer, R. Estimating the prevalence of limb loss in the United States: 2005 to 2050. *Arch. Phys. Med. Rehabil.* **2008**, *89*, 422–429. [CrossRef] [PubMed]
30. Faglia, E.; Clerici, G.; Clerissi, J.; Gabrielli, L.; Losa, S.; Mantero, M.; Caminiti, M.; Curci, V.; Quarantiello, A.; Lupattelli, T.; et al. Long-term prognosis of diabetic patients with critical limb ischemia: A population-based cohort study. *Diabetes Care* **2009**, *32*, 822–827. [CrossRef] [PubMed]
31. Santulli, G.; Lombardi, A.; Sorriento, D.; Anastasio, A.; Del Giudice, C.; Formisano, P.; Beguinot, F.; Trimarco, B.; Miele, C.; Iaccarino, G. Age-related impairment in insulin release: The essential role of beta(2)-adrenergic receptor. *Diabetes* **2012**, *61*, 692–701. [CrossRef] [PubMed]
32. Rosengren, A.H.; Jokubka, R.; Tojjar, D.; Granhall, C.; Hansson, O.; Li, D.Q.; Nagaraj, V.; Reinbothe, T.M.; Tuncel, J.; Eliasson, L.; et al. Overexpression of alpha2A-adrenergic receptors contributes to type 2 diabetes. *Science* **2010**, *327*, 217–220. [CrossRef] [PubMed]
33. Nevzorova, J.; Evans, B.A.; Bengtsson, T.; Summers, R.J. Multiple signalling pathways involved in beta2-adrenoceptor-mediated glucose uptake in rat skeletal muscle cells. *Br. J. Pharmacol.* **2006**, *147*, 446–454. [CrossRef] [PubMed]
34. Hutchinson, D.S.; Bengtsson, T. alpha1A-adrenoceptors activate glucose uptake in L6 muscle cells through a phospholipase C-phosphatidylinositol-3 kinase-, and atypical protein kinase C.-dependent pathway. *Endocrinology* **2005**, *146*, 901–912. [CrossRef] [PubMed]
35. Lembo, G.; Capaldo, B.; Rendina, V.; Iaccarino, G.; Napoli, R.; Guida, R.; Trimarco, B.; Sacca, L. Acute noradrenergic activation induces insulin resistance in human skeletal muscle. *Am. J. Physiol.* **1994**, *266*, E242–E247. [CrossRef] [PubMed]
36. Cipolletta, E.; Del Giudice, C.; Santulli, G.; Trimarco, B.; Iaccarino, G. Opposite effects of beta2-adrenoceptor gene deletion on insulin signaling in liver and skeletal muscle. *Nutr. Metab. Cardiovasc. Dis.* **2017**, *27*, 615–623. [CrossRef] [PubMed]
37. Basu, R.; Breda, E.; Oberg, A.L.; Powell, C.C.; Dalla Man, C.; Basu, A.; Vittone, J.L.; Klee, G.G.; Arora, P.; Jensen, M.D.; et al. Mechanisms of the age-associated deterioration in glucose tolerance: Contribution of alterations in insulin secretion, action, and clearance. *Diabetes* **2003**, *52*, 1738–1748. [CrossRef] [PubMed]
38. Iozzo, P.; Beck-Nielsen, H.; Laakso, M.; Smith, U.; Yki-Jarvinen, H.; Ferrannini, E. Independent influence of age on basal insulin secretion in nondiabetic humans. European Group for the Study of Insulin Resistance. *J. Clin. Endocrinol. Metab.* **1999**, *84*, 863–868. [CrossRef] [PubMed]
39. Ciccarelli, M.; Santulli, G.; Campanile, A.; Galasso, G.; Cervero, P.; Altobelli, G.G.; Cimini, V.; Pastore, L.; Piscione, F.; Trimarco, B.; et al. Endothelial alpha1-adrenoceptors regulate neo-angiogenesis. *Br. J. Pharmacol.* **2008**, *153*, 936–946. [CrossRef] [PubMed]
40. Ciccarelli, M.; Sorriento, D.; Cipolletta, E.; Santulli, G.; Fusco, A.; Zhou, R.H.; Eckhart, A.D.; Peppel, K.; Koch, W.J.; Trimarco, B.; et al. Impaired neoangiogenesis in beta(2)-adrenoceptor gene-deficient mice: Restoration by intravascular human beta(2)-adrenoceptor gene transfer and role of NFkappaB and CREB transcription factors. *Br. J. Pharmacol.* **2011**, *162*, 712–721. [CrossRef] [PubMed]

41. Centers for Disease Control and Prevention. *National Diabetes Statistics Report, 2017*; Centers for Disease Control and Prevention, US Department of Health and Human Services: Atlanta, GA, USA, 2017.
42. Grant, P.J. Diabetes mellitus as a prothrombotic condition. *J. Intern. Med.* **2007**, *262*, 157–172. [CrossRef] [PubMed]
43. Blonde, L.; Klein, E.J.; Han, J.; Zhang, B.; Mac, S.M.; Poon, T.H.; Taylor, K.L.; Trautmann, M.E.; Kim, D.D.; Kendall, D.M. Interim analysis of the effects of exenatide treatment on A1C, weight and cardiovascular risk factors over 82 weeks in 314 overweight patients with type 2 diabetes. *Diabetes Obes. Metab.* **2006**, *8*, 436–447. [CrossRef] [PubMed]
44. Chehade, J.M.; Alcalde, R.; Naem, E.; Mooradian, A.D.; Wong, N.C.; Haas, M.J. Induction of apolipoprotein A-I gene expression by glucagon-like peptide-1 and exendin-4 in hepatocytes but not intestinal cells. *Metabolism* **2013**, *62*, 265–274. [CrossRef] [PubMed]
45. Irwin, N.; McClean, P.L.; Hunter, K.; Flatt, P.R. Metabolic effects of sustained activation of the GLP-1 receptor alone and in combination with background GIP receptor antagonism in high fat-fed mice. *Diabetes Obes. Metab.* **2009**, *11*, 603–610. [CrossRef] [PubMed]
46. Parlevliet, E.T.; Schroder-van der Elst, J.P.; Corssmit, E.P.; Picha, K.; O'Neil, K.; Stojanovic-Susulic, V.; Ort, T.; Havekes, L.M.; Romijn, J.A.; Pijl, H. CNTO736, a novel glucagon-like peptide-1 receptor agonist, ameliorates insulin resistance and inhibits very low-density lipoprotein production in high-fat-fed mice. *J. Pharmacol. Exp. Ther.* **2009**, *328*, 240–248. [CrossRef] [PubMed]
47. Qin, X.; Shen, H.; Liu, M.; Yang, Q.; Zheng, S.; Sabo, M.; D'Alessio, D.A.; Tso, P. GLP-1 reduces intestinal lymph flow, triglyceride absorption, and apolipoprotein production in rats. *Am. J. Physiol. Gastrointest. Liver Physiol.* **2005**, *288*, G943–G949. [CrossRef] [PubMed]
48. Vanderweele, D.A.; Geiselman, P.J.; Novin, D. Pancreatic glucagon, food deprivation and feeding in intact and vagotomized rabbits. *Physiol. Behav.* **1979**, *23*, 155–158. [CrossRef]
49. Drucker, D.J.; Nauck, M.A. The incretin system: Glucagon-like peptide-1 receptor agonists and dipeptidyl peptidase-4 inhibitors in type 2 diabetes. *Lancet* **2006**, *368*, 1696–1705. [CrossRef]
50. Kirino, Y.; Sei, M.; Kawazoe, K.; Minakuchi, K.; Sato, Y. Plasma dipeptidyl peptidase 4 activity correlates with body mass index and the plasma adiponectin concentration in healthy young people. *Endocr. J.* **2012**, *59*, 949–953. [CrossRef] [PubMed]
51. Lamers, D.; Famulla, S.; Wronkowitz, N.; Hartwig, S.; Lehr, S.; Ouwens, D.M.; Eckardt, K.; Kaufman, J.M.; Ryden, M.; Muller, S.; et al. Dipeptidyl peptidase 4 is a novel adipokine potentially linking obesity to the metabolic syndrome. *Diabetes* **2011**, *60*, 1917–1925. [CrossRef] [PubMed]
52. Gupta, N.A.; Mells, J.; Dunham, R.M.; Grakoui, A.; Handy, J.; Saxena, N.K.; Anania, F.A. Glucagon-like peptide-1 receptor is present on human hepatocytes and has a direct role in decreasing hepatic steatosis in vitro by modulating elements of the insulin signaling pathway. *Hepatology* **2010**, *51*, 1584–1592. [CrossRef] [PubMed]
53. Bullock, B.P.; Heller, R.S.; Habener, J.F. Tissue distribution of messenger ribonucleic acid encoding the rat glucagon-like peptide-1 receptor. *Endocrinology* **1996**, *137*, 2968–2978. [CrossRef] [PubMed]
54. D'Alessio, D.A.; Kahn, S.E.; Leusner, C.R.; Ensinck, J.W. Glucagon-like peptide 1 enhances glucose tolerance both by stimulation of insulin release and by increasing insulin-independent glucose disposal. *J. Clin. Investig.* **1994**, *93*, 2263–2266. [CrossRef] [PubMed]
55. Seghieri, M.; Rebelos, E.; Gastaldelli, A.; Astiarraga, B.D.; Casolaro, A.; Barsotti, E.; Pocai, A.; Nauck, M.; Muscelli, E.; Ferrannini, E. Direct effect of GLP-1 infusion on endogenous glucose production in humans. *Diabetologia* **2013**, *56*, 156–161. [CrossRef] [PubMed]
56. Iltz, J.L.; Baker, D.E.; Setter, S.M.; Keith Campbell, R. Exenatide: An incretin mimetic for the treatment of type 2 diabetes mellitus. *Clin. Ther.* **2006**, *28*, 652–665. [CrossRef] [PubMed]
57. Eng, J.; Kleinman, W.A.; Singh, L.; Singh, G.; Raufman, J.P. Isolation and characterization of exendin-4, an exendin-3 analogue, from Heloderma suspectum venom. Further evidence for an exendin receptor on dispersed acini from guinea pig pancreas. *J. Biol. Chem.* **1992**, *267*, 7402–7405. [PubMed]
58. Dhanesha, N.; Joharapurkar, A.; Shah, G.; Dhote, V.; Kshirsagar, S.; Bahekar, R.; Jain, M. Exendin-4 reduces glycemia by increasing liver glucokinase activity: An insulin independent effect. *Pharmacol. Rep.* **2012**, *64*, 140–149. [CrossRef]
59. Kolterman, O.G.; Buse, J.B.; Fineman, M.S.; Gaines, E.; Heintz, S.; Bicsak, T.A.; Taylor, K.; Kim, D.; Aisporna, M.; Wang, Y.; et al. Synthetic exendin-4 (exenatide) significantly reduces postprandial and

fasting plasma glucose in subjects with type 2 diabetes. *J. Clin. Endocrinol. Metab.* **2003**, *88*, 3082–3089. [CrossRef] [PubMed]

60. Degn, K.B.; Brock, B.; Juhl, C.B.; Djurhuus, C.B.; Grubert, J.; Kim, D.; Han, J.; Taylor, K.; Fineman, M.; Schmitz, O. Effect of intravenous infusion of exenatide (synthetic exendin-4) on glucose-dependent insulin secretion and counterregulation during hypoglycemia. *Diabetes* **2004**, *53*, 2397–2403. [CrossRef] [PubMed]
61. Gedulin, B.R.; Nikoulina, S.E.; Smith, P.A.; Gedulin, G.; Nielsen, L.L.; Baron, A.D.; Parkes, D.G.; Young, A.A. Exenatide (exendin-4) improves insulin sensitivity and {beta}-cell mass in insulin-resistant obese fa/fa Zucker rats independent of glycemia and body weight. *Endocrinology* **2005**, *146*, 2069–2076. [CrossRef] [PubMed]
62. Guo, C.; Huang, T.; Chen, A.; Chen, X.; Wang, L.; Shen, F.; Gu, X. Glucagon-like peptide 1 improves insulin resistance in vitro through anti-inflammation of macrophages. *Braz. J. Med. Biol. Res.* **2016**, *49*, e5826. [CrossRef] [PubMed]
63. Idris, I.; Patiag, D.; Gray, S.; Donnelly, R. Exendin-4 increases insulin sensitivity via a PI-3-kinase-dependent mechanism: Contrasting effects of GLP-1. *Biochem. Pharmacol.* **2002**, *63*, 993–996. [CrossRef]
64. Wang, A.; Li, T.; An, P.; Yan, W.; Zheng, H.; Wang, B.; Mu, Y. Exendin-4 Upregulates Adiponectin Level in Adipocytes via Sirt1/Foxo-1 Signaling Pathway. *PLoS ONE* **2017**, *12*, e0169469. [CrossRef] [PubMed]
65. Ban, K.; Noyan-Ashraf, M.H.; Hoefer, J.; Bolz, S.S.; Drucker, D.J.; Husain, M. Cardioprotective and vasodilatory actions of glucagon-like peptide 1 receptor are mediated through both glucagon-like peptide 1 receptor-dependent and -independent pathways. *Circulation* **2008**, *117*, 2340–2350. [CrossRef] [PubMed]
66. Du, X.L.; Edelstein, D.; Dimmeler, S.; Ju, Q.; Sui, C.; Brownlee, M. Hyperglycemia inhibits endothelial nitric oxide synthase activity by posttranslational modification at the Akt site. *J. Clin. Investig.* **2001**, *108*, 1341–1348. [CrossRef] [PubMed]
67. Guzik, T.J.; Mussa, S.; Gastaldi, D.; Sadowski, J.; Ratnatunga, C.; Pillai, R.; Channon, K.M. Mechanisms of increased vascular superoxide production in human diabetes mellitus: Role of NAD(P)H oxidase and endothelial nitric oxide synthase. *Circulation* **2002**, *105*, 1656–1662. [CrossRef] [PubMed]
68. Wenzel, P.; Daiber, A.; Oelze, M.; Brandt, M.; Closs, E.; Xu, J.; Thum, T.; Bauersachs, J.; Ertl, G.; Zou, M.H.; et al. Mechanisms underlying recoupling of eNOS by HMG-CoA reductase inhibition in a rat model of streptozotocin-induced diabetes mellitus. *Atherosclerosis* **2008**, *198*, 65–76. [CrossRef] [PubMed]
69. Shah, Z.; Pineda, C.; Kampfrath, T.; Maiseyeu, A.; Ying, Z.; Racoma, I.; Deiuliis, J.; Xu, X.; Sun, Q.; Moffatt-Bruce, S.; et al. Acute DPP-4 inhibition modulates vascular tone through GLP-1 independent pathways. *Vasc. Pharmacol.* **2011**, *55*, 2–9. [CrossRef] [PubMed]
70. Qi, S.Y.; Riviere, P.J.; Trojnar, J.; Junien, J.L.; Akinsanya, K.O. Cloning and characterization of dipeptidyl peptidase 10, a new member of an emerging subgroup of serine proteases. *Biochem. J.* **2003**, *373*, 179–189. [CrossRef] [PubMed]
71. Polgar, L. The prolyl oligopeptidase family. *Cell. Mol. Life Sci.* **2002**, *59*, 349–362. [CrossRef] [PubMed]
72. Rawlings, N.D.; Polgar, L.; Barrett, A.J. A new family of serine-type peptidases related to prolyl oligopeptidase. *Biochem. J.* **1991**, *279 Pt 3*, 907–908. [CrossRef]
73. Sedo, A.; Malik, R. Dipeptidyl peptidase IV-like molecules: Homologous proteins or homologous activities? *Biochim. Biophys. Acta* **2001**, *1550*, 107–116. [CrossRef]
74. Niedermeyer, J.; Enenkel, B.; Park, J.E.; Lenter, M.; Rettig, W.J.; Damm, K.; Schnapp, A. Mouse fibroblast-activation protein—Conserved Fap gene organization and biochemical function as a serine protease. *Eur. J. Biochem.* **1998**, *254*, 650–654. [CrossRef] [PubMed]
75. Jacotot, E.; Callebaut, C.; Blanco, J.; Krust, B.; Neubert, K.; Barth, A.; Hovanessian, A.G. Dipeptidyl-peptidase IV-beta, a novel form of cell-surface-expressed protein with dipeptidyl-peptidase IV activity. *Eur. J. Biochem.* **1996**, *239*, 248–258. [CrossRef] [PubMed]
76. Wada, K.; Yokotani, N.; Hunter, C.; Doi, K.; Wenthold, R.J.; Shimasaki, S. Differential expression of two distinct forms of mRNA encoding members of a dipeptidyl aminopeptidase family. *Proc. Natl. Acad. Sci. USA* **1992**, *89*, 197–201. [CrossRef] [PubMed]
77. Fukasawa, K.M.; Fukasawa, K.; Higaki, K.; Shiina, N.; Ohno, M.; Ito, S.; Otogoto, J.; Ota, N. Cloning and functional expression of rat kidney dipeptidyl peptidase II. *Biochem. J.* **2001**, *353*, 283–290. [CrossRef] [PubMed]

78. Abbott, C.A.; Yu, D.M.; Woollatt, E.; Sutherland, G.R.; McCaughan, G.W.; Gorrell, M.D. Cloning, expression and chromosomal localization of a novel human dipeptidyl peptidase (DPP) IV homolog, DPP8. *Eur. J. Biochem.* **2000**, *267*, 6140–6150. [CrossRef] [PubMed]
79. Wang, Z.; Grigo, C.; Steinbeck, J.; von Horsten, S.; Amann, K.; Daniel, C. Soluble DPP4 originates in part from bone marrow cells and not from the kidney. *Peptides* **2014**, *57*, 109–117. [CrossRef] [PubMed]
80. Mentlein, R. Dipeptidyl-peptidase IV (CD26)—Role in the inactivation of regulatory peptides. *Regul. Pept.* **1999**, *85*, 9–24. [CrossRef]
81. Zhong, J.; Rao, X.; Deiuliis, J.; Braunstein, Z.; Narula, V.; Hazey, J.; Mikami, D.; Needleman, B.; Satoskar, A.R.; Rajagopalan, S. A potential role for dendritic cell/macrophage-expressing DPP4 in obesity-induced visceral inflammation. *Diabetes* **2013**, *62*, 149–157. [CrossRef] [PubMed]
82. Morimoto, C.; Schlossman, S.F. The structure and function of CD26 in the T-cell immune response. *Immunol. Rev.* **1998**, *161*, 55–70. [CrossRef] [PubMed]
83. Shah, Z.; Kampfrath, T.; Deiuliis, J.A.; Zhong, J.; Pineda, C.; Ying, Z.; Xu, X.; Lu, B.; Moffatt-Bruce, S.; Durairaj, R.; et al. Long-term dipeptidyl-peptidase 4 inhibition reduces atherosclerosis and inflammation via effects on monocyte recruitment and chemotaxis. *Circulation* **2011**, *124*, 2338–2349. [CrossRef] [PubMed]
84. Sueyoshi, R.; Woods Ignatoski, K.M.; Okawada, M.; Hartmann, B.; Holst, J.; Teitelbaum, D.H. Stimulation of intestinal growth and function with DPP4 inhibition in a mouse short bowel syndrome model. *Am. J. Physiol. Gastrointest. Liver Physiol.* **2014**, *307*, G410–G419. [CrossRef] [PubMed]
85. Ben-Shlomo, S.; Zvibel, I.; Shnell, M.; Shlomai, A.; Chepurko, E.; Halpern, Z.; Barzilai, N.; Oren, R.; Fishman, S. Glucagon-like peptide-1 reduces hepatic lipogenesis via activation of AMP-activated protein kinase. *J. Hepatol.* **2011**, *54*, 1214–1223. [CrossRef] [PubMed]
86. Richard, E.; Arredondo-Vega, F.X.; Santisteban, I.; Kelly, S.J.; Patel, D.D.; Hershfield, M.S. The binding site of human adenosine deaminase for CD26/Dipeptidyl peptidase IV: The Arg142Gln mutation impairs binding to cd26 but does not cause immune deficiency. *J. Exp. Med.* **2000**, *192*, 1223–1236. [CrossRef] [PubMed]
87. Masur, K.; Schwartz, F.; Entschladen, F.; Niggemann, B.; Zaenker, K.S. DPPIV inhibitors extend GLP-2 mediated tumour promoting effects on intestinal cancer cells. *Regul. Pept.* **2006**, *137*, 147–155. [CrossRef] [PubMed]
88. Ahren, B.; Hughes, T.E. Inhibition of dipeptidyl peptidase-4 augments insulin secretion in response to exogenously administered glucagon-like peptide-1, glucose-dependent insulinotropic polypeptide, pituitary adenylate cyclase-activating polypeptide, and gastrin-releasing peptide in mice. *Endocrinology* **2005**, *146*, 2055–2059. [CrossRef] [PubMed]
89. Zhong, J.; Rao, X.; Rajagopalan, S. An emerging role of dipeptidyl peptidase 4 (DPP4) beyond glucose control: Potential implications in cardiovascular disease. *Atherosclerosis* **2013**, *226*, 305–314. [CrossRef] [PubMed]
90. Devin, J.K.; Pretorius, M.; Nian, H.; Yu, C.; Billings FTt and Brown, N.J. Dipeptidyl-peptidase 4 inhibition and the vascular effects of glucagon-like peptide-1 and brain natriuretic peptide in the human forearm. *J. Am. Heart. Assoc.* **2014**, *3*. [CrossRef] [PubMed]
91. Busek, P.; Stremenova, J.; Krepela, E.; Sedo, A. Modulation of substance P signaling by dipeptidyl peptidase-IV enzymatic activity in human glioma cell lines. *Physiol. Res.* **2008**, *57*, 443–449. [PubMed]
92. Reinehr, T.; Roth, C.L.; Enriori, P.J.; Masur, K. Changes of dipeptidyl peptidase IV (DPP-IV) in obese children with weight loss: Relationships to peptide, Y.Y.; pancreatic peptide, and insulin sensitivity. *J. Pediatr. Endocrinol. Metab.* **2010**, *23*, 101–108. [CrossRef] [PubMed]
93. Wagner, L.; Kaestner, F.; Wolf, R.; Stiller, H.; Heiser, U.; Manhart, S.; Hoffmann, T.; Rahfeld, J.U.; Demuth, H.U.; Rothermundt, M.; et al. Identifying neuropeptide Y (NPY) as the main stress-related substrate of dipeptidyl peptidase 4 (DPP4) in blood circulation. *Neuropeptides* **2016**, *57*, 21–34. [CrossRef] [PubMed]
94. Ajami, K.; Pitman, M.R.; Wilson, C.H.; Park, J.; Menz, R.I.; Starr, A.E.; Cox, J.H.; Abbott, C.A.; Overall, C.M.; Gorrell, M.D. Stromal cell-derived factors 1alpha and 1beta, inflammatory protein-10 and interferon-inducible T cell chemo-attractant are novel substrates of dipeptidyl peptidase 8. *FEBS Lett.* **2008**, *582*, 819–825. [CrossRef] [PubMed]
95. Nieto-Fontarigo, J.J.; Gonzalez-Barcala, F.J.; San-Jose, M.E.; Cruz, M.J.; Linares, T.; Soto-Mera, M.T.; Valdes-Cuadrado, L.; Garcia-Gonzalez, M.A.; Andrade-Bulos, L.J.; Arias, P.; et al. Expansion of a CD26low Effector TH Subset and Reduction in Circulating Levels of sCD26 in Stable Allergic Asthma in Adults. *J. Investig. Allergol. Clin. Immunol.* **2018**, *28*, 113–125. [CrossRef] [PubMed]

96. Proost, P.; Schutyser, E.; Menten, P.; Struyf, S.; Wuyts, A.; Opdenakker, G.; Detheux, M.; Parmentier, M.; Durinx, C.; Lambeir, A.M.; et al. Amino-terminal truncation of CXCR3 agonists impairs receptor signaling and lymphocyte chemotaxis, while preserving antiangiogenic properties. *Blood* **2001**, *98*, 3554–3561. [CrossRef] [PubMed]
97. Mulvihill, E.E.; Drucker, D.J. Pharmacology, physiology, and mechanisms of action of dipeptidyl peptidase-4 inhibitors. *Endocr. Rev.* **2014**, *35*, 992–1019. [CrossRef] [PubMed]
98. Iwata, S.; Yamaguchi, N.; Munakata, Y.; Ikushima, H.; Lee, J.F.; Hosono, O.; Schlossman, S.F.; Morimoto, C. CD26/dipeptidyl peptidase IV differentially regulates the chemotaxis of T cells and monocytes toward RANTES: Possible mechanism for the switch from innate to acquired immune response. *Int. Immunol.* **1999**, *11*, 417–426. [CrossRef] [PubMed]
99. Broxmeyer, H.E.; Hoggatt, J.; O'Leary, H.A.; Mantel, C.; Chitteti, B.R.; Cooper, S.; Messina-Graham, S.; Hangoc, G.; Farag, S.; Rohrabaugh, S.L.; et al. Dipeptidylpeptidase 4 negatively regulates colony-stimulating factor activity and stress hematopoiesis. *Nat. Med.* **2012**, *18*, 1786–1796. [CrossRef] [PubMed]
100. Pacheco, R.; Martinez-Navio, J.M.; Lejeune, M.; Climent, N.; Oliva, H.; Gatell, J.M.; Gallart, T.; Mallol, J.; Lluis, C.; Franco, R. CD26, adenosine deaminase, and adenosine receptors mediate costimulatory signals in the immunological synapse. *Proc. Natl. Acad. Sci. USA* **2005**, *102*, 9583–9588. [CrossRef] [PubMed]
101. Ohnuma, K.; Uchiyama, M.; Yamochi, T.; Nishibashi, K.; Hosono, O.; Takahashi, N.; Kina, S.; Tanaka, H.; Lin, X.; Dang, N.H.; et al. Caveolin-1 triggers T-cell activation via CD26 in association with CARMA1. *J. Biol. Chem.* **2007**, *282*, 10117–10131. [CrossRef] [PubMed]
102. Ikushima, H.; Munakata, Y.; Ishii, T.; Iwata, S.; Terashima, M.; Tanaka, H.; Schlossman, S.F.; Morimoto, C. Internalization of CD26 by mannose 6-phosphate/insulin-like growth factor II receptor contributes to T. cell activation. *Proc. Natl. Acad. Sci. USA* **2000**, *97*, 8439–8444. [CrossRef] [PubMed]
103. Salgado, F.J.; Lojo, J.; Alonso-Lebrero, J.L.; Lluis, C.; Franco, R.; Cordero, O.J.; Nogueira, M. A role for interleukin-12 in the regulation of T cell plasma membrane compartmentation. *J. Biol. Chem.* **2003**, *278*, 24849–24857. [CrossRef] [PubMed]
104. Ghersi, G.; Zhao, Q.; Salamone, M.; Yeh, Y.; Zucker, S.; Chen, W.T. The protease complex consisting of dipeptidyl peptidase, I.V.; seprase plays a role in the migration and invasion of human endothelial cells in collagenous matrices. *Cancer Res.* **2006**, *66*, 4652–4661. [CrossRef] [PubMed]
105. Ohnuma, K.; Yamochi, T.; Uchiyama, M.; Nishibashi, K.; Yoshikawa, N.; Shimizu, N.; Iwata, S.; Tanaka, H.; Dang, N.H.; Morimoto, C. CD26 up-regulates expression of CD86 on antigen-presenting cells by means of caveolin-1. *Proc. Natl. Acad. Sci. USA* **2004**, *101*, 14186–14191. [CrossRef] [PubMed]
106. Girardi, A.C.; Degray, B.C.; Nagy, T.; Biemesderfer, D.; Aronson, P.S. Association of Na(+)-H(+) exchanger isoform NHE3 and dipeptidyl peptidase IV in the renal proximal tubule. *J. Biol. Chem.* **2001**, *276*, 46671–46677. [CrossRef] [PubMed]
107. Weihofen, W.A.; Liu, J.; Reutter, W.; Saenger, W.; Fan, H. Crystal structures of HIV-1 Tat-derived nonapeptides Tat-(1-9) and Trp2-Tat-(1-9) bound to the active site of dipeptidyl-peptidase IV (CD26). *J. Biol. Chem.* **2005**, *280*, 14911–14917. [CrossRef] [PubMed]
108. Askari, A.T.; Unzek, S.; Popovic, Z.B.; Goldman, C.K.; Forudi, F.; Kiedrowski, M.; Rovner, A.; Ellis, S.G.; Thomas, J.D.; DiCorleto, P.E.; et al. Effect of stromal-cell-derived factor 1 on stem-cell homing and tissue regeneration in ischaemic cardiomyopathy. *Lancet* **2003**, *362*, 697–703. [CrossRef]
109. Deglurkar, I.; Mal, N.; Mills, W.R.; Popovic, Z.B.; McCarthy, P.; Blackstone, E.H.; Laurita, K.R.; Penn, M.S. Mechanical and electrical effects of cell-based gene therapy for ischemic cardiomyopathy are independent. *Hum. Gene Ther.* **2006**, *17*, 1144–1151. [CrossRef] [PubMed]
110. Sundararaman, S.; Miller, T.J.; Pastore, J.M.; Kiedrowski, M.; Aras, R.; Penn, M.S. Plasmid-based transient human stromal cell-derived factor-1 gene transfer improves cardiac function in chronic heart failure. *Gene Ther.* **2011**, *18*, 867–873. [CrossRef] [PubMed]
111. Zhang, M.; Mal, N.; Kiedrowski, M.; Chacko, M.; Askari, A.T.; Popovic, Z.B.; Koc, O.N.; Penn, M.S. SDF-1 expression by mesenchymal stem cells results in trophic support of cardiac myocytes after myocardial infarction. *FASEB J.* **2007**, *21*, 3197–3207. [CrossRef] [PubMed]
112. Christopherson, K.W.; Hangoc, G.; Mantel, C.R.; Broxmeyer, H.E. Modulation of hematopoietic stem cell homing and engraftment by CD26. *Science* **2004**, *305*, 1000–1003. [CrossRef] [PubMed]

113. Zaruba, M.M.; Theiss, H.D.; Vallaster, M.; Mehl, U.; Brunner, S.; David, R.; Fischer, R.; Krieg, L.; Hirsch, E.; Huber, B.; et al. Synergy between CD26/DPP-IV inhibition and G-CSF improves cardiac function after acute myocardial infarction. *Cell Stem Cell* **2009**, *4*, 313–323. [CrossRef] [PubMed]
114. Dingenouts, C.K.E.; Bakker, W.; Lodder, K.; Wiesmeijer, K.C.; Moerkamp, A.T.; Maring, J.A.; Arthur, H.M.; Smits, A.M.; Goumans, M.J. Inhibiting DPP4 in a mouse model of HHT1 results in a shift towards regenerative macrophages and reduces fibrosis after myocardial infarction. *PLoS ONE* **2017**, *12*, e0189805. [CrossRef] [PubMed]
115. Haverslag, R.T.; de Groot, D.; Grundmann, S.; Meder, B.; Goumans, M.J.; Pasterkamp, G.; Hoefer, I.E.; de Kleijn, D.P. CD26 inhibition enhances perfusion recovery in ApoE-/-mice. *Curr. Vasc. Pharmacol.* **2013**, *11*, 21–28. [CrossRef] [PubMed]
116. Peled, A.; Kollet, O.; Ponomaryov, T.; Petit, I.; Franitza, S.; Grabovsky, V.; Slav, M.M.; Nagler, A.; Lider, O.; Alon, R.; et al. The chemokine SDF-1 activates the integrins LFA-1, VLA-4, and VLA-5 on immature human CD34(+) cells: Role in transendothelial/stromal migration and engraftment of NOD/SCID mice. *Blood* **2000**, *95*, 3289–3296. [PubMed]
117. Ganju, R.K.; Brubaker, S.A.; Meyer, J.; Dutt, P.; Yang, Y.; Qin, S.; Newman, W.; Groopman, J.E. The alpha-chemokine, stromal cell-derived factor-1alpha, binds to the transmembrane G-protein-coupled CXCR-4 receptor and activates multiple signal transduction pathways. *J. Biol. Chem.* **1998**, *273*, 23169–23175. [CrossRef] [PubMed]
118. Thomas, M.N.; Kalnins, A.; Andrassy, M.; Wagner, A.; Klussmann, S.; Rentsch, M.; Habicht, A.; Pratschke, S.; Stangl, M.; Bazhin, A.V.; et al. SDF-1/CXCR4/CXCR7 is pivotal for vascular smooth muscle cell proliferation and chronic allograft vasculopathy. *Transpl. Int.* **2015**, *28*, 1426–1435. [CrossRef] [PubMed]
119. De Groot, D.; Haverslag, R.T.; Pasterkamp, G.; de Kleijn, D.P.; Hoefer, I.E. Targeted deletion of the inhibitory NF-kappaB p50 subunit in bone marrow-derived cells improves collateral growth after arterial occlusion. *Cardiovasc. Res.* **2010**, *88*, 179–185. [CrossRef] [PubMed]
120. Eitenmuller, I.; Volger, O.; Kluge, A.; Troidl, K.; Barancik, M.; Cai, W.J.; Heil, M.; Pipp, F.; Fischer, S.; Horrevoets, A.J.; et al. The range of adaptation by collateral vessels after femoral artery occlusion. *Circ. Res.* **2006**, *99*, 656–662. [CrossRef] [PubMed]
121. Hoefer, I.E.; van Royen, N.; Rectenwald, J.E.; Bray, E.J.; Abouhamze, Z.; Moldawer, L.L.; Voskuil, M.; Piek, J.J.; Buschmann, I.R.; Ozaki, C.K. Direct evidence for tumor necrosis factor-alpha signaling in arteriogenesis. *Circulation* **2002**, *105*, 1639–1641. [CrossRef] [PubMed]
122. Van Royen, N.; Hoefer, I.; Buschmann, I.; Heil, M.; Kostin, S.; Deindl, E.; Vogel, S.; Korff, T.; Augustin, H.; Bode, C.; et al. Exogenous application of transforming growth factor beta 1 stimulates arteriogenesis in the peripheral circulation. *FASEB J.* **2002**. [CrossRef] [PubMed]
123. Krieger, J.R.; Ogle, M.E.; McFaline-Figueroa, J.; Segar, C.E.; Temenoff, J.S.; Botchwey, E.A. Spatially localized recruitment of anti-inflammatory monocytes by SDF-1alpha-releasing hydrogels enhances microvascular network remodeling. *Biomaterials* **2015**, *77*, 280–290. [CrossRef] [PubMed]
124. Troidl, C.; Jung, G.; Troidl, K.; Hoffmann, J.; Mollmann, H.; Nef, H.; Schaper, W.; Hamm, C.W.; Schmitz-Rixen, T. The temporal and spatial distribution of macrophage subpopulations during arteriogenesis. *Curr. Vasc. Pharmacol.* **2013**, *11*, 5–12. [CrossRef] [PubMed]
125. Brenner, C.; Franz, W.M.; Kuhlenthal, S.; Kuschnerus, K.; Remm, F.; Gross, L.; Theiss, H.D.; Landmesser, U.; Krankel, N. DPP-4 inhibition ameliorates atherosclerosis by priming monocytes into M2 macrophages. *Int. J. Cardiol.* **2015**, *199*, 163–169. [CrossRef] [PubMed]
126. Lee, Y.S.; Shin, S.; Shigihara, T.; Hahm, E.; Liu, M.J.; Han, J.; Yoon, J.W.; Jun, H.S. Glucagon-like peptide-1 gene therapy in obese diabetic mice results in long-term cure of diabetes by improving insulin sensitivity and reducing hepatic gluconeogenesis. *Diabetes* **2007**, *56*, 1671–1679. [CrossRef] [PubMed]
127. Van Weel, V.; de Vries, M.; Voshol, P.J.; Verloop, R.E.; Eilers, P.H.; van Hinsbergh, V.W.; van Bockel, J.H.; Quax, P.H. Hypercholesterolemia reduces collateral artery growth more dominantly than hyperglycemia or insulin resistance in mice. *Arterioscler. Thromb. Vasc. Biol.* **2006**, *26*, 1383–1390. [CrossRef] [PubMed]
128. Buschmann, I.R.; Hoefer, I.E.; van Royen, N.; Katzer, E.; Braun-Dulleaus, R.; Heil, M.; Kostin, S.; Bode, C.; Schaper, W. GM-CSF: A strong arteriogenic factor acting by amplification of monocyte function. *Atherosclerosis* **2001**, *159*, 343–356. [CrossRef]

129. Deindl, E.; Zaruba, M.M.; Brunner, S.; Huber, B.; Mehl, U.; Assmann, G.; Hoefer, I.E.; Mueller-Hoecker, J.; Franz, W.M. G-CSF administration after myocardial infarction in mice attenuates late ischemic cardiomyopathy by enhanced arteriogenesis. *FASEB J.* **2006**, *20*, 956–958. [CrossRef] [PubMed]
130. Meier, P.; Hemingway, H.; Lansky, A.J.; Knapp, G.; Pitt, B.; Seiler, C. The impact of the coronary collateral circulation on mortality: A meta-analysis. *Eur. Heart. J.* **2012**, *33*, 614–621. [CrossRef] [PubMed]
131. Fazel, S.; Cimini, M.; Chen, L.; Li, S.; Angoulvant, D.; Fedak, P.; Verma, S.; Weisel, R.D.; Keating, A.; Li, R.K. Cardioprotective c-kit+ cells are from the bone marrow and regulate the myocardial balance of angiogenic cytokines. *J. Clin. Investig.* **2006**, *116*, 1865–1877. [CrossRef] [PubMed]
132. Green, J.B.; Bethel, M.A.; Armstrong, P.W.; Buse, J.B.; Engel, S.S.; Garg, J.; Josse, R.; Kaufman, K.D.; Koglin, J.; Korn, S.; et al. Effect of Sitagliptin on Cardiovascular Outcomes in Type 2 Diabetes. *N. Engl. J. Med.* **2015**, *373*, 232–242. [CrossRef] [PubMed]
133. Scirica, B.M.; Bhatt, D.L.; Braunwald, E.; Steg, P.G.; Davidson, J.; Hirshberg, B.; Ohman, P.; Frederich, R.; Wiviott, S.D.; Hoffman, E.B.; et al. Saxagliptin and cardiovascular outcomes in patients with type 2 diabetes mellitus. *N. Engl. J. Med.* **2013**, *369*, 1317–1326. [CrossRef] [PubMed]
134. Boucaud-Maitre, D. Inclusion of the EXAMINE study in a meta-analysis of the addition of dipeptidyl peptidase-4 inhibitors to sulphonylureas and risk of hypoglycaemia. *BMJ* **2016**, *353*, i3186. [CrossRef] [PubMed]
135. Scheen, A.J. Cardiovascular Effects of New Oral Glucose-Lowering Agents: DPP-4 and SGLT-2 Inhibitors. *Circ. Res.* **2018**, *122*, 1439–1459. [CrossRef] [PubMed]
136. Rosenstock, J.; Marx, N.; Kahn, S.E.; Zinman, B.; Kastelein, J.J.; Lachin, J.M.; Bluhmki, E.; Patel, S.; Johansen, O.E.; Woerle, H.J. Cardiovascular outcome trials in type 2 diabetes and the sulphonylurea controversy: Rationale for the active-comparator CAROLINA trial. *Diabetes Vasc. Dis. Res.* **2013**, *10*, 289–301. [CrossRef] [PubMed]
137. Costa, P.Z.; Soares, R. Neovascularization in diabetes and its complications. Unraveling the angiogenic paradox. *Life Sci.* **2013**, *92*, 1037–1045. [CrossRef] [PubMed]
138. Jawa, A.; Kcomt, J.; Fonseca, V.A. Diabetic nephropathy and retinopathy. *Med. Clin. North Am.* **2004**, *88*, 1001–1036. [CrossRef] [PubMed]
139. Rao Kondapally Seshasai, S.; Kaptoge, S.; Thompson, A.; Di Angelantonio, E.; Gao, P.; Sarwar, N.; Whincup, P.H.; Mukamal, K.J.; Gillum, R.F.; Holme, I.; et al. Diabetes mellitus, fasting glucose, and risk of cause-specific death. *N. Engl. J. Med.* **2011**, *364*, 829–841. [CrossRef] [PubMed]
140. Chao, C.T.; Wang, J.; Wu, H.Y.; Chien, K.L.; Hung, K.Y. Dipeptidyl peptidase 4 inhibitor use is associated with a lower risk of incident acute kidney injury in patients with diabetes. *Oncotarget* **2017**, *8*, 53028–53040. [CrossRef] [PubMed]
141. Chung, Y.R.; Park, S.W.; Kim, J.W.; Kim, J.H.; Lee, K. Protective Effects of Dipeptidyl Peptidase-4 Inhibitors on Progression of Diabetic Retinopathy in Patients with Type 2 Diabetes. *Retina* **2016**, *36*, 2357–2363. [CrossRef] [PubMed]
142. Goncalves, A.; Almeida, L.; Silva, A.P.; Fontes-Ribeiro, C.; Ambrosio, A.F.; Cristovao, A.; Fernandes, R. The dipeptidyl peptidase-4 (DPP-4) inhibitor sitagliptin ameliorates retinal endothelial cell dysfunction triggered by inflammation. *Biomed. Pharmacother.* **2018**, *102*, 833–838. [CrossRef] [PubMed]
143. Kanozawa, K.; Noguchi, Y.; Sugahara, S.; Nakamura, S.; Yamamoto, H.; Kaneko, K.; Kono, R.; Sato, S.; Ogawa, T.; Hasegawa, H.; et al. The renoprotective effect and safety of a DPP-4 inhibitor, sitagliptin, at a small dose in type 2 diabetic patients with a renal dysfunction when changed from other DPP-4 inhibitors: REAL trial. *Clin. Exp. Nephrol.* **2018**, *22*, 825–834. [CrossRef] [PubMed]
144. Li, H.; Wang, Y.S. An angiotensin-converting enzyme inhibitor modulates stromal-derived factor-1 through CD26/dipeptidyl peptidase IV to inhibit laser-induced choroidal neovascularization. *Mol. Vis.* **2013**, *19*, 1107–1121. [PubMed]
145. Theiss, H.D.; Gross, L.; Vallaster, M.; David, R.; Brunner, S.; Brenner, C.; Nathan, P.; Assmann, G.; Mueller-Hoecker, J.; Vogeser, M.; et al. Antidiabetic gliptins in combination with G-CSF enhances myocardial function and survival after acute myocardial infarction. *Int. J. Cardiol.* **2013**, *168*, 3359–3369. [CrossRef] [PubMed]
146. Remm, F.; Krankel, N.; Lener, D.; Drucker, D.J.; Sopper, S.; Brenner, C. Sitagliptin Accelerates Endothelial Regeneration after Vascular Injury Independent from GLP1 Receptor Signaling. *Stem Cells Int.* **2018**, *2018*, 5284963. [CrossRef] [PubMed]

147. Moraes, F.; Paye, J.; Mac Gabhann, F.; Zhuang, Z.W.; Zhang, J.; Lanahan, A.A.; Simons, M. Endothelial cell-dependent regulation of arteriogenesis. *Circ. Res.* **2013**, *113*, 1076–1086. [CrossRef] [PubMed]
148. Ghorpade, D.S.; Ozcan, L.; Zheng, Z.; Nicoloro, S.M.; Shen, Y.; Chen, E.; Bluher, M.; Czech, M.P.; Tabas, I. Hepatocyte-secreted DPP4 in obesity promotes adipose inflammation and insulin resistance. *Nature* **2018**, *555*, 673–677. [CrossRef] [PubMed]
149. Aschner, P.; Kipnes, M.S.; Lunceford, J.K.; Sanchez, M.; Mickel, C.; Williams-Herman, D.E. Effect of the dipeptidyl peptidase-4 inhibitor sitagliptin as monotherapy on glycemic control in patients with type 2 diabetes. *Diabetes Care* **2006**, *29*, 2632–2637. [CrossRef] [PubMed]
150. Jung, C.H.; Park, C.Y.; Ahn, K.J.; Kim, N.H.; Jang, H.C.; Lee, M.K.; Park, J.Y.; Chung, C.H.; Min, K.W.; Sung, Y.A.; et al. A randomized, double-blind, placebo-controlled, phase II clinical trial to investigate the efficacy and safety of oral DA-1229 in patients with type 2 diabetes mellitus who have inadequate glycaemic control with diet and exercise. *Diabetes Metab. Res. Rev.* **2015**, *31*, 295–306. [CrossRef] [PubMed]
151. Kadowaki, T.; Kondo, K. Efficacy, safety and dose-response relationship of teneligliptin, a dipeptidyl peptidase-4 inhibitor, in Japanese patients with type 2 diabetes mellitus. *Diabetes Obes. Metab.* **2013**, *15*, 810–818. [CrossRef] [PubMed]
152. Kutoh, E.; Ukai, Y. Alogliptin as an initial therapy in patients with newly diagnosed, drug naive type 2 diabetes: A randomized, control trial. *Endocrine* **2012**, *41*, 435–441. [CrossRef] [PubMed]
153. Raz, I.; Hanefeld, M.; Xu, L.; Caria, C.; Williams-Herman, D.; Khatami, H. Efficacy and safety of the dipeptidyl peptidase-4 inhibitor sitagliptin as monotherapy in patients with type 2 diabetes mellitus. *Diabetologia* **2006**, *49*, 2564–2571. [CrossRef] [PubMed]
154. Ristic, S.; Byiers, S.; Foley, J.; Holmes, D. Improved glycaemic control with dipeptidyl peptidase-4 inhibition in patients with type 2 diabetes: Vildagliptin (LAF237) dose response. *Diabetes Obes. Metab.* **2005**, *7*, 692–698. [CrossRef] [PubMed]
155. Syed, Y.Y.; McCormack, P.L. Exenatide Extended-Release: An Updated Review of Its Use in Type 2 Diabetes Mellitus. *Drugs* **2015**, *75*, 1141–1152. [CrossRef] [PubMed]
156. Tan, X.; Cao, X.; Zhou, M.; Zou, P.; Hu, J. Efficacy and safety of once-weekly semaglutide for the treatment of type 2 diabetes. *Expert Opin. Investig. Drugs* **2017**, *26*, 1083–1089. [CrossRef] [PubMed]

3

An Emerging Role for isomiRs and the microRNA Epitranscriptome in Neovascularization

Reginald V.C.T. van der Kwast [1], Paul H. A. Quax [1] and A. Yaël Nossent [1,2,*]

[1] Department of Surgery and Einthoven Laboratory for Experimental Vascular Medicine, Leiden University Medical Center, 2333 ZA Leiden, The Netherlands; rvdkwast@lumc.nl (R.V.C.T.v.d.K.); P.H.A.Quax@lumc.nl (P.H.A.Q.)

[2] Department of Laboratory Medicine and Department of Internal Medicine II, Medical University of Vienna, 1090 Vienna, Austria

* Correspondence: a.y.nossent@lumc.nl

Abstract: Therapeutic neovascularization can facilitate blood flow recovery in patients with ischemic cardiovascular disease, the leading cause of death worldwide. Neovascularization encompasses both angiogenesis, the sprouting of new capillaries from existing vessels, and arteriogenesis, the maturation of preexisting collateral arterioles into fully functional arteries. Both angiogenesis and arteriogenesis are highly multifactorial processes that require a multifactorial regulator to be stimulated simultaneously. MicroRNAs can regulate both angiogenesis and arteriogenesis due to their ability to modulate expression of many genes simultaneously. Recent studies have revealed that many microRNAs have variants with altered terminal sequences, known as isomiRs. Additionally, endogenous microRNAs have been identified that carry biochemically modified nucleotides, revealing a dynamic microRNA epitranscriptome. Both types of microRNA alterations were shown to be dynamically regulated in response to ischemia and are able to influence neovascularization by affecting the microRNA's biogenesis, or even its silencing activity. Therefore, these novel regulatory layers influence microRNA functioning and could provide new opportunities to stimulate neovascularization. In this review we will highlight the formation and function of isomiRs and various forms of microRNA modifications, and discuss recent findings that demonstrate that both isomiRs and microRNA modifications directly affect neovascularization and vascular remodeling.

Keywords: microRNA; isomiRs; epitranscriptome; neovascularization; angiogenesis; arteriogenesis; A-to-I editing; m6A; RNA modifications; RNA methylation

---

1. Introduction

Ischemic cardiovascular disease (CVD) is the leading cause of death in worldwide and was responsible for approximately 17.8 million deaths in 2017 [1,2]. Additionally, it is estimated that current standard therapies are unsuitable or insufficient for 30% of patients [3,4]. Therefore, there is a critical need for new therapeutic treatments for ischemic CVD.

A potential strategy to treat patients with ischemia is to stimulate neovascularization, which is the body's natural repair mechanism to restore blood flow to ischemic tissues. Postnatal neovascularization is comprised of angiogenesis, the sprouting of new capillaries from existing vessels, and arteriogenesis, the maturation of preexisting collateral arterioles into fully functional arteries. Both angiogenesis and arteriogenesis are highly multifactorial processes that involve multiple types of vascular and immune cells. In order to improve neovascularization as a whole, therapeutic strategies which simultaneously target both angiogenesis and arteriogenesis are needed [5,6].

During the last decade, microRNAs have emerged as multifactorial regulators of neovascularization [7–9]. MicroRNAs are short non-coding RNAs of approximately 22 nucleotides that inhibit translation of messenger RNAs (mRNAs). A single microRNA can have hundreds of mRNAs in its 'targetome', often regulating an entire network or pathway simultaneously [10]. MicroRNAs are typically defined as one specific sequence of RNA nucleotides, however, recent studies have shown that this 'canonical' microRNA sequence is often altered. These microRNA alterations can be grouped into two types: (i) isomiRs, which are microRNAs with altered terminal sequences and (ii) biochemical modifications of specific nucleotides within microRNAs, which collectively are referred to as the microRNA epitranscriptome. Both types of microRNA variations appear actively regulated in response to ischemia and can directly influence neovascularization associated processes, as we will discuss below. The microRNA epitranscriptome unveils a whole new regulatory layer that could provide novel therapeutic options for ischemic CVD. In this review we will first briefly introduce the processes involved in angiogenesis and arteriogenesis, after which we will highlight various ways in which a microRNA can be altered, and discuss recent findings which demonstrate that these microRNA alterations can affect neovascularization associated processes.

2. Neovascularization—Angiogenesis and Arteriogenesis

After the occlusion of a large artery, blood flow to the downstream tissues is hampered, causing ischemia. Blood flow towards the ischemic tissue can be restored by a process called arteriogenesis. Arteriogenesis is the growth and maturation of collateral arteries from a pre-existing arteriole network, which connects all major arteries in the body [5]. Arteriogenesis is triggered by an increase in shear stress in the arterioles, which occurs after an arterial occlusion causes redirection of blood flow through the arterioles. The increased shear stress causes endothelial cells (ECs) in the arteriole wall to express adhesion molecules and secrete cytokines, leading to the attraction of circulating monocytes and other immune cells [11–15]. These inflammatory cells produce and secrete proteases, growth factors, and cytokines which enable remodeling of the vessel wall and stimulate migration and proliferation of vascular ECs and smooth muscle cells (SMCs) [16–18]. This results in an increase in vessel diameter, until fluid sheer stress decreases which halts the arteriogenic process. Finally, the vascular SMCs and fibroblasts secrete matrix components to reconstitute the vessel wall [19,20].

The process of angiogenesis, on the other hand, is the sprouting of a new capillary from the existing vasculature in order to redistribute local blood flow towards ischemic areas. Unlike arteriogenesis, angiogenesis is driven by the hypoxia caused by ischemia, and revolves around resolving local ischemia rather than restoring arterial blood flow after the occlusion of a vessel. Angiogenesis is initiated when an angiogenic stimulus, produced by hypoxic cells, activates the vascular endothelial layer. Activated ECs will start to proliferate and migrate towards the stimulus, such as vascular endothelial growth factor (VEGF), resulting in a new capillary [21]. Next to ECs, other cell types are important regulators of angiogenesis. Vascular SMCs, pericytes, fibroblasts and immune cells play key roles by supporting and modulating EC function and secreting the proangiogenic stimuli to start the process [22–24].

Since both angiogenesis and arteriogenesis are highly multifactorial processes, the simultaneous stimulation of both processes requires a multifactorial regulator, like microRNAs [7,8].

3. MicroRNAs

MicroRNAs are endogenous, small non-coding RNA molecules that inhibit translation of mRNAs. The microRNA's target selection is predominantly determined by the microRNA's 'seed sequence', nucleotides 2–8 at the 5′-end of a microRNA [25,26], which bind their target mRNAs via Watson–Crick base-pairing. Due to this relatively small targeting sequence, a single microRNA's 'targetome' can consist of hundreds of mRNAs, enabling microRNAs to regulate multifactorial processes [10].

The biogenesis of microRNAs starts with the transcription of the microRNA containing gene, yielding a primary microRNA (pri-miR) which then undergoes several steps of maturation to form the mature and functional microRNA (Figure 1) [27]. First, the pri-miR is cleaved in the nucleus by Drosha to generate a hairpin-shaped precursor microRNA (pre-miR) [28]. The pre-miR is then translocated to the cytoplasm where a final cleavage is performed by Dicer, yielding a microRNA duplex [29]. Either side of the duplex can associate with Argonaute proteins and become a functional mature microRNA after incorporation into the RNA-induced silencing complex (RISC) [30]. Mature microRNAs are named after their side, 5′ or 3′, in the pri-miR hairpin (e.g., miR-#-5p or -3p).

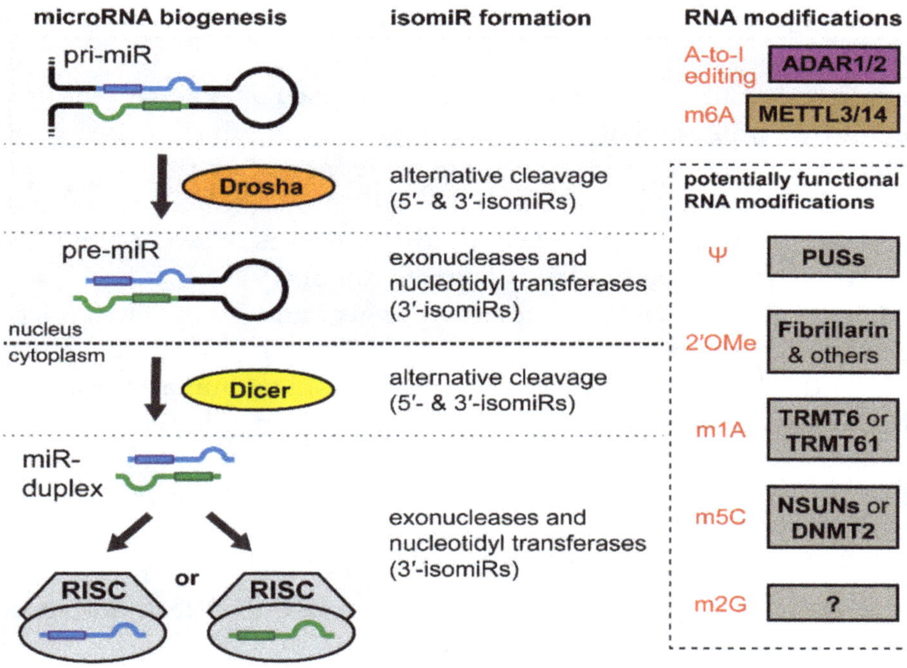

Figure 1. MicroRNA biogenesis and alterations that induce isomiR formation or microRNA nucleotide modifications. Transcription of the microRNA containing gene forms the primary microRNA (pri-miR). Drosha cleaves the pri-miR to generate the precursor microRNA (pre-miR). The pre-miR cleaved by Dicer in the cytoplasm yielding the microRNA duplex. Either side of the duplex can be incorporated into the RNA-induced silencing complex (RISC) to become a functional mature microRNA. IsomiRs can be formed during microRNA biogenesis when Drosha or Dicer cleave in alternative locations, or when exonucleases or nucleotidyl transferases remove or add nucleotides to the 3′-end of the pre-miR or the mature microRNA. RNA nucleotide modifications with known or potential functional implications on microRNA biogenesis or functioning are shown in red with their 'writers' next to them.

MicroRNA biogenesis is strictly regulated, even at a microRNA-specific level, by numerous factors, including DNA methylation, activity modulation of key maturation proteins and many RNA-binding proteins [29,31–33]. As a result, microRNA expression is often highly tissue specific and is dynamically regulated during key physiological processes, including the response to ischemia [29,34].

In 2007, the importance of microRNAs in neovascularization was demonstrated for the first time when several studies showed that Dicer-dependent microRNAs were required for angiogenesis [35–37]. Since then, microRNAs have been shown to play a functional role in all processes involved in neovascularization, including production and secretion of angiogenic stimuli, as well as EC, SMC, fibroblast and immune cell proliferation, migration and activation, which have recently been reviewed in references [8,38–40]. Several of these vasoactive microRNAs have also been well described to play an important role in vascular remodeling during ischemic cardiovascular diseases [8,41].

For example, Bonauer et al. showed that miR-92a is highly expressed in human ECs and functions as negative regulator of angiogenesis [42]. Inhibition of miR-92a increased angiogenesis in vivo and improved blood flow recovery after hindlimb ischemia [42]. Furthermore, administration of miR-92a inhibitors in porcine models for myocardial infarction demonstrated that miR-92 inhibition prevents adverse infarct remodeling and ischemia/reperfusion injury [43,44]. Phase 1 trials aimed to improve wound healing with a future potential clinical application towards heart failure treatment have recently been completed for miR-92a inhibitor MRG 110 (NCT03603431) [45].

Both miR-126-3p and -5p are also highly expressed in ECs where they promote angiogenesis by stimulating EC proliferation and VEGF signaling and regulating leukocyte adhesion [46–49]. Inhibition of miR-126-3p was shown to decrease recovery after myocardial infarction and hindlimb ischemia in mice [47,50,51]. Furthermore, miR-126 levels are decreased in patients with ischemic coronary artery disease [52]. Similarly, miR-10a also stimulates angiogenesis by promoting VEGF signaling in ECs and regulating their inflammatory phenotype [53–57].

MiR-21-5p regulates proliferation and apoptosis of vascular wall smooth muscle cells [58,59] and promotes fibrosis by stimulating fibroblast survival and growth factor secretion [60]. Preclinical studies have shown that inhibition of miR-21-5p can prevent maladaptive vascular remodeling and heart failure [59,60]. These findings suggest that the miR-21-5p inhibitor RG-012, which is currently being tested in a phase 2 clinical trial to prevent kidney fibrosis in patients with Alport syndrome (NCT02855268), could potentially be used for the treatment of CVD.

Additionally, it is noteworthy that several groups of genomically clustered microRNAs have been identified that are able to broadly regulate neovascularization in response to ischemia: Knockout of the miR-17/92 gene cluster (located on chromosome 14 in mice and on human chromosome 13) increased both angiogenesis and arteriogenesis [61,62], while the inhibition of individual microRNAs from the 14q32 microRNA cluster (located on chromosome 12F1 in mice and on human chromosome 14) was shown to independently stimulate both angiogenesis and arteriogenesis [9].

4. IsomiRs and the microRNA Epitranscriptome

Typically, microRNAs have been defined as a single sequence of RNA nucleotides, and are listed as such in the principle public microRNA database, miRbase [63]. However, recent studies have shown that this 'canonical' microRNA sequence can be altered. These microRNA alterations can be separated into two types: isomiRs and RNA nucleotide modifications.

IsomiRs are microRNA sequence variants that have one or more nucleotides added or deleted at their 5′- and/or 3′-ends compared to the canonical microRNA sequence.

RNA nucleotide modifications are biochemical modifications of the standard RNA nucleotides, which are performed by enzymes present in all living organisms. Recent studies have demonstrated that these RNA nucleotide modifications have a functional regulatory role and form what has been named the 'epitranscriptome' [64]. While many different RNA nucleotide modifications exist, only a few have been studied in the context of microRNAs: Adenosine-to-inosine editing (A-to-I editing) and N6-adenosine methylation (m6A) and 2′-*O*-methylation (2′OMe).

Below, we will discuss those studies that demonstrate that isomiRs and microRNA A-to-I editing and m6A can be actively regulated and play a directing role in neovascularization, as well as other modifications (including 2′OMe) that are likely to have a similar role.

5. IsomiRs

5.1. IsomiRs

IsomiRs were discovered when microRNA sequencing studies observed that many microRNAs had sequence variants with one or more nucleotides added or deleted from the 5′- and/or 3′-ends compared to the 'canonical' microRNA sequence [65,66]. While initially dismissed as errors or artifacts, isomiRs have since been shown to be functional microRNAs which actively associate with the RISC complex and inhibit mRNA translation of their targets [67–70]. Furthermore, sequencing studies have shown that isomiRs are widespread and represent approximately 50% of the microRNA transcripts present in cells and tissue [71,72].

IsomiRs are primarily generated by cleavage variations of either DROSHA or DICER during microRNA biogenesis (Figure 1) [68,73]. IsomiRs with altered 3′-end sequences, 3′-isomiRs, can also be created by exonucleases which remove 3′ nucleotides, or by nucleotidyl transferases, which catalyze the addition of 3′ nucleotides. The number and type of isomiRs that arise from a single locus varies per microRNA, but approximately 75% of microRNA loci give rise to at least one isomiR [74].

In general, 3′-isomiRs are more abundant than 5′-isomiRs, however, a number of microRNAs do have prevalent 5′-isomiRs [75–78]. Since a microRNA's 5′-end determines its seed sequence, 5′-isomiRs have an altered targetome compared to the canonical microRNA sequence and are thus functionally different (Figure 2) [67,79–81]. While 3′-isomiRs do not have an altered seed sequence, their 3′-end variability has been associated with altered microRNA stability and turnover [82–86]. Furthermore, recent findings have shown that changes in microRNA length due to 3′-end variation can affect microRNA targeting strength and activity in specific cases [87,88]. Combined, these findings highlight the importance to take isomiRs into account during microRNA research.

pri-miR-21 sequence	CGGGUAGCUUAUCAGACUGAUGUUGACUGU	Mechanisms of formation	Potential effects
canonical miR-21-5p	5′ UAGCUUAUCAGACUGAUGUUGA 3′	• canonical biogenesis	• canonical function
5′-isomiRs	AGCUUAUCAGACUGAUGUUGA GUAGCUUAUCAGACUGAUGUUGA	• alternative cleavage by Dicer or Drosha	• altered targetome • length-dependent effects
3′-isomiRs	UAGCUUAUCAGACUGAUGUUGAC UAGCUUAUCAGACUGAUG UAGCUUAUCAGACUGAUGUUGAA	• alternative cleavage by Dicer or Drosha • exonuclease or nucleotidyl transferase activity	• altered stability and/or turnover • length-dependent effects
5′- & 3′-isomiRs	AGCUUAUCAGACUGAUGUUGAC UAGCUUAUCAGACUGAUGUUGACA AGCUUAUCAGACUGAUGUUGACA	• alternative cleavage by Dicer and/or Drosha • exonuclease or nucleotidyl transferase activity	• altered targetome • altered stability and/or turnover • length-dependent effects

Figure 2. Different types of isomiRs, their mechanism of formation and their potential functional effects. The sequence of miR-21 and some of its isomiRs are shown to exemplify the different isomiR types. In each case, the seed sequence is underlined (red if altered) and red nucleotides are due to nucleotidyl transferase activity. Relative to the canonical microRNA, 5′-isomiRs generally have an altered targetome due to shift in seed sequence whereas 3′-isomiRs can affect the microRNAs stability or turnover. Both types of isomiRs affect the length of the microRNA and can thus incur length-dependent effects.

5.2. IsomiRs in Neovascularization Associated Cells and Processes

Due to the prevalence of isomiRs, most microRNAs that are known regulators of neovascularization have isomiRs. In fact, the microRNA loci with the most known isomiRs are miR-21-5p (Figure 2) and miR-10a-5p, two microRNAs with well-established roles in vascular biology and neovascularization [53–57], which have at least 40 isomiRs each [74]. MiR-21-5p isomiRs were found to be highly expressed in endothelial cells, as well as, miR-126-5p and -3p and their isomiRs, which are also well-established vasoactive microRNAs [8,89–91]. Combined, the miR-21-5p and miR-126 transcripts accounted for almost 40% of the total endothelial microRNA transcripts detected, including at least two 5′-isomiRs with physiologically relevant abundance [89,91]. One of these studies reported that approximately 55% of the total microRNA transcripts detected in human umbilical vein endothelial cells (HUVECs) were in fact isomiRs originating from 230 distinct microRNA loci [89]. For 33 of these microRNA loci, the isomiR variant was the most abundant form, rather than the canonical sequence. Since isomiRs often have altered stability and turnover [83–86], these abundant isomiRs could help regulate vasoactive microRNA expression. Furthermore, abundant 5′-isomiRs are likely to be functionally important due to their altered seed sequence and thus targetome.

IsomiR expression profiles can vary based on cell type and in response to biological stimuli, including stimuli associated with neovascularization [75,76,78,92]. For example, Voellenke et al. examined isomiR expression of normoxic and hypoxic human umbilical vein endothelial cells (HUVECs) using deep sequencing [89]. While the study lacked the power to identify any statistically significant patterns, the authors did observe that hypoxic conditions altered isomiR expression. Furthermore, Nejad et al. demonstrated that treating fibroblasts with interferon-beta, a regulatory factor in both angiogenesis and arteriogenesis [93–95], specifically decreased expression of the longer 3′-isomiRs from 13 microRNA loci, while the shorter isomiRs were generally upregulated [96]. Among the regulated microRNAs was miR-222-3p, which has been shown to regulate angiogenesis and inflammation-mediated vascular remodeling [97,98]. Interestingly, the longer 3′-isomiRs of miR-222-3p (>22 nt) were previously found to increase apoptotic activity, whereas the shorter isomiRs did not, suggesting the altered 3′-isomiR profiles could also be functionally important [88]. However, the exact factors that mediate the isomiR-specific regulation remain to be uncovered. It is likely that, similar to canonical microRNA biogenesis, isomiR biogenesis is regulated by a multitude of factors, including factors which specifically regulate individual isomiRs [29,31,68].

We have recently performed a focused study on the 5′-isomiR of miR-411-5p from the vasoactive 14q32 microRNA cluster in order to collect direct evidence that isomiRs are actively regulated during ischemia-induced neovascularization [99]. We found that miR-411's isomiR expression profile was tissue-specific and that canonical miR-411-5p was less abundant than its 5′-isomiR in human vascular ECs, fibroblasts and in whole human venous tissue. We discovered that the expression of the 5′-isomiR is decreased relative to canonical miR-411-5p expression in response to acute ischemia, both in cells and in a murine model for effective neovascularization after ischemia [99]. Strikingly, the relative 5′-isomiR expression was upregulated instead in ischemic veins from patients with critical limb ischemia due to peripheral artery disease (PAD). We demonstrated that the 5′-isomiR has a different targetome than the canonical miR-411-5p and inhibits translation of, among others, the pro-angiogenic Angiopoietin-1. Finally, we showed that the 5′-isomiR decreases vascular cell migration while the canonical miR-411-5p does not [99]. Combined these data show that isomiR formation is indeed a functional pathway, which is actively regulated during ischemia, with direct implications for neovascularization.

Table 1 presents a summary of the key studies that demonstrate the prevalence and importance of isomiRs.

Table 1. Key studies demonstrating the prevalence and importance of isomiRs.

Topic	Key Findings	References
Prevalence of isomiRs	• Generally, isomiRs represent ~50% of microRNA transcripts in cells and tissues (~55% in HUVECs)	[71,72,89,91]
	• ~75% of microRNA loci can produce at least 1 isomiR	[74]
Potential functional effect of isomiRs	• 5′-isomiRs have altered targetome due to a shifted seed sequence compared to the cannonical microRNA	[67,79–81,99]
	• 3′-isomiRs can have altered microRNA stability and turnover	[82–86]
	• isomiRs with different length can have altered targeting strength and activity	[87,88]
Abundant vasoactive microRNAs with isomiRs	• miR-21-5p (at least 43 potential isomiRs, also in HUVECs)	[74,89,91]
	• miR-10a-5p (at least 41 isomiRs)	[74]
	• miR-126 (highly abundant in HUVECs together with miR-21-5p and its isomiRs)	[89,91]
	• miR-222-3p (has functionally different 3′-isomiRs)	[88,96]
	• miR-411-5p (5′-isomiR has altered functionality and anti-angiogenic properties)	[99]
Regulation of isomiRs	• IsomiR expression profiles can vary based on cell type and in response to biological stimuli	[75,76,78,92]
	• Hypoxic HUVECs display altered isomiR expression	[89]
	• Independent regulation of miR-411-5p and its 5′-isomiR in response to ischemia	[99]

HUVECs: human umbilical vein endothelial cells.

6. Adenosine-to-Inosine Editing

6.1. Adenosine-to-Inosine Editing

A-to-I editing is the biochemical modification of adenosines into inosines by deamination. Unlike adenosine, inosine preferentially binds to cytidine and is therefore generally interpreted as guanosine by the cellular machinery [100]. This form of RNA editing can have a number of consequences on RNA functioning, ranging from destabilizing the RNA molecules' secondary structure to altering a protein amino acid sequence due to editing of the mRNA's coding sequence [101–103]. In mammals, A-to-I editing accounts for more than 90% of all RNA editing events and is catalyzed by either ADAR1 or ADAR2 (adenosine deaminase acting on RNA 1 or 2), which are expressed throughout the body [104–106]. The removal of the editing activity of either ADAR1 or ADAR2 in mice leads to premature lethality, demonstrating that A-to-I editing is of vital importance [107–109]. However, the precise regulatory mechanisms governing this critical cellular process have yet to be fully elucidated [110]. Changes to ADAR levels or its activity were shown to affect global editing, but these observations do not always correlate well with frequencies of individual editing events [111,112]. Therefore, it is evident that additional regulatory mechanisms exist that modulate A-to-I editing in a site-specific manner.

ADARs specifically target double stranded RNA structures, including those found in pri-miRs (Figure 1). The editing of a pri-miR can profoundly influence microRNA maturation, resulting in changes in mature microRNA expression [113–115]. However, when editing alters the microRNA's seed sequence, this can completely change the mature microRNA's target selection, resulting in the regulation of a different targetome [116].

6.2. MicroRNA A-to-I Editing in Neovascularization

MicroRNA editing is a widespread phenomenon which also affects many vasoactive microRNAs, as demonstrated recently in a study by Li et al. The authors mapped microRNA A-to-I editing at an unprecedented scale and found 2711 potential pri-miR editing sites within approximately 80% of all human pri-miRs [117]. MicroRNA editing profiles were also found to be tissue-specific, which is in agreement with previous findings [113,115,118]. Furthermore, 367 potential editing sites were found within human mature microRNAs, often located in the seed sequence [117].

In the field of cancer research, several microRNA editing events were shown to have a functional effect on cell migration and/or proliferation [119–121], which are also crucial processes in both angiogenesis and arteriogenesis [20,21]. For example, seed sequence editing of miR-455-5p was shown to alter its targetome, causing edited miR-455-5p to decrease tumor cell proliferation and migration, while the unedited version had the opposite effect [122]. Furthermore, editing of the seed sequence of miR-200b enhanced tumor cell proliferation and migration, in contrast to the unedited version [120]. Interestingly, higher miR-200b editing levels were associated with a poorer prognosis in cancer patients, highlighting the possibility that microRNA editing can be clinically relevant as a biomarker or therapeutic target.

We have recently demonstrated that microRNA-editing can also directly regulate neovascularization. We showed that A-to-I-editing of miR-487b-3p, another microRNA from the vasoactive 14q32 microRNA cluster, is increased in ischemic muscle tissues undergoing neovascularization after induction of hindlimb ischemia [123]. MiR-487b-3p editing was also found in all human vascular ECs, SMCs, and fibroblasts. The edited mature miR-487b-3p has a unique targetome and promotes angiogenesis, in contrast to the canonical miR-487b-3p [123]. In a follow-up study, we demonstrate that vasoactive microRNA editing is a widespread phenomenon that enhances neovascularization in response to ischemia (manuscript submitted).

7. N6-Adenosine Methylation

7.1. N6-Adenosine Methylation

The modification of adenosine to N^6-methyladenosine (m6A) is perhaps the most prevalent RNA nucleotide modification in eukaryotic cells and is present in more than 25% of human transcripts [124,125]. m6A is installed by the methyltransferase complex containing 'writer' METTL3 (Methyltransferase Like 3) and RNA-binding platform METTL14 [126], supported by cofactors WTAP (Wilms' tumor 1-associating protein) and KIAA1429 [127,128]. Strikingly, m6A levels are dynamically regulated throughout all stages of life, with the help of m6A demethylases, or 'erasers', FTO (fat mass and obesity-associated protein), and ALKBH5 (alkB homolog 5) [129,130]. m6A methylation has been shown to affect almost every aspect of RNA metabolism, from expression and processing in the nucleus to translation and degradation in the cytoplasm [131–133]. The importance of its functions is illustrated by studies that demonstrate that individual knockout of either METTL3, METTL14 or WTAP causes prenatal lethality in mice [134–136]. While m6A can alter RNA folding and structure [137,138], most of m6A's biological functions are mediated through a group of 'reader' proteins that specifically recognize the methylated adenosine on RNA, including the YTHD (YT521-B homology domain) and the IGF2BP (insulin-like growth factor-2 mRNA-binding protein) families [127,139–141].

While most m6A research has focused predominantly on mRNAs, several studies have demonstrated that m6A is important for microRNA biogenesis. Alarcon et al. demonstrated that pri-miRs are marked by the METTL3-dependent m6A (Figure 1). Pri-miR m6A marks are read by m6A-binding protein hnRNPA2B1 that, in turn, stimulates initiation of DICER-mediated processing through recruitment of DICER's cofactor DGCR8 [142,143]. Intriguingly, a study by Berulava et al. demonstrated that well over 200 mature microRNAs contain m6A in a human embryonic kidney cell line (HEK293). While m6A does not affect canonical base pairing, several studies have suggested that it may block the noncanonical A:G base pairing, which could affect mRNA-microRNA interaction strength [138,144]. This is supported by a recent study that found that an m6A modified miR-200c-3p resulted in significantly less suppression of its target genes than unmethylated miR-200c-3p [145]. Furthermore, recent studies also suggest that m6A of mRNAs can influence their 'targetability' by microRNAs by promoting or preventing the binding of certain RNA-binding proteins that block microRNA-mediated transcript destabilization [141,146].

7.2. *Importance of m6A in the Cardio-Vasculature and in Vasoactive MicroRNAs*

Two recent studies have demonstrated the importance of m6A in cardiovascular homeostasis. Dorn et al. demonstrates that METTL3-dependant m6A helps modulate cardiac homeostasis and hypertrophic stress responses in mice [147]. The overexpression of METTL3 was shown to cause spontaneous hypertrophy, whereas METTL3 knockdown leads to maladaptive remodeling and signs of heart failure. Mathiyalagan et al. demonstrated that m6A is increased in failing mammalian hearts and in hypoxic cardiomyocytes [148]. Furthermore, increasing the expression of m6A eraser FTO in ischemic mouse hearts attenuates the ischemia-induced increase in m6A and decrease in cardiac contractile function. These findings highlight a key role for m6A in ischemic cardiovascular disease.

Pri-miR m6A marks were shown to be required for the appropriate processing of most pri-miRs to mature miRNAs, including vasoactive microRNAs [142,143]. Furthermore, m6A of the above mentioned vasoactive miR-126 and miR-222 was shown to affect cell migration and/or proliferation in cancer cells. A study by Ma et al., demonstrated that the pri-miR of miR-126 undergoes METTL14-dependent m6A, which facilitates its processing to mature miR-126 [149]. Decreased METTL14-dependent m6A of pri-miR-126 led to the reduced expression of miR-126, which in turn increased cancer cell migration and invasion [149]. Han et al. showed that METTL3-dependant m6A of pri-miR-222 increases its maturation to mature miR-222, resulting in the reduction of PTEN, and ultimately leading to the proliferation of bladder cancer [150]. Furthermore, METTL3 was increased in bladder cancer and correlated with poor patient prognosis [150].

Combined, the abundance of m6A, its importance in microRNA biogenesis and functioning, and the dysregulation of m6A during ischemia and cardiovascular disease, suggest that m6A of microRNAs could play an important role in ischemic cardiovascular disease and neovascularization.

8. Other Modifications in the microRNA Epitranscriptome

As mentioned above, numerous other RNA nucleotide modifications exist, however, their presence and function in small RNAs (16–28 nucleotides long), which consist mostly of microRNAs [151], remains understudied [152]. An important reason for this is that conventional methods to detect RNA modifications are often unsuitable for small RNAs [152,153]. Recently, Lan et al. optimized a screening based on mass spectrometry which allowed them to provide the first overview of RNA nucleotide modifications in mammalian small RNAs using human HEK293T cells [154]. Besides inosine and m6A, 22 additional distinct nucleotide modifications were found, 13 of which consisted of different types or combinations of RNA methylations [154]. While little is known about the effect of these RNA nucleotide modifications on the functioning of small RNA, and thus microRNA, several have been studied in other RNA types.

Below, we will report the key findings of these studied RNA modifications and highlight which properties could potentially affect microRNA function. Furthermore, the discussed nucleotide modifications and their potential effects on microRNAs are summarized in Table 2.

Table 2. Known or postulated effects of nucleotide modification within microRNAs.

Nucleotide Modification	Abbreviation	Writers	Erasers	Potential Effects on microRNAs
Adenosine-to-inosine editing	A-to-I editing	ADAR1 or ADAR2	-	• pri-miR editing can profoundly influence maturation • seed sequence editing can alter targetome
N6-methyl-adenosine	m6A	METTL3/14	ALKBH5 FTO	• regulates pri-miR processing • hampered nonstandard A:G base pairing may affect silencing activity
Pseudouridine	Ψ	PUSs	-	• stronger base pairing with adenosine might affect silencing activity *
2′-*O*-methyl-nucleosides	2′OMe	Methyl-transferases	-	• may protect from A-to-I editing * • may affect stability and turnover * • enhanced RNA-RNA duplex stability might affect silencing activity *
N1-methyl-adenosine	m1A	TRMT6 & 61	ALKBH3	• positive charge can dramatically alter interactions with proteins * • disrupts RNA base pairing which can affect silencing activity *
N5-methyl-cytosine	m5C	NSUNs DNMT2	-	• may enhance stability *
N2-methyl-guanosine	m2G	unclear	-	• allows noncanonical base pairing which may affect silencing activity *

* effects are postulated effects based on observations in other RNA types.

8.1. *Pseudouridine (Ψ)*

Pseudouridine (Ψ) is one of the most abundant RNA modifications [155,156]. Ψ is highly conserved and is generated from isomerization of uridine, catalyzed by pseudouridine synthases (PUSs) [155,156]. Recent advances in high-resolution detection methods have demonstrated that Ψ-nucleotides are found in many, if not all, species of RNA [156,157]. Pseudouridylation was shown to be important for ribosomal RNA biogenesis, pre-mRNA splicing, and translation fidelity [155,156]. Compared to a uracil, Ψ forms a stronger base pairing interaction with adenosine, which allows it to alter RNA secondary structures, suggesting that microRNA pseudouridylation could affect mRNA silencing [158,159]. Furthermore, transcriptome wide pseudouridylation was shown to increase under stress conditions, including serum deprivation, a key component of ischemia [160].

8.2. 2′-O-Methylnucleosides

It is known that 2′-O-methylation (2′OMe) can reside on all four ribonucleosides and is widely conserved [161,162]. Furthermore, 2′OMe is performed by methyltransferases like Fibrillarin and many, if not all, 2′OMe-events are directed by small nucleolar RNAs [64,163,164]. 2′OMe appears essential in processing ribosomal RNAs, small nuclear RNAs, and transfer RNAs, but it has also been found in mRNAs and even in microRNAs, by our group among others [123,161,165]. While the precise location and function of 2′OMe sites in many RNA types are currently unclear, 2′OMe in general has a stabilizing effect and can influence interactions with proteins or other RNAs [161,162]. 2′OMe may in fact protect adenosine residues from A-to-I editing [165–167]. Interestingly, we found that both 2′OMe and A-to-I editing of the same adenosine residue in pri-miR-487b are increased simultaneously under ischemia [123]. However, further studies are required to examine whether both RNA modifications can be found on a single copy of miR-487b-3p. Finally, 2′OMe also greatly enhances the stability of RNA-RNA duplexes, a quality that is often utilized to enhance the stability and specificity of synthetic antisense RNA-oligonucleotides, with similar implications for 2′OMe of microRNAs [168–171].

8.3. N1-Methyladenosine (m1A)

Recent methodological advances have demonstrated that m1A is a transcriptome-wide modification [172,173]. Several members of the TRMT family (tRNA methyltransferase family) have already been shown to be m1A writers and additional writers are thought to exist [172–174]. Similar to m6A, m1A is reversible and can be demethylated by erasers ALKBH1 and 3 (alkB homolog 1 and 3) [173,175]. Furthermore, m1A levels are dynamically regulated by various types of cellular stress and correlate with upregulation of translation in general [172,173]. This modification carries a positive charge and can therefore alter both protein–RNA interactions and RNA secondary structures dramatically [131], which can potentially lead to disruption of microRNA biogenesis [29]. Furthermore, m1A appears to disrupts RNA base-pairing and induces local RNA duplex melting, suggesting that m1A may also affect microRNA-target interactions [132,176].

8.4. N5-Methylcytosine (m5C)

While best known as a DNA modification in the epigenome, m5C can be installed on RNAs too by members from the NSUN family (nucleolar protein/sun RNA methyltransferase family) and by DNMT2 (DNA methyltransferase-2) and is therefore also part of the epitranscriptome [177–181]. m5C has been found in both noncoding and coding RNAs in mammals and a few studies have shown that m5C has functional implications [177,182,183]. For example, m5C of tRNAs was shown to protect tRNAs against stress-induced cleavage [180,184,185]. Furthermore, the depletion of m5C methyltransferase Nsun7 in mice resulted in a concomitant decrease of expression of specific non-coding RNAs, suggesting m5C marks can enhance RNA stability [186].

8.5. N2-Methylguanosine (m2G)

In tRNAs and rRNAs, m2G is a relatively common RNA modification, however, which m2G writers are responsible in humans remains unclear [187,188]. Interestingly, the study by Lan et al. demonstrated that m2G is also relatively common in small RNAs [154]. Our knowledge about this RNA modification is still very limited due to a lack of high-throughput detection methods [188,189]. However, studies have shown that m2G can form both canonical and non-canonical Watson–Crick base pairing interactions, allowing m2G to regulate the stability of tRNA tertiary structures and potentially influence microRNA silencing activity [188,190].

9. Dynamic Regulation of the Epitranscriptome

The epitranscriptome is dynamically regulated. This is abundantly clear for m6A modifications due to the discovery of both m6A writers and erasers [147,148]. Not all modifications may be reversible like m6A, but most, if not all, other modifications do appear to be regulated. Several studies have shown that RNA alterations are modulated under stress and pathological conditions [64,191,192]. For example, the deposition and distribution of m6A were increased in response to heat shock and DNA damage [193–195]. Total transcriptomic pseudourydilation increased in response to heat shock, nutrient deprivation, and serum deprivation [157,160]. Further, m1A levels in mammalian cells also increased in response to heat shock, but decreased after nutrient starvation [172]. Furthermore, cellular m5C levels are decreased in response external stress and cytotoxic stress which affects protein translation rates [196,197]. Additionally, the expression of methyltransferase Fibrillarin is increased in many cancers to facilitate additional 2′OMe of ribosomal RNAs [162,198,199], while mRNA A-to-I editing is induced by both hypoxia and inflammation [200]. Importantly, we have shown that both A-to-I editing and 2′OMe also increase in microRNAs during ischemia [123,201]. These findings suggest that the microRNA epitranscriptome is likely to also be dynamically regulated and functional in pathological conditions, and could provide novel targets for therapeutic intervention.

Several studies have also indicated that certain RNA nucleotide modifications regulate each other. As mentioned previously, 2′OMe was found to protect adenosine residues from A-to-I editing [165–167]. A different study demonstrated that replacing an adenosine which can be A-to-I edited by m6A also prevents editing almost completely in an in vitro assay [202]. Furthermore, it was recently demonstrated that transcript m6A levels are negatively correlated with the A-to-I editing levels of the transcript, even when they are not competing for the same nucleotide [203]. The depletion of m6A resulted in upregulated A-to-I editing on the m6A-depleted transcripts, confirming a transcriptome wide interplay between m6A and A-to-I editing [203]. These findings highlight the complexity of the epitranscriptome and the importance of studying multiple RNA modifications simultaneously in order to examine known interactions and to identify novel interactions.

10. Concluding Remarks

During the past decade, both isomiRs and the epitranscriptome have emerged as novel and dynamic layers of regulation of gene expression. Both types of microRNA alterations have been shown to modulate key physiological responses, including neovascularization by affecting the microRNA's biogenesis, stability and function. MicroRNAs have already been established as multifactorial regulators of both angiogenesis and arteriogenesis [7–9], and therefore this additional regulatory layer may provide new options for therapeutic neovascularization. The therapeutic potential of both isomiRs and the microRNA epitranscriptome is highlighted by the findings that 5′-isomiR formation of miR-411-5p and A-to-I editing of miR-487b-3p are actively regulated in response to ischemia in vivo, resulting in novel microRNAs with anti- or pro-angiogenic properties, respectively [99,123]. Therefore, altered microRNAs could provide novel targets for therapeutic inhibition or overexpression to stimulate neovascularization after ischemic CVD.

The first therapeutic small RNA (Patisiran) was granted FDA approval in 2018 and the first phase 2 clinical trials with microRNA-oriented RNA therapeutics are currently ongoing, highlighting that microRNA therapeutics are on their way to clinical practice [45]. Over the last decade, important advances have been made in development of microRNA therapeutics, however, several key issues remain, which have been expertly reviewed in the studies by Lucas et al. and Rupaimoole et al. [41,204]. These issues include maximizing the effect of the therapeutics' effect on the diseased tissue, while minimizing the off-target binding and toxicity. Now that the prevalence and functionality of microRNA alterations are becoming clear, further research is warranted to understand which altered microRNAs could pose off-target risks during design and development of microRNA-based therapeutics. However, uncovering the intricate mechanisms which govern regulation of microRNA alterations could also reveal novel therapeutic targets to modulate microRNA functioning.

Alternatively, tissue- and pathology-specific regulation of the microRNA alterations could potentially be used as a biomarker for cardiovascular disease, considering that isomiR expression profiles were found sufficient to distinguish between cancer subtypes [205].

Finally, while the abundance and function of many nucleotide modifications have not been studied in microRNAs yet, it is likely that most, if not all, will prove clinically relevant. The unique properties of certain nucleotide modifications, like for example m6A, could be exploited to enhance the specificity of microRNA-therapeutics when targeting microRNAs carrying such modifications. It is important to note that further advances in technology and methodology are required to expand our knowledge of the microRNA epitranscriptome [154,206]. However, given the surge of interest in this field, we expect many more clinically relevant microRNA alteration events to be discovered in the near future.

Author Contributions: Conceptualization—R.V.C.T.v.d.K., P.H.A.Q. and A.Y.N.; Writing—Original Draft—R.V.C.T.v.d.K.; Writing—Review & Editing—R.V.C.T.v.d.K., P.H.A.Q. and A.Y.N.; Funding Acquisition—A.Y.N. All authors have read and agreed to the published version of the manuscript.

References

1. Timmis, A.; Townsend, N.; Gale, C.; Grobbee, R.; Maniadakis, N.; Flather, M.; Wilkins, E.; Wright, L.; Vos, R.; Bax, J.; et al. European Society of Cardiology: Cardiovascular Disease Statistics 2017. *Eur Heart J.* **2018**, *39*, 508–579. [CrossRef] [PubMed]
2. Kaptoge, S.; Pennells, L.; De Bacquer, D.; Cooney, M.T.; Kavousi, M.; Stevens, G.; Riley, L.M.; Savin, S.; Khan, T.; Altay, S.; et al. World Health Organization cardiovascular disease risk charts: Revised models to estimate risk in 21 global regions. *Lancet Glob. Health* **2019**, *7*, e1332–e1345. [CrossRef]
3. Dormandy, J.; Heeck, L.; Vig, S. Acute limb ischemia. *Semin. Vasc. Surg.* **1999**, *12*, 148–153. [PubMed]
4. Powell, R.J.; Comerota, A.J.; Berceli, S.A.; Guzman, R.; Henry, T.D.; Tzeng, E.; Velazquez, O.; Marston, W.A.; Bartel, R.L.; Longcore, A.; et al. Interim analysis results from the RESTORE-CLI, a randomized, double-blind multicenter phase II trial comparing expanded autologous bone marrow-derived tissue repair cells and placebo in patients with critical limb ischemia. *J. Vasc. Surg.* **2011**, *54*, 1032–1041. [CrossRef] [PubMed]
5. Van Oostrom, M.C.; van Oostrom, O.; Quax, P.H.; Verhaar, M.C.; Hoefer, I.E. Insights into mechanisms behind arteriogenesis: What does the future hold? *J. Leukoc. Biol.* **2008**, *84*, 1379–1391. [CrossRef] [PubMed]
6. Raval, Z.; Losordo, D.W. Cell Therapy of Peripheral Arterial Disease: From Experimental Findings to Clinical Trials. *Circ. Res.* **2013**, *112*, 1288–1302. [CrossRef]
7. Weber, C. MicroRNAs: From basic mechanisms to clinical application in cardiovascular medicine. *Arterioscler. Thromb. Vasc. Biol.* **2013**, *33*, 168–169. [CrossRef]
8. Welten, S.M.; Goossens, E.A.; Quax, P.H.; Nossent, A.Y. The multifactorial nature of microRNAs in vascular remodelling. *Cardiovasc. Res.* **2016**, *110*, 6–22. [CrossRef]
9. Welten, S.M.; Bastiaansen, A.J.; de Jong, R.C.; de Vries, M.R.; Peters, E.H.; Boonstra, M.; Sheikh, S.P.; La, M.N.; Kandimalla, E.R.; Quax, P.H.; et al. Inhibition of 14q32 MicroRNAs miR-329, miR-487b, miR-494 and miR-495 Increases Neovascularization and Blood Flow Recovery after Ischemia. *Circ. Res.* **2014**, *115*, 696–708. [CrossRef]
10. Friedman, R.C.; Farh, K.K.; Burge, C.B.; Bartel, D.P. Most mammalian mRNAs are conserved targets of microRNAs. *Genome Res.* **2009**, *19*, 92–105. [CrossRef]
11. Heil, M.; Schaper, W. Pathophysiology of collateral development. *Coron. Artery Dis.* **2004**, *15*, 373–378. [CrossRef] [PubMed]
12. Hoefer, I.E.; van Royen, N.; Rectenwald, J.E.; Deindl, E.; Hua, J.; Jost, M.; Grundmann, S.; Voskuil, M.; Ozaki, C.K.; Piek, J.J.; et al. Arteriogenesis proceeds via ICAM-1/Mac-1- mediated mechanisms. *Circ. Res.* **2004**, *94*, 1179–1185. [CrossRef] [PubMed]
13. Scholz, D.; Ito, W.; Fleming, I.; Deindl, E.; Sauer, A.; Wiesnet, M.; Busse, R.; Schaper, J.; Schaper, W. Ultrastructure and molecular histology of rabbit hind-limb collateral artery growth (arteriogenesis). *Virchows Arch.* **2000**, *436*, 257–270. [CrossRef] [PubMed]
14. Hoefer, I.E.; van Royen, N.; Rectenwald, J.E.; Bray, E.J.; Abouhamze, Z.; Moldawer, L.L.; Voskuil, M.; Piek, J.J.; Buschmann, I.R.; Ozaki, C.K. Direct evidence for tumor necrosis factor-alpha signaling in arteriogenesis. *Circulation* **2002**, *105*, 1639–1641. [CrossRef] [PubMed]

15. Kosaki, K.; Ando, J.; Korenaga, R.; Kurokawa, T.; Kamiya, A. Fluid shear stress increases the production of granulocyte-macrophage colony-stimulating factor by endothelial cells via mRNA stabilization. *Circ. Res.* **1998**, *82*, 794–802. [CrossRef] [PubMed]
16. Bergmann, C.E.; Hoefer, I.E.; Meder, B.; Roth, H.; van Royen, N.; Breit, S.M.; Jost, M.M.; Aharinejad, S.; Hartmann, S.; Buschmann, I.R. Arteriogenesis depends on circulating monocytes and macrophage accumulation and is severely depressed in op/op mice. *J. Leukoc. Biol.* **2006**, *80*, 59–65. [CrossRef] [PubMed]
17. Stabile, E.; Burnett, M.S.; Watkins, C.; Kinnaird, T.; Bachis, A.; la Sala, A.; Miller, J.M.; Shou, M.; Epstein, S.E.; Fuchs, S. Impaired arteriogenic response to acute hindlimb ischemia in CD4-knockout mice. *Circulation* **2003**, *108*, 205–210. [CrossRef]
18. Van Weel, V.; Toes, R.E.; Seghers, L.; Deckers, M.M.; de Vries, M.R.; Eilers, P.H.; Sipkens, J.; Schepers, A.; Eefting, D.; van Hinsbergh, V.W.; et al. Natural killer cells and CD4+ T-cells modulate collateral artery development. *Arterioscler. Thromb. Vasc. Biol.* **2007**, *27*, 2310–2318. [CrossRef]
19. Wolf, C.; Cai, W.J.; Vosschulte, R.; Koltai, S.; Mousavipour, D.; Scholz, D.; Afsah-Hedjri, A.; Schaper, W.; Schaper, J. Vascular remodeling and altered protein expression during growth of coronary collateral arteries. *J. Mol. Cell. Cardiol.* **1998**, *30*, 2291–2305. [CrossRef]
20. Buschmann, I.; Schaper, W. Arteriogenesis Versus Angiogenesis: Two Mechanisms of Vessel Growth. *News Physiol Sci.* **1999**, *14*, 121–125. [CrossRef]
21. Carmeliet, P. Mechanisms of angiogenesis and arteriogenesis. *Nat. Med.* **2000**, *6*, 389–395. [CrossRef] [PubMed]
22. Schwartz, C.J.; Mitchell, J.R. Cellular infiltration of the human arterial adventitia associated with atheromatous plaques. *Circulation* **1962**, *26*, 73–78. [CrossRef] [PubMed]
23. Newman, A.C.; Nakatsu, M.N.; Chou, W.; Gershon, P.D.; Hughes, C.C.W. The requirement for fibroblasts in angiogenesis: Fibroblast-derived matrix proteins are essential for endothelial cell lumen formation. *Mol. Biol. Cell* **2011**, *22*, 3791–3800. [CrossRef] [PubMed]
24. Noonan, D.M.; De Lerma Barbaro, A.; Vannini, N.; Mortara, L.; Albini, A. Inflammation, inflammatory cells and angiogenesis: Decisions and indecisions. *Cancer Metastasis Rev.* **2008**, *27*, 31–40. [CrossRef] [PubMed]
25. Brennecke, J.; Stark, A.; Russell, R.B.; Cohen, S.M. Principles of microRNA-target recognition. *PLoS Biol.* **2005**, *3*, e85. [CrossRef]
26. Lewis, B.P.; Shih, I.H.; Jones-Rhoades, M.W.; Bartel, D.P.; Burge, C.B. Prediction of mammalian microRNA targets. *Cell* **2003**, *115*, 787–798. [CrossRef]
27. Lee, Y.; Jeon, K.; Lee, J.T.; Kim, S.; Kim, V.N. MicroRNA maturation: Stepwise processing and subcellular localization. *EMBO J.* **2002**, *21*, 4663–4670. [CrossRef]
28. Lee, Y.; Ahn, C.; Han, J.; Choi, H.; Kim, J.; Yim, J.; Lee, J.; Provost, P.; Radmark, O.; Kim, S.; et al. The nuclear RNase III Drosha initiates microRNA processing. *Nature* **2003**, *425*, 415–419. [CrossRef]
29. Ha, M.; Kim, V.N. Regulation of microRNA biogenesis. *Nat. Rev. Mol. Cell Biol.* **2014**, *15*, 509–524. [CrossRef]
30. Kobayashi, H.; Tomari, Y. RISC assembly: Coordination between small RNAs and Argonaute proteins. *Biochim. Biophys. Acta* **2016**, *1859*, 71–81. [CrossRef]
31. Treiber, T.; Treiber, N.; Plessmann, U.; Harlander, S.; Daiss, J.L.; Eichner, N.; Lehmann, G.; Schall, K.; Urlaub, H.; Meister, G. A Compendium of RNA-Binding Proteins that Regulate MicroRNA Biogenesis. *Mol. Cell* **2017**, *66*, 270. [CrossRef] [PubMed]
32. Saito, Y.; Liang, G.; Egger, G.; Friedman, J.M.; Chuang, J.C.; Coetzee, G.A.; Jones, P.A. Specific activation of microRNA-127 with downregulation of the proto-oncogene BCL6 by chromatin-modifying drugs in human cancer cells. *Cancer Cell* **2006**, *9*, 435–443. [CrossRef] [PubMed]
33. Vrba, L.; Munoz-Rodriguez, J.L.; Stampfer, M.R.; Futscher, B.W. miRNA gene promoters are frequent targets of aberrant DNA methylation in human breast cancer. *PLoS ONE* **2013**, *8*, e54398. [CrossRef] [PubMed]
34. Downie Ruiz Velasco, A.; Welten, S.M.J.; Goossens, E.A.C.; Quax, P.H.A.; Rappsilber, J.; Michlewski, G.; Nossent, A.Y. Posttranscriptional Regulation of 14q32 MicroRNAs by the CIRBP and HADHB during Vascular Regeneration after Ischemia. *Mol. Ther. Nucleic Acids* **2019**, *14*, 329–338. [CrossRef] [PubMed]

35. Kuehbacher, A.; Urbich, C.; Zeiher, A.M.; Dimmeler, S. Role of Dicer and Drosha for endothelial microRNA expression and angiogenesis. *Circ. Res.* **2007**, *101*, 59–68. [CrossRef]
36. Suarez, Y.; Fernandez-Hernando, C.; Pober, J.S.; Sessa, W.C. Dicer dependent microRNAs regulate gene expression and functions in human endothelial cells. *Circ. Res.* **2007**, *100*, 1164–1173. [CrossRef]
37. Suarez, Y.; Fernandez-Hernando, C.; Yu, J.; Gerber, S.A.; Harrison, K.D.; Pober, J.S.; Iruela-Arispe, M.L.; Merkenschlager, M.; Sessa, W.C. Dicer-dependent endothelial microRNAs are necessary for postnatal angiogenesis. *Proc. Natl. Acad. Sci. USA* **2008**, *105*, 14082–14087. [CrossRef]
38. Kir, D.; Schnettler, E.; Modi, S.; Ramakrishnan, S. Regulation of angiogenesis by microRNAs in cardiovascular diseases. *Angiogenesis* **2018**, *21*, 699–710. [CrossRef]
39. Lin, X.; Zhan, J.K.; Wang, Y.J.; Tan, P.; Chen, Y.Y.; Deng, H.Q.; Liu, Y.S. Function, Role, and Clinical Application of MicroRNAs in Vascular Aging. *BioMed Res. Int.* **2016**, *2016*, 6021394. [CrossRef]
40. Sun, L.L.; Li, W.D.; Lei, F.R.; Li, X.Q. The regulatory role of microRNAs in angiogenesis-related diseases. *J. Cell Mol. Med.* **2018**, *22*, 4568–4587. [CrossRef]
41. Lucas, T.; Bonauer, A.; Dimmeler, S. RNA Therapeutics in Cardiovascular Disease. *Circ. Res.* **2018**, *123*, 205–220. [CrossRef] [PubMed]
42. Bonauer, A.; Carmona, G.; Iwasaki, M.; Mione, M.; Koyanagi, M.; Fischer, A.; Burchfield, J.; Fox, H.; Doebele, C.; Ohtani, K.; et al. MicroRNA-92a controls angiogenesis and functional recovery of ischemic tissues in mice. *Science* **2009**, *324*, 1710–1713. [CrossRef] [PubMed]
43. Hinkel, R.; Penzkofer, D.; Zuhlke, S.; Fischer, A.; Husada, W.; Xu, Q.F.; Baloch, E.; van Rooij, E.; Zeiher, A.M.; Kupatt, C.; et al. Inhibition of microRNA-92a protects against ischemia/reperfusion injury in a large-animal model. *Circulation* **2013**, *128*, 1066–1075. [CrossRef] [PubMed]
44. Bellera, N.; Barba, I.; Rodriguez-Sinovas, A.; Ferret, E.; Asin, M.A.; Gonzalez-Alujas, M.T.; Perez-Rodon, J.; Esteves, M.; Fonseca, C.; Toran, N.; et al. Single intracoronary injection of encapsulated antagomir-92a promotes angiogenesis and prevents adverse infarct remodeling. *J. Am. Heart Assoc.* **2014**, *3*, e000946. [CrossRef] [PubMed]
45. Hanna, J.; Hossain, G.S.; Kocerha, J. The Potential for microRNA Therapeutics and Clinical Research. *Front. Genet.* **2019**, *10*, 478. [CrossRef] [PubMed]
46. Fish, J.E.; Santoro, M.M.; Morton, S.U.; Yu, S.; Yeh, R.F.; Wythe, J.D.; Ivey, K.N.; Bruneau, B.G.; Stainier, D.Y.; Srivastava, D. miR-126 regulates angiogenic signaling and vascular integrity. *Dev. Cell* **2008**, *15*, 272–284. [CrossRef] [PubMed]
47. Wang, S.; Aurora, A.B.; Johnson, B.A.; Qi, X.; McAnally, J.; Hill, J.A.; Richardson, J.A.; Bassel-Duby, R.; Olson, E.N. The endothelial-specific microRNA miR-126 governs vascular integrity and angiogenesis. *Dev. Cell* **2008**, *15*, 261–271. [CrossRef]
48. Schober, A.; Nazari-Jahantigh, M.; Wei, Y.; Bidzhekov, K.; Gremse, F.; Grommes, J.; Megens, R.T.; Heyll, K.; Noels, H.; Hristov, M.; et al. MicroRNA-126-5p promotes endothelial proliferation and limits atherosclerosis by suppressing Dlk1. *Nat. Med.* **2014**, *20*, 368–376. [CrossRef]
49. Harris, T.A.; Yamakuchi, M.; Ferlito, M.; Mendell, J.T.; Lowenstein, C.J. MicroRNA-126 regulates endothelial expression of vascular cell adhesion molecule 1. *Proc. Natl. Acad. Sci. USA* **2008**, *105*, 1516–1521. [CrossRef]
50. Van Solingen, C.; Seghers, L.; Bijkerk, R.; Duijs, J.M.; Roeten, M.K.; van Oeveren-Rietdijk, A.M.; Baelde, H.J.; Monge, M.; Vos, J.B.; de Boer, H.C.; et al. Antagomir-mediated silencing of endothelial cell specific microRNA-126 impairs ischemia-induced angiogenesis. *J. Cell Mol. Med.* **2009**, *13*, 1577–1585. [CrossRef]
51. Katare, R.; Rawal, S.; Munasinghe, P.E.; Tsuchimochi, H.; Inagaki, T.; Fujii, Y.; Dixit, P.; Umetani, K.; Kangawa, K.; Shirai, M.; et al. Ghrelin Promotes Functional Angiogenesis in a Mouse Model of Critical Limb Ischemia Through Activation of Proangiogenic MicroRNAs. *Endocrinology* **2016**, *157*, 432–445. [CrossRef] [PubMed]
52. Fichtlscherer, S.; De Rosa, S.; Fox, H.; Schwietz, T.; Fischer, A.; Liebetrau, C.; Weber, M.; Hamm, C.W.; Roxe, T.; Muller-Ardogan, M.; et al. Circulating microRNAs in patients with coronary artery disease. *Circ. Res.* **2010**, *107*, 677–684. [CrossRef] [PubMed]
53. Wang, X.; Ling, C.C.; Li, L.; Qin, Y.; Qi, J.; Liu, X.; You, B.; Shi, Y.; Zhang, J.; Jiang, Q.; et al. MicroRNA-10a/10b represses a novel target gene mib1 to regulate angiogenesis. *Cardiovasc. Res.* **2016**, *110*, 140–150. [CrossRef] [PubMed]

54. Hergenreider, E.; Heydt, S.; Treguer, K.; Boettger, T.; Horrevoets, A.J.; Zeiher, A.M.; Scheffer, M.P.; Frangakis, A.S.; Yin, X.; Mayr, M.; et al. Atheroprotective communication between endothelial cells and smooth muscle cells through miRNAs. *Nat. Cell Biol.* **2012**, *14*, 249–256. [CrossRef] [PubMed]
55. Fang, Y.; Shi, C.; Manduchi, E.; Civelek, M.; Davies, P.F. MicroRNA-10a regulation of proinflammatory phenotype in athero-susceptible endothelium in vivo and in vitro. *Proc. Natl. Acad Sci. USA* **2010**, *107*, 13450–13455. [CrossRef]
56. Hassel, D.; Cheng, P.; White, M.P.; Ivey, K.N.; Kroll, J.; Augustin, H.G.; Katus, H.A.; Stainier, D.Y.; Srivastava, D. MicroRNA-10 regulates the angiogenic behavior of zebrafish and human endothelial cells by promoting vascular endothelial growth factor signaling. *Circ. Res.* **2012**, *111*, 1421–1433. [CrossRef]
57. Liu, L.Z.; Li, C.; Chen, Q.; Jing, Y.; Carpenter, R.; Jiang, Y.; Kung, H.F.; Lai, L.; Jiang, B.H. MiR-21 induced angiogenesis through AKT and ERK activation and HIF-1alpha expression. *PLoS ONE* **2011**, *6*, e19139. [CrossRef]
58. Maegdefessel, L.; Azuma, J.; Toh, R.; Deng, A.; Merk, D.R.; Raiesdana, A.; Leeper, N.J.; Raaz, U.; Schoelmerich, A.M.; McConnell, M.V.; et al. MicroRNA-21 blocks abdominal aortic aneurysm development and nicotine-augmented expansion. *Sci. Transl. Med.* **2012**, *4*, 122ra122. [CrossRef]
59. Ji, R.; Cheng, Y.; Yue, J.; Yang, J.; Liu, X.; Chen, H.; Dean, D.B.; Zhang, C. MicroRNA expression signature and antisense-mediated depletion reveal an essential role of MicroRNA in vascular neointimal lesion formation. *Circ. Res.* **2007**, *100*, 1579–1588. [CrossRef]
60. Thum, T.; Gross, C.; Fiedler, J.; Fischer, T.; Kissler, S.; Bussen, M.; Galuppo, P.; Just, S.; Rottbauer, W.; Frantz, S.; et al. MicroRNA-21 contributes to myocardial disease by stimulating MAP kinase signalling in fibroblasts. *Nature* **2008**, *456*, 980–984. [CrossRef]
61. Kaluza, D.; Kroll, J.; Gesierich, S.; Manavski, Y.; Boeckel, J.N.; Doebele, C.; Zelent, A.; Rossig, L.; Zeiher, A.M.; Augustin, H.G.; et al. Histone deacetylase 9 promotes angiogenesis by targeting the antiangiogenic microRNA-17-92 cluster in endothelial cells. *Arterioscler. Thromb. Vasc. Biol.* **2013**, *33*, 533–543. [CrossRef] [PubMed]
62. Landskroner-Eiger, S.; Qiu, C.; Perrotta, P.; Siragusa, M.; Lee, M.Y.; Ulrich, V.; Luciano, A.K.; Zhuang, Z.W.; Corti, F.; Simons, M.; et al. Endothelial miR-17 approximately 92 cluster negatively regulates arteriogenesis via miRNA-19 repression of WNT signaling. *Proc. Natl. Acad. Sci. USA* **2015**, *112*, 12812–12817. [CrossRef] [PubMed]
63. Kozomara, A.; Birgaoanu, M.; Griffiths-Jones, S. miRBase: From microRNA sequences to function. *Nucleic Acids Res.* **2019**, *47*, D155–D162. [CrossRef] [PubMed]
64. Hoernes, T.P.; Erlacher, M.D. Translating the epitranscriptome. *Wiley Interdiscip. Rev. RNA* **2017**, 8. [CrossRef] [PubMed]
65. Landgraf, P.; Rusu, M.; Sheridan, R.; Sewer, A.; Iovino, N.; Aravin, A.; Pfeffer, S.; Rice, A.; Kamphorst, A.O.; Landthaler, M.; et al. A mammalian microRNA expression atlas based on small RNA library sequencing. *Cell* **2007**, *129*, 1401–1414. [CrossRef]
66. Blow, M.J.; Grocock, R.J.; van Dongen, S.; Enright, A.J.; Dicks, E.; Futreal, P.A.; Wooster, R.; Stratton, M.R. RNA editing of human microRNAs. *Genome Biol.* **2006**, *7*, R27. [CrossRef]
67. Cloonan, N.; Wani, S.; Xu, Q.; Gu, J.; Lea, K.; Heater, S.; Barbacioru, C.; Steptoe, A.L.; Martin, H.C.; Nourbakhsh, E.; et al. MicroRNAs and their isomiRs function cooperatively to target common biological pathways. *Genome Biol.* **2011**, *12*, R126. [CrossRef]
68. Neilsen, C.T.; Goodall, G.J.; Bracken, C.P. IsomiRs—The overlooked repertoire in the dynamic microRNAome. *Trends Genet.* **2012**, *28*, 544–549. [CrossRef]
69. Llorens, F.; Banez-Coronel, M.; Pantano, L.; del Rio, J.A.; Ferrer, I.; Estivill, X.; Marti, E. A highly expressed miR-101 isomiR is a functional silencing small RNA. *BMC Genom.* **2013**, *14*, 104. [CrossRef]
70. Loher, P.; Londin, E.R.; Rigoutsos, I. IsomiR expression profiles in human lymphoblastoid cell lines exhibit population and gender dependencies. *Oncotarget* **2014**, *5*, 8790–8802. [CrossRef]
71. McCall, M.N.; Kim, M.S.; Adil, M.; Patil, A.H.; Lu, Y.; Mitchell, C.J.; Leal-Rojas, P.; Xu, J.; Kumar, M.; Dawson, V.L.; et al. Toward the human cellular microRNAome. *Genome Res.* **2017**, *27*, 1769–1781. [CrossRef] [PubMed]
72. Tan, G.C.; Chan, E.; Molnar, A.; Sarkar, R.; Alexieva, D.; Isa, I.M.; Robinson, S.; Zhang, S.; Ellis, P.; Langford, C.F.; et al. 5′ isomiR variation is of functional and evolutionary importance. *Nucleic Acids Res.* **2014**, *42*, 9424–9435. [CrossRef] [PubMed]

73. Bofill-De Ros, X.; Yang, A.; Gu, S. IsomiRs: Expanding the miRNA repression toolbox beyond the seed. *Biochim. Biophys. Acta Gene Regul. Mech.* **2019**. [CrossRef] [PubMed]
74. Telonis, A.G.; Loher, P.; Jing, Y.; Londin, E.; Rigoutsos, I. Beyond the one-locus-one-miRNA paradigm: microRNA isoforms enable deeper insights into breast cancer heterogeneity. *Nucleic Acids Res.* **2015**, *43*, 9158–9175. [CrossRef] [PubMed]
75. Burroughs, A.M.; Ando, Y.; de Hoon, M.J.; Tomaru, Y.; Nishibu, T.; Ukekawa, R.; Funakoshi, T.; Kurokawa, T.; Suzuki, H.; Hayashizaki, Y.; et al. A comprehensive survey of 3′ animal miRNA modification events and a possible role for 3′ adenylation in modulating miRNA targeting effectiveness. *Genome Res.* **2010**, *20*, 1398–1410. [CrossRef] [PubMed]
76. Wyman, S.K.; Knouf, E.C.; Parkin, R.K.; Fritz, B.R.; Lin, D.W.; Dennis, L.M.; Krouse, M.A.; Webster, P.J.; Tewari, M. Post-transcriptional generation of miRNA variants by multiple nucleotidyl transferases contributes to miRNA transcriptome complexity. *Genome Res.* **2011**, *21*, 1450–1461. [CrossRef]
77. Lee, L.W.; Zhang, S.; Etheridge, A.; Ma, L.; Martin, D.; Galas, D.; Wang, K. Complexity of the microRNA repertoire revealed by next-generation sequencing. *RNA* **2010**, *16*, 2170–2180. [CrossRef]
78. Newman, M.A.; Mani, V.; Hammond, S.M. Deep sequencing of microRNA precursors reveals extensive 3′ end modification. *RNA* **2011**, *17*, 1795–1803. [CrossRef]
79. Mercey, O.; Popa, A.; Cavard, A.; Paquet, A.; Chevalier, B.; Pons, N.; Magnone, V.; Zangari, J.; Brest, P.; Zaragosi, L.E.; et al. Characterizing isomiR variants within the microRNA-34/449 family. *FEBS Lett.* **2017**, *591*, 693–705. [CrossRef]
80. Karali, M.; Persico, M.; Mutarelli, M.; Carissimo, A.; Pizzo, M.; Singh Marwah, V.; Ambrosio, C.; Pinelli, M.; Carrella, D.; Ferrari, S.; et al. High-resolution analysis of the human retina miRNome reveals isomiR variations and novel microRNAs. *Nucleic Acids Res.* **2016**, *44*, 1525–1540. [CrossRef]
81. Manzano, M.; Forte, E.; Raja, A.N.; Schipma, M.J.; Gottwein, E. Divergent target recognition by coexpressed 5′-isomiRs of miR-142-3p and selective viral mimicry. *RNA* **2015**, *21*, 1606–1620. [CrossRef] [PubMed]
82. Marzi, M.J.; Ghini, F.; Cerruti, B.; de Pretis, S.; Bonetti, P.; Giacomelli, C.; Gorski, M.M.; Kress, T.; Pelizzola, M.; Muller, H.; et al. Degradation dynamics of microRNAs revealed by a novel pulse-chase approach. *Genome Res.* **2016**, *26*, 554–565. [CrossRef] [PubMed]
83. Guo, Y.; Liu, J.; Elfenbein, S.J.; Ma, Y.; Zhong, M.; Qiu, C.; Ding, Y.; Lu, J. Characterization of the mammalian miRNA turnover landscape. *Nucleic Acids Res.* **2015**, *43*, 2326–2341. [CrossRef] [PubMed]
84. Gutierrez-Vazquez, C.; Enright, A.J.; Rodriguez-Galan, A.; Perez-Garcia, A.; Collier, P.; Jones, M.R.; Benes, V.; Mizgerd, J.P.; Mittelbrunn, M.; Ramiro, A.R.; et al. 3′ Uridylation controls mature microRNA turnover during CD4 T-cell activation. *RNA* **2017**, *23*, 882–891. [CrossRef] [PubMed]
85. Katoh, T.; Hojo, H.; Suzuki, T. Destabilization of microRNAs in human cells by 3′ deadenylation mediated by PARN and CUGBP1. *Nucleic Acids Res.* **2015**, *43*, 7521–7534. [CrossRef]
86. Katoh, T.; Sakaguchi, Y.; Miyauchi, K.; Suzuki, T.; Kashiwabara, S.; Baba, T.; Suzuki, T. Selective stabilization of mammalian microRNAs by 3′ adenylation mediated by the cytoplasmic poly(A) polymerase GLD-2. *Genes Dev.* **2009**, *23*, 433–438. [CrossRef]
87. Yamane, D.; Selitsky, S.R.; Shimakami, T.; Li, Y.; Zhou, M.; Honda, M.; Sethupathy, P.; Lemon, S.M. Differential hepatitis C virus RNA target site selection and host factor activities of naturally occurring miR-122 3 variants. *Nucleic Acids Res.* **2017**, *45*, 4743–4755. [CrossRef]
88. Yu, F.; Pillman, K.A.; Neilsen, C.T.; Toubia, J.; Lawrence, D.M.; Tsykin, A.; Gantier, M.P.; Callen, D.F.; Goodall, G.J.; Bracken, C.P. Naturally existing isoforms of miR-222 have distinct functions. *Nucleic Acids Res.* **2017**, *45*, 11371–11385. [CrossRef]
89. Voellenkle, C.; Rooij, J.; Guffanti, A.; Brini, E.; Fasanaro, P.; Isaia, E.; Croft, L.; David, M.; Capogrossi, M.C.; Moles, A.; et al. Deep-sequencing of endothelial cells exposed to hypoxia reveals the complexity of known and novel microRNAs. *RNA* **2012**, *18*, 472–484. [CrossRef]
90. Chistiakov, D.A.; Orekhov, A.N.; Bobryshev, Y.V. The role of miR-126 in embryonic angiogenesis, adult vascular homeostasis, and vascular repair and its alterations in atherosclerotic disease. *J. Mol. Cell. Cardiol.* **2016**, *97*, 47–55. [CrossRef]
91. Guduric-Fuchs, J.; O'Connor, A.; Cullen, A.; Harwood, L.; Medina, R.J.; O'Neill, C.L.; Stitt, A.W.; Curtis, T.M.; Simpson, D.A. Deep sequencing reveals predominant expression of miR-21 amongst the small non-coding RNAs in retinal microvascular endothelial cells. *J. Cell. Biochem.* **2012**, *113*, 2098–2111. [CrossRef] [PubMed]

92. Fernandez-Valverde, S.L.; Taft, R.J.; Mattick, J.S. Dynamic isomiR regulation in Drosophila development. *RNA* **2010**, *16*, 1881–1888. [CrossRef] [PubMed]
93. Schirmer, S.H.; Fledderus, J.O.; Bot, P.T.; Moerland, P.D.; Hoefer, I.E.; Baan, J., Jr.; Henriques, J.P.; van der Schaaf, R.J.; Vis, M.M.; Horrevoets, A.J.; et al. Interferon-beta signaling is enhanced in patients with insufficient coronary collateral artery development and inhibits arteriogenesis in mice. *Circ. Res.* **2008**, *102*, 1286–1294. [CrossRef] [PubMed]
94. Yildirim, C.; Nieuwenhuis, S.; Teunissen, P.F.; Horrevoets, A.J.; van Royen, N.; van der Pouw Kraan, T.C. Interferon-Beta, a Decisive Factor in Angiogenesis and Arteriogenesis. *J. Interferon Cytokine Res. Off. J. Int. Soc. Interferon Cytokine Res.* **2015**, *35*, 411–420. [CrossRef] [PubMed]
95. Schirmer, S.H.; Bot, P.T.; Fledderus, J.O.; van der Laan, A.M.; Volger, O.L.; Laufs, U.; Bohm, M.; de Vries, C.J.; Horrevoets, A.J.; Piek, J.J.; et al. Blocking interferon-beta stimulates vascular smooth muscle cell proliferation and arteriogenesis. *J. Biol. Chem.* **2010**, *285*, 34677–34685. [CrossRef] [PubMed]
96. Nejad, C.; Pillman, K.A.; Siddle, K.J.; Pepin, G.; Anko, M.L.; McCoy, C.E.; Beilharz, T.H.; Quintana-Murci, L.; Goodall, G.J.; Bracken, C.P.; et al. miR-222 isoforms are differentially regulated by type-I interferon. *RNA* **2018**, *24*, 332–341. [CrossRef] [PubMed]
97. Poliseno, L.; Tuccoli, A.; Mariani, L.; Evangelista, M.; Citti, L.; Woods, K.; Mercatanti, A.; Hammond, S.; Rainaldi, G. MicroRNAs modulate the angiogenic properties of HUVECs. *Blood* **2006**, *108*, 3068–3071. [CrossRef]
98. Dentelli, P.; Rosso, A.; Orso, F.; Olgasi, C.; Taverna, D.; Brizzi, M.F. microRNA-222 controls neovascularization by regulating signal transducer and activator of transcription 5A expression. *Arterioscler. Thromb. Vasc. Biol.* **2010**, *30*, 1562–1568. [CrossRef]
99. Van der Kwast, R.; Woudenberg, T.; Quax, P.H.A.; Nossent, A.Y. MicroRNA-411 and Its 5′-IsomiR Have Distinct Targets and Functions and Are Differentially Regulated in the Vasculature under Ischemia. *Mol. Ther. J. Am. Soc. Gene Ther.* **2019**. [CrossRef]
100. Wagner, R.W.; Smith, J.E.; Cooperman, B.S.; Nishikura, K. A double-stranded RNA unwinding activity introduces structural alterations by means of adenosine to inosine conversions in mammalian cells and Xenopus eggs. *Proc. Natl. Acad. Sci. USA* **1989**, *86*, 2647–2651. [CrossRef]
101. Gommans, W.M. A-to-I editing of microRNAs: Regulating the regulators? *Semin. Cell Dev. Biol.* **2012**, *23*, 251–257. [CrossRef] [PubMed]
102. Kume, H.; Hino, K.; Galipon, J.; Ui-Tei, K. A-to-I editing in the miRNA seed region regulates target mRNA selection and silencing efficiency. *Nucleic Acids Res.* **2014**, *42*, 10050–10060. [CrossRef] [PubMed]
103. Savva, Y.A.; Rieder, L.E.; Reenan, R.A. The ADAR protein family. *Genome Biol.* **2012**, *13*, 252. [CrossRef] [PubMed]
104. Nishikura, K. A-to-I editing of coding and non-coding RNAs by ADARs. *Nat. Rev. Mol. Cell Biol.* **2016**, *17*, 83–96. [CrossRef]
105. Mallela, A.; Nishikura, K. A-to-I editing of protein coding and noncoding RNAs. *Crit. Rev. Biochem. Mol. Biol.* **2012**, *47*, 493–501. [CrossRef]
106. Nigita, G.; Veneziano, D.; Ferro, A. A-to-I RNA Editing: Current Knowledge Sources and Computational Approaches with Special Emphasis on Non-Coding RNA Molecules. *Front. Bioeng. Biotechnol.* **2015**, 3. [CrossRef]
107. Wang, Q.; Khillan, J.; Gadue, P.; Nishikura, K. Requirement of the RNA editing deaminase ADAR1 gene for embryonic erythropoiesis. *Science* **2000**, *290*, 1765–1768. [CrossRef]
108. Higuchi, M.; Maas, S.; Single, F.N.; Hartner, J.; Rozov, A.; Burnashev, N.; Feldmeyer, D.; Sprengel, R.; Seeburg, P.H. Point mutation in an AMPA receptor gene rescues lethality in mice deficient in the RNA-editing enzyme ADAR2. *Nature* **2000**, *406*, 78–81. [CrossRef]
109. Brusa, R.; Zimmermann, F.; Koh, D.S.; Feldmeyer, D.; Gass, P.; Seeburg, P.H.; Sprengel, R. Early-onset epilepsy and postnatal lethality associated with an editing-deficient GluR-B allele in mice. *Science* **1995**, *270*, 1677–1680. [CrossRef]
110. Hong, H.; Lin, J.; Chen, L. Regulatory factors governing adenosine-to-inosine (A-to-I) RNA editing. *Biosci Rep.* **2015**, 35. [CrossRef]
111. Lai, F.; Chen, C.X.; Lee, V.M.; Nishikura, K. Dramatic increase of the RNA editing for glutamate receptor subunits during terminal differentiation of clonal human neurons. *J. Neurochem.* **1997**, *69*, 43–52. [CrossRef] [PubMed]

112. Liu, Y.; Emeson, R.B.; Samuel, C.E. Serotonin-2C receptor pre-mRNA editing in rat brain and in vitro by splice site variants of the interferon-inducible double-stranded RNA-specific adenosine deaminase ADAR1. *J. Biol. Chem.* **1999**, *274*, 18351–18358. [CrossRef] [PubMed]
113. Yang, W.; Chendrimada, T.P.; Wang, Q.; Higuchi, M.; Seeburg, P.H.; Shiekhattar, R.; Nishikura, K. Modulation of microRNA processing and expression through RNA editing by ADAR deaminases. *Nat. Struct. Mol. Biol.* **2006**, *13*, 13–21. [CrossRef] [PubMed]
114. Kawahara, Y.; Zinshteyn, B.; Chendrimada, T.P.; Shiekhattar, R.; Nishikura, K. RNA editing of the microRNA-151 precursor blocks cleavage by the Dicer-TRBP complex. *EMBO Rep.* **2007**, *8*, 763–769. [CrossRef]
115. Kawahara, Y.; Megraw, M.; Kreider, E.; Iizasa, H.; Valente, L.; Hatzigeorgiou, A.G.; Nishikura, K. Frequency and fate of microRNA editing in human brain. *Nucleic Acids Res.* **2008**, *36*, 5270–5280. [CrossRef]
116. Kawahara, Y.; Zinshteyn, B.; Sethupathy, P.; Iizasa, H.; Hatzigeorgiou, A.G.; Nishikura, K. Redirection of silencing targets by adenosine-to-inosine editing of miRNAs. *Science* **2007**, *315*, 1137–1140. [CrossRef]
117. Li, L.; Song, Y.; Shi, X.; Liu, J.; Xiong, S.; Chen, W.; Fu, Q.; Huang, Z.; Gu, N.; Zhang, R. The landscape of miRNA editing in animals and its impact on miRNA biogenesis and targeting. *Genome Res.* **2018**, *28*, 132–143. [CrossRef]
118. Vitsios, D.M.; Davis, M.P.; van Dongen, S.; Enright, A.J. Large-scale analysis of microRNA expression, epi-transcriptomic features and biogenesis. *Nucleic Acids Res.* **2016**. [CrossRef]
119. Wang, Y.; Liang, H. When MicroRNAs Meet RNA Editing in Cancer: A Nucleotide Change Can Make a Difference. *Bioessays News Rev. Mol. Cell. Dev. Biol.* **2018**, 40. [CrossRef]
120. Wang, Y.; Xu, X.; Yu, S.; Jeong, K.J.; Zhou, Z.; Han, L.; Tsang, Y.H.; Li, J.; Chen, H.; Mangala, L.S.; et al. Systematic characterization of A-to-I RNA editing hotspots in microRNAs across human cancers. *Genome Res.* **2017**, *27*, 1112–1125. [CrossRef]
121. Cho, C.J.; Myung, S.J.; Chang, S. ADAR1 and MicroRNA.; A Hidden Crosstalk in Cancer. *Int. J. Mol. Sci.* **2017**, *18*, 799. [CrossRef] [PubMed]
122. Shoshan, E.; Mobley, A.K.; Braeuer, R.R.; Kamiya, T.; Huang, L.; Vasquez, M.E.; Salameh, A.; Lee, H.J.; Kim, S.J.; Ivan, C.; et al. Reduced adenosine-to-inosine miR-455-5p editing promotes melanoma growth and metastasis. *Nat. Cell Biol.* **2015**, *17*, 311–321. [CrossRef] [PubMed]
123. Van der Kwast, R.V.C.T.; van Ingen, E.; Parma, L.; Peters, H.A.B.; Quax, P.H.A.; Nossent, A.Y. Adenosine-to-Inosine Editing of MicroRNA-487b Alters Target Gene Selection After Ischemia and Promotes Neovascularization. *Circ. Res.* **2018**, *122*, 444–456. [CrossRef] [PubMed]
124. Dominissini, D.; Moshitch-Moshkovitz, S.; Schwartz, S.; Salmon-Divon, M.; Ungar, L.; Osenberg, S.; Cesarkas, K.; Jacob-Hirsch, J.; Amariglio, N.; Kupiec, M.; et al. Topology of the human and mouse m6A RNA methylomes revealed by m6A-seq. *Nature* **2012**, *485*, 201–206. [CrossRef]
125. Meyer, K.D.; Saletore, Y.; Zumbo, P.; Elemento, O.; Mason, C.E.; Jaffrey, S.R. Comprehensive analysis of mRNA methylation reveals enrichment in 3′ UTRs and near stop codons. *Cell* **2012**, *149*, 1635–1646. [CrossRef]
126. Wang, P.; Doxtader, K.A.; Nam, Y. Structural Basis for Cooperative Function of Mettl3 and Mettl14 Methyltransferases. *Mol. Cell* **2016**, *63*, 306–317. [CrossRef]
127. Yang, Y.; Hsu, P.J.; Chen, Y.S.; Yang, Y.G. Dynamic transcriptomic m(6)A decoration: Writers, erasers, readers and functions in RNA metabolism. *Cell Res.* **2018**, *28*, 616–624. [CrossRef]
128. Schwartz, S.; Mumbach, M.R.; Jovanovic, M.; Wang, T.; Maciag, K.; Bushkin, G.G.; Mertins, P.; Ter-Ovanesyan, D.; Habib, N.; Cacchiarelli, D.; et al. Perturbation of m6A writers reveals two distinct classes of mRNA methylation at internal and 5′ sites. *Cell Rep.* **2014**, *8*, 284–296. [CrossRef]
129. Zheng, G.; Dahl, J.A.; Niu, Y.; Fedorcsak, P.; Huang, C.M.; Li, C.J.; Vagbo, C.B.; Shi, Y.; Wang, W.L.; Song, S.H.; et al. ALKBH5 is a mammalian RNA demethylase that impacts RNA metabolism and mouse fertility. *Mol. Cell* **2013**, *49*, 18–29. [CrossRef]
130. Jia, G.; Fu, Y.; Zhao, X.; Dai, Q.; Zheng, G.; Yang, Y.; Yi, C.; Lindahl, T.; Pan, T.; Yang, Y.G.; et al. N6-methyladenosine in nuclear RNA is a major substrate of the obesity-associated FTO. *Nat. Chem. Biol.* **2011**, *7*, 885–887. [CrossRef]
131. Roundtree, I.A.; Evans, M.E.; Pan, T.; He, C. Dynamic RNA Modifications in Gene Expression Regulation. *Cell* **2017**, *169*, 1187–1200. [CrossRef] [PubMed]
132. Zhao, B.S.; Roundtree, I.A.; He, C. Post-transcriptional gene regulation by mRNA modifications. *Nat. Rev. Mol. Cell Biol.* **2017**, *18*, 31–42. [CrossRef] [PubMed]

133. Nachtergaele, S.; He, C. The emerging biology of RNA post-transcriptional modifications. *RNA Biol.* **2017**, *14*, 156–163. [CrossRef] [PubMed]
134. Yoon, K.J.; Ringeling, F.R.; Vissers, C.; Jacob, F.; Pokrass, M.; Jimenez-Cyrus, D.; Su, Y.; Kim, N.S.; Zhu, Y.; Zheng, L.; et al. Temporal Control of Mammalian Cortical Neurogenesis by m(6)A Methylation. *Cell* **2017**, *171*, 877–889. [CrossRef] [PubMed]
135. Wang, Y.; Li, Y.; Toth, J.I.; Petroski, M.D.; Zhang, Z.; Zhao, J.C. N6-methyladenosine modification destabilizes developmental regulators in embryonic stem cells. *Nat. Cell Biol.* **2014**, *16*, 191–198. [CrossRef] [PubMed]
136. Horiuchi, K.; Umetani, M.; Minami, T.; Okayama, H.; Takada, S.; Yamamoto, M.; Aburatani, H.; Reid, P.C.; Housman, D.E.; Hamakubo, T.; et al. Wilms' tumor 1-associating protein regulates G2/M transition through stabilization of cyclin A2 mRNA. *Proc. Natl. Acad. Sci. USA* **2006**, *103*, 17278–17283. [CrossRef]
137. Liu, N.; Zhou, K.I.; Parisien, M.; Dai, Q.; Diatchenko, L.; Pan, T. N6-methyladenosine alters RNA structure to regulate binding of a low-complexity protein. *Nucleic Acids Res.* **2017**, *45*, 6051–6063. [CrossRef]
138. Liu, N.; Dai, Q.; Zheng, G.; He, C.; Parisien, M.; Pan, T. N(6)-methyladenosine-dependent RNA structural switches regulate RNA-protein interactions. *Nature* **2015**, *518*, 560–564. [CrossRef]
139. Huang, H.; Weng, H.; Sun, W.; Qin, X.; Shi, H.; Wu, H.; Zhao, B.S.; Mesquita, A.; Liu, C.; Yuan, C.L.; et al. Recognition of RNA N(6)-methyladenosine by IGF2BP proteins enhances mRNA stability and translation. *Nat. Cell Biol.* **2018**, *20*, 285–295. [CrossRef]
140. Wang, X.; Zhao, B.S.; Roundtree, I.A.; Lu, Z.; Han, D.; Ma, H.; Weng, X.; Chen, K.; Shi, H.; He, C. N(6)-methyladenosine Modulates Messenger RNA Translation Efficiency. *Cell* **2015**, *161*, 1388–1399. [CrossRef]
141. Wang, X.; Lu, Z.; Gomez, A.; Hon, G.C.; Yue, Y.; Han, D.; Fu, Y.; Parisien, M.; Dai, Q.; Jia, G.; et al. N6-methyladenosine-dependent regulation of messenger RNA stability. *Nature* **2014**, *505*, 117–120. [CrossRef] [PubMed]
142. Alarcon, C.R.; Goodarzi, H.; Lee, H.; Liu, X.; Tavazoie, S.; Tavazoie, S.F. HNRNPA2B1 Is a Mediator of m(6)A-Dependent Nuclear RNA Processing Events. *Cell* **2015**, *162*, 1299–1308. [CrossRef] [PubMed]
143. Alarcon, C.R.; Lee, H.; Goodarzi, H.; Halberg, N.; Tavazoie, S.F. N6-methyladenosine marks primary microRNAs for processing. *Nature* **2015**, *519*, 482–485. [CrossRef] [PubMed]
144. Dai, Q.; Fong, R.; Saikia, M.; Stephenson, D.; Yu, Y.T.; Pan, T.; Piccirilli, J.A. Identification of recognition residues for ligation-based detection and quantitation of pseudouridine and N6-methyladenosine. *Nucleic Acids Res.* **2007**, *35*, 6322–6329. [CrossRef]
145. Konno, M.; Koseki, J.; Asai, A.; Yamagata, A.; Shimamura, T.; Motooka, D.; Okuzaki, D.; Kawamoto, K.; Mizushima, T.; Eguchi, H.; et al. Distinct methylation levels of mature microRNAs in gastrointestinal cancers. *Nat. Commun.* **2019**, *10*, 3888. [CrossRef]
146. Muller, S.; Glass, M.; Singh, A.K.; Haase, J.; Bley, N.; Fuchs, T.; Lederer, M.; Dahl, A.; Huang, H.; Chen, J.; et al. IGF2BP1 promotes SRF-dependent transcription in cancer in a m6A- and miRNA-dependent manner. *Nucleic Acids Res.* **2019**, *47*, 375–390. [CrossRef]
147. Dorn, L.E.; Lasman, L.; Chen, J.; Xu, X.; Hund, T.J.; Medvedovic, M.; Hanna, J.H.; van Berlo, J.H.; Accornero, F. The N(6)-Methyladenosine mRNA Methylase METTL3 Controls Cardiac Homeostasis and Hypertrophy. *Circulation* **2019**, *139*, 533–545. [CrossRef]
148. Mathiyalagan, P.; Adamiak, M.; Mayourian, J.; Sassi, Y.; Liang, Y.; Agarwal, N.; Jha, D.; Zhang, S.; Kohlbrenner, E.; Chepurko, E.; et al. FTO-Dependent N(6)-Methyladenosine Regulates Cardiac Function During Remodeling and Repair. *Circulation* **2019**, *139*, 518–532. [CrossRef]
149. Ma, J.Z.; Yang, F.; Zhou, C.C.; Liu, F.; Yuan, J.H.; Wang, F.; Wang, T.T.; Xu, Q.G.; Zhou, W.P.; Sun, S.H. METTL14 suppresses the metastatic potential of hepatocellular carcinoma by modulating N(6)-methyladenosine-dependent primary MicroRNA processing. *Hepatology* **2017**, *65*, 529–543. [CrossRef]
150. Han, J.; Wang, J.Z.; Yang, X.; Yu, H.; Zhou, R.; Lu, H.C.; Yuan, W.B.; Lu, J.C.; Zhou, Z.J.; Lu, Q.; et al. METTL3 promote tumor proliferation of bladder cancer by accelerating pri-miR221/222 maturation in m6A-dependent manner. *Mol. Cancer* **2019**, *18*, 110. [CrossRef]
151. Cech, T.R.; Steitz, J.A. The noncoding RNA revolution-trashing old rules to forge new ones. *Cell* **2014**, *157*, 77–94. [CrossRef] [PubMed]
152. Kim, Y.K.; Heo, I.; Kim, V.N. Modifications of small RNAs and their associated proteins. *Cell* **2010**, *143*, 703–709. [CrossRef] [PubMed]

153. Zhang, X.; Cozen, A.E.; Liu, Y.; Chen, Q.; Lowe, T.M. Small RNA Modifications: Integral to Function and Disease. *Trends Mol. Med.* **2016**, *22*, 1025–1034. [CrossRef] [PubMed]
154. Lan, M.D.; Xiong, J.; You, X.J.; Weng, X.C.; Zhou, X.; Yuan, B.F.; Feng, Y.Q. Existence of Diverse Modifications in Small-RNA Species Composed of 16-28 Nucleotides. *Chem. Eur. J.* **2018**, *24*, 9949–9956. [CrossRef] [PubMed]
155. Charette, M.; Gray, M.W. Pseudouridine in RNA: What, where, how, and why. *Iubmb Life* **2000**, *49*, 341–351. [CrossRef] [PubMed]
156. Karijolich, J.; Yi, C.; Yu, Y.T. Transcriptome-wide dynamics of RNA pseudouridylation. *Nat. Rev. Mol. Cell Biol.* **2015**, *16*, 581–585. [CrossRef]
157. Schwartz, S.; Bernstein, D.A.; Mumbach, M.R.; Jovanovic, M.; Herbst, R.H.; Leon-Ricardo, B.X.; Engreitz, J.M.; Guttman, M.; Satija, R.; Lander, E.S.; et al. Transcriptome-wide mapping reveals widespread dynamic-regulated pseudouridylation of ncRNA and mRNA. *Cell* **2014**, *159*, 148–162. [CrossRef]
158. Arnez, J.G.; Steitz, T.A. Crystal structure of unmodified tRNA(Gln) complexed with glutaminyl-tRNA synthetase and ATP suggests a possible role for pseudo-uridines in stabilization of RNA structure. *Biochemistry* **1994**, *33*, 7560–7567. [CrossRef]
159. Cohn, W.E. Pseudouridine, a carbon-carbon linked ribonucleoside in ribonucleic acids: Isolation, structure, and chemical characteristics. *J. Biol. Chem.* **1960**, *235*, 1488–1498.
160. Carlile, T.M.; Rojas-Duran, M.F.; Zinshteyn, B.; Shin, H.; Bartoli, K.M.; Gilbert, W.V. Pseudouridine profiling reveals regulated mRNA pseudouridylation in yeast and human cells. *Nature* **2014**, *515*, 143–146. [CrossRef]
161. Ayadi, L.; Galvanin, A.; Pichot, F.; Marchand, V.; Motorin, Y. RNA ribose methylation (2′-O-methylation): Occurrence, biosynthesis and biological functions. *Biochim. Biophys. Acta Gene Regul. Mech.* **2018**. [CrossRef] [PubMed]
162. Dimitrova, D.G.; Teysset, L.; Carre, C. RNA 2′-O-Methylation (Nm) Modification in Human Diseases. *Genes* **2019**, *10*, 117. [CrossRef] [PubMed]
163. Bachellerie, J.P.; Cavaille, J.; Huttenhofer, A. The expanding snoRNA world. *Biochimie* **2002**, *84*, 775–790. [CrossRef]
164. Cavaille, J.; Buiting, K.; Kiefmann, M.; Lalande, M.; Brannan, C.I.; Horsthemke, B.; Bachellerie, J.P.; Brosius, J.; Huttenhofer, A. Identification of brain-specific and imprinted small nucleolar RNA genes exhibiting an unusual genomic organization. *Proc. Natl. Acad. Sci. USA* **2000**, *97*, 14311–14316. [CrossRef]
165. Vitali, P.; Basyuk, E.; Le, M.E.; Bertrand, E.; Muscatelli, F.; Cavaille, J.; Huttenhofer, A. ADAR2-mediated editing of RNA substrates in the nucleolus is inhibited by C/D small nucleolar RNAs. *J. Cell Biol.* **2005**, *169*, 745–753. [CrossRef]
166. Yi-Brunozzi, H.Y.; Easterwood, L.M.; Kamilar, G.M.; Beal, P.A. Synthetic substrate analogs for the RNA-editing adenosine deaminase ADAR-2. *Nucleic Acids Res.* **1999**, *27*, 2912–2917. [CrossRef]
167. Mizrahi, R.A.; Phelps, K.J.; Ching, A.Y.; Beal, P.A. Nucleoside analog studies indicate mechanistic differences between RNA-editing adenosine deaminases. *Nucleic Acids Res.* **2012**, *40*, 9825–9835. [CrossRef]
168. Inoue, H.; Hayase, Y.; Imura, A.; Iwai, S.; Miura, K.; Ohtsuka, E. Synthesis and hybridization studies on two complementary nona(2′-O-methyl)ribonucleotides. *Nucleic Acids Res.* **1987**, *15*, 6131–6148. [CrossRef]
169. Majlessi, M.; Nelson, N.C.; Becker, M.M. Advantages of 2′-O-methyl oligoribonucleotide probes for detecting RNA targets. *Nucleic Acids Res.* **1998**, *26*, 2224–2229. [CrossRef]
170. Tsourkas, A.; Behlke, M.A.; Bao, G. Hybridization of 2′-O-methyl and 2′-deoxy molecular beacons to RNA and DNA targets. *Nucleic Acids Res.* **2002**, *30*, 5168–5174. [CrossRef]
171. Yu, B.; Yang, Z.; Li, J.; Minakhina, S.; Yang, M.; Padgett, R.W.; Steward, R.; Chen, X. Methylation as a crucial step in plant microRNA biogenesis. *Science* **2005**, *307*, 932–935. [CrossRef] [PubMed]
172. Dominissini, D.; Nachtergaele, S.; Moshitch-Moshkovitz, S.; Peer, E.; Kol, N.; Ben-Haim, M.S.; Dai, Q.; Di Segni, A.; Salmon-Divon, M.; Clark, W.C.; et al. The dynamic N1-methyladenosine methylome in eukaryotic messenger RNA. *Nature* **2016**, *530*, 441–446. [CrossRef] [PubMed]
173. Li, X.; Xiong, X.; Wang, K.; Wang, L.; Shu, X.; Ma, S.; Yi, C. Transcriptome-wide mapping reveals reversible and dynamic N(1)-methyladenosine methylome. *Nat. Chem. Biol.* **2016**, *12*, 311–316. [CrossRef] [PubMed]
174. Zhang, C.; Jia, G. Reversible RNA Modification N(1)-methyladenosine (m(1)A) in mRNA and tRNA. *Genom. Proteom. Bioinform.* **2018**, *16*, 155–161. [CrossRef]
175. Liu, F.; Clark, W.; Luo, G.; Wang, X.; Fu, Y.; Wei, J.; Wang, X.; Hao, Z.; Dai, Q.; Zheng, G.; et al. ALKBH1-Mediated tRNA Demethylation Regulates Translation. *Cell* **2016**, *167*, 816–828. [CrossRef]

176. Zhou, H.; Kimsey, I.J.; Nikolova, E.N.; Sathyamoorthy, B.; Grazioli, G.; McSally, J.; Bai, T.; Wunderlich, C.H.; Kreutz, C.; Andricioaei, I.; et al. m(1)A and m(1)G disrupt A-RNA structure through the intrinsic instability of Hoogsteen base pairs. *Nat. Struct. Mol. Biol.* **2016**, *23*, 803–810. [CrossRef]
177. Squires, J.E.; Patel, H.R.; Nousch, M.; Sibbritt, T.; Humphreys, D.T.; Parker, B.J.; Suter, C.M.; Preiss, T. Widespread occurrence of 5-methylcytosine in human coding and non-coding RNA. *Nucleic Acids Res.* **2012**, *40*, 5023–5033. [CrossRef]
178. Van Haute, L.; Dietmann, S.; Kremer, L.; Hussain, S.; Pearce, S.F.; Powell, C.A.; Rorbach, J.; Lantaff, R.; Blanco, S.; Sauer, S.; et al. Deficient methylation and formylation of mt-tRNA(Met) wobble cytosine in a patient carrying mutations in NSUN3. *Nat. Commun.* **2016**, *7*, 12039. [CrossRef]
179. Nakano, S.; Suzuki, T.; Kawarada, L.; Iwata, H.; Asano, K.; Suzuki, T. NSUN3 methylase initiates 5-formylcytidine biogenesis in human mitochondrial tRNA(Met). *Nat. Chem. Biol.* **2016**, *12*, 546–551. [CrossRef]
180. Goll, M.G.; Kirpekar, F.; Maggert, K.A.; Yoder, J.A.; Hsieh, C.L.; Zhang, X.; Golic, K.G.; Jacobsen, S.E.; Bestor, T.H. Methylation of tRNAAsp by the DNA methyltransferase homolog Dnmt2. *Science* **2006**, *311*, 395–398. [CrossRef]
181. Trixl, L.; Lusser, A. The dynamic RNA modification 5-methylcytosine and its emerging role as an epitranscriptomic mark. *Wiley Interdiscip. Rev. RNA* **2019**, *10*, e1510. [CrossRef] [PubMed]
182. Hussain, S.; Sajini, A.A.; Blanco, S.; Dietmann, S.; Lombard, P.; Sugimoto, Y.; Paramor, M.; Gleeson, J.G.; Odom, D.T.; Ule, J.; et al. NSun2-mediated cytosine-5 methylation of vault noncoding RNA determines its processing into regulatory small RNAs. *Cell Rep.* **2013**, *4*, 255–261. [CrossRef] [PubMed]
183. Khoddami, V.; Cairns, B.R. Identification of direct targets and modified bases of RNA cytosine methyltransferases. *Nat. Biotechnol.* **2013**, *31*, 458–464. [CrossRef] [PubMed]
184. Jurkowski, T.P.; Meusburger, M.; Phalke, S.; Helm, M.; Nellen, W.; Reuter, G.; Jeltsch, A. Human DNMT2 methylates tRNA(Asp) molecules using a DNA methyltransferase-like catalytic mechanism. *RNA* **2008**, *14*, 1663–1670. [CrossRef] [PubMed]
185. Schaefer, M.; Pollex, T.; Hanna, K.; Tuorto, F.; Meusburger, M.; Helm, M.; Lyko, F. RNA methylation by Dnmt2 protects transfer RNAs against stress-induced cleavage. *Genes Dev.* **2010**, *24*, 1590–1595. [CrossRef]
186. Aguilo, F.; Li, S.; Balasubramaniyan, N.; Sancho, A.; Benko, S.; Zhang, F.; Vashisht, A.; Rengasamy, M.; Andino, B.; Chen, C.H.; et al. Deposition of 5-Methylcytosine on Enhancer RNAs Enables the Coactivator Function of PGC-1alpha. *Cell Rep.* **2016**, *14*, 479–492. [CrossRef]
187. Sergiev, P.V.; Bogdanov, A.A.; Dontsova, O.A. Ribosomal RNA guanine-(N2)-methyltransferases and their targets. *Nucleic Acids Res.* **2007**, *35*, 2295–2301. [CrossRef]
188. Chen, W.; Song, X.; Lv, H.; Lin, H. iRNA-m2G: Identifying N(2)-methylguanosine Sites Based on Sequence-Derived Information. *Mol. Ther. Nucleic Acids* **2019**, *18*, 253–258. [CrossRef]
189. Bavi, R.S.; Kamble, A.D.; Kumbhar, N.M.; Kumbhar, B.V.; Sonawane, K.D. Conformational preferences of modified nucleoside N(2)-methylguanosine (m(2)G) and its derivative N(2), N(2)-dimethylguanosine (m(2)(2)G) occur at 26th position (hinge region) in tRNA. *Cell Biochem. Biophys.* **2011**, *61*, 507–521. [CrossRef]
190. Bavi, R.S.; Sambhare, S.B.; Sonawane, K.D. MD simulation studies to investigate iso-energetic conformational behaviour of modified nucleosides m(2)G and m(2) 2G present in tRNA. *Comput. Struct. Biotechnol. J.* **2013**, *5*, e201302015. [CrossRef]
191. Pinto, Y.; Buchumenski, I.; Levanon, E.Y.; Eisenberg, E. Human cancer tissues exhibit reduced A-to-I editing of miRNAs coupled with elevated editing of their targets. *Nucleic Acids Res.* **2018**, *46*, 71–82. [CrossRef] [PubMed]
192. Esteller, M.; Pandolfi, P.P. The Epitranscriptome of Noncoding RNAs in Cancer. *Cancer Discov.* **2017**, *7*, 359–368. [CrossRef] [PubMed]
193. Meyer, K.D.; Patil, D.P.; Zhou, J.; Zinoviev, A.; Skabkin, M.A.; Elemento, O.; Pestova, T.V.; Qian, S.B.; Jaffrey, S.R. 5′ UTR m(6)A Promotes Cap-Independent Translation. *Cell* **2015**, *163*, 999–1010. [CrossRef] [PubMed]
194. Xiang, Y.; Laurent, B.; Hsu, C.H.; Nachtergaele, S.; Lu, Z.; Sheng, W.; Xu, C.; Chen, H.; Ouyang, J.; Wang, S.; et al. RNA m(6)A methylation regulates the ultraviolet-induced DNA damage response. *Nature* **2017**, *543*, 573–576. [CrossRef]
195. Zhou, J.; Wan, J.; Gao, X.; Zhang, X.; Jaffrey, S.R.; Qian, S.B. Dynamic m(6)A mRNA methylation directs translational control of heat shock response. *Nature* **2015**, *526*, 591–594. [CrossRef]

196. Blanco, S.; Bandiera, R.; Popis, M.; Hussain, S.; Lombard, P.; Aleksic, J.; Sajini, A.; Tanna, H.; Cortes-Garrido, R.; Gkatza, N.; et al. Stem cell function and stress response are controlled by protein synthesis. *Nature* **2016**, *534*, 335–340. [CrossRef]
197. Blanco, S.; Dietmann, S.; Flores, J.V.; Hussain, S.; Kutter, C.; Humphreys, P.; Lukk, M.; Lombard, P.; Treps, L.; Popis, M.; et al. Aberrant methylation of tRNAs links cellular stress to neuro-developmental disorders. *EMBO J.* **2014**, *33*, 2020–2039. [CrossRef]
198. Krogh, N.; Jansson, M.D.; Hafner, S.J.; Tehler, D.; Birkedal, U.; Christensen-Dalsgaard, M.; Lund, A.H.; Nielsen, H. Profiling of 2′-O-Me in human rRNA reveals a subset of fractionally modified positions and provides evidence for ribosome heterogeneity. *Nucleic Acids Res.* **2016**, *44*, 7884–7895. [CrossRef]
199. Marcel, V.; Ghayad, S.E.; Belin, S.; Therizols, G.; Morel, A.P.; Solano-Gonzalez, E.; Vendrell, J.A.; Hacot, S.; Mertani, H.C.; Albaret, M.A.; et al. p53 acts as a safeguard of translational control by regulating fibrillarin and rRNA methylation in cancer. *Cancer Cell* **2013**, *24*, 318–330. [CrossRef]
200. Gatsiou, A.; Stellos, K. Dawn of Epitranscriptomic Medicine. *Circ. Genom. Precis. Med.* **2018**, *11*, e001927. [CrossRef]
201. Stellos, K.; Gatsiou, A.; Stamatelopoulos, K.; Perisic Matic, L.; John, D.; Lunella, F.F.; Jae, N.; Rossbach, O.; Amrhein, C.; Sigala, F.; et al. Adenosine-to-inosine RNA editing controls cathepsin S expression in atherosclerosis by enabling HuR-mediated post-transcriptional regulation. *Nat. Med.* **2016**, *22*, 1140–1150. [CrossRef] [PubMed]
202. Veliz, E.A.; Easterwood, L.M.; Beal, P.A. Substrate analogues for an RNA-editing adenosine deaminase: Mechanistic investigation and inhibitor design. *J. Am. Chem. Soc.* **2003**, *125*, 10867–10876. [CrossRef] [PubMed]
203. Xiang, J.F.; Yang, Q.; Liu, C.X.; Wu, M.; Chen, L.L.; Yang, L. N(6)-Methyladenosines Modulate A-to-I RNA Editing. *Mol. Cell* **2018**, *69*, 126–135.e126. [CrossRef] [PubMed]
204. Rupaimoole, R.; Slack, F.J. MicroRNA therapeutics: Towards a new era for the management of cancer and other diseases. *Nat. Rev. Drug Discov.* **2017**, *16*, 203–222. [CrossRef]
205. Telonis, A.G.; Magee, R.; Loher, P.; Chervoneva, I.; Londin, E.; Rigoutsos, I. Knowledge about the presence or absence of miRNA isoforms (isomiRs) can successfully discriminate amongst 32 TCGA cancer types. *Nucleic Acids Res.* **2017**, *45*, 2973–2985. [CrossRef]
206. Schaefer, M.; Kapoor, U.; Jantsch, M.F. Understanding RNA modifications: The promises and technological bottlenecks of the 'epitranscriptome'. *Open Biol.* **2017**, *7*, 170077. [CrossRef]

4

Insulin Treatment Forces Arteriogenesis in Diabetes Mellitus by Upregulation of the Early Growth Response-1 (Egr-1) Pathway in Mice

Senthilkumar Thulasingam [1], Sundar Krishnasamy , David Raj C. [1], Manuel Lasch [2,3], Srinivasan Vedantham [1,†] and Elisabeth Deindl [3,*,†]

1 School of Chemical and Biotechnology, SASTRA Deemed to be University, Thanjavur 613401, India
2 Department of Otorhinolaryngology, Head & Neck Surgery, University Hospital, LMU Munich, 81377 Munich, Germany
3 Walter-Brendel-Centre of Experimental Medicine, University Hospital, LMU Munich, 81377 Munich, Germany
* Correspondence: Elisabeth.Deindl@med.uni-muenchen.de
† These authors contributed equally to this work.

Abstract: The process of arteriogenesis is severely compromised in patients with diabetes mellitus (DM). Earlier studies have reported the importance of *Egr-1* in promoting collateral outward remodeling. However, the role of *Egr-1* in the presence of DM in outward vessel remodeling was not studied. We hypothesized that *Egr-1* expression may be compromised in DM which may lead to impaired collateral vessel growth. Here, we investigated the relevance of the transcription factor *Egr-1* for the process of collateral artery growth in diabetic mice. Induction of arteriogenesis by femoral artery ligation resulted in an increased expression of Egr-1 on mRNA and protein level but was severely compromised in streptozotocin-induced diabetic mice. Diabetes mellitus mice showed a significantly reduced expression of *Egr-1* endothelial downstream genes Intercellular Adhesion Molecule-1 (*ICAM-1*) and urokinase Plasminogen Activator (*uPA*), relevant for extravasation of leukocytes which promote arteriogenesis. Fluorescent-activated cell sorting analyses confirmed reduced leukocyte recruitment. Diabetes mellitus mice showed a reduced expression of the proliferation marker Ki-67 in growing collaterals whose luminal diameters were also reduced. The Splicing Factor-1 (SF-1), which is critical for smooth muscle cell proliferation and phenotype switch, was found to be elevated in collaterals of DM mice. Treatment of DM mice with insulin normalized the expression of *Egr-1* and its downstream targets and restored leukocyte recruitment. SF-1 expression and the diameter of growing collaterals were normalized by insulin treatment as well. In summary, our results showed that Egr-1 signaling was impaired in DM mice; however, it can be rescued by insulin treatment.

Keywords: arteriogenesis; endothelial cells; smooth muscle cells; diabetes mellitus; Egr-1; streptozotocin; collateral arteries; insulin

---

1. Introduction

Peripheral artery disease (PAD) is one of the common vascular complications in diabetes mellitus [1]. Patients with PAD exhibit poor lower extremity function and develop critical limb ischemia and ulceration, ultimately leading to limb amputation [2–4]. Moreover, compared to healthy individuals, diabetic patients with PAD exhibit cardiovascular co-morbidities, neuropathy, and higher mortality [5–8]. Patients with PAD show poorer outcomes after leg bypass surgery with higher incidence of restenosis, longer hospitalization, and reduced amputation-free survival [8–11].

Arteriogenesis, which is an endothelial dependent process [12], is characterized by outward remodeling of pre-existing anastomoses in conducting arteries, and through this process, the blood flow to peripheral tissues can largely be restored. The process of collateral artery growth is strongly dependent on perivascular recruitment and accumulation of leukocytes, particularly macrophages, which supply growth factors and cytokines to the growing vessel [13]. In addition, lymphocytes accumulate in the perivascular space [14]; however, little is known about their function. It is well established that the presence of DM limits the process of arteriogenesis [15]. Indeed, it has been previously shown by van Weel et al. [16] that reperfusion recovery after femoral artery ligation (FAL) was significantly reduced in streptozotocin (STZ)-induced diabetic mice, as shown by laser Doppler perfusion measurements. The exact mechanisms through which impairment of arteriogenesis in DM occurs are not clear. Elevated vasomotor function attenuating the sensing of shear stress and defects in downstream monocyte signaling are reported as major contributors to the vascular impairments seen in arteriogenesis [17].

Early growth response-1 (*Egr-1*) is a zinc finger transcription factor, which is expressed after exposure of cells to mediators associated with growth and differentiation [18]. Several studies have shown a link between the activation of *Egr-1* through hypoxia, ischemia/reperfusion, mechanical stress, shear stress, emphysema, atherosclerosis, and acute vascular injury [19]. Early growth response-1 has been reported to play a critical role in a hind limb ischemia model [20], and in a separate study, it was shown that adenoviral-mediated *Egr-1* delivery improved perfusion recovery [21]. Early growth response-1 is important for leukocyte recruitment and vascular cell proliferation during arteriogenesis in vivo in mice subjected to FAL [22]. Thus, with increased *Egr-1* expression playing a critical role in both arteriogenesis and regulation under hyperglycemic conditions, the present study was performed to understand the influence of DM on *Egr-1* expression and its consequent biological events. We hypothesized that *Egr-1* expression may be compromised in DM which may lead to impaired collateral vessel growth. In the present study, we investigated the role of *Egr-1* in collateral artery growth in vivo in streptozotocin-induced diabetic mice employing a hind limb model in which arteriogenesis was induced by FAL.

2. Results

C57Bl6J mice were made diabetic using streptozotocin. The diabetic mice showed a significant rise in blood glucose levels (328 ± 38 mg/dL) compared to non-diabetic mice (144 ± 10 mg/dl) 24 h post-ligation. In accordance with this, diabetic mice treated with insulin showed a significant decrease in glucose levels (216 ± 35 mg/dL) compared to the diabetic group (Table 1) at the same timepoint.

Table 1. Plasma glucose levels measured 24 h post-Femoral Artery Ligation prior to sacrifice ($n = 7$ in each group).

Group	Random Plasma Glucose (mg/dL)
Control	144 ± 10
Streptozotocin	328 ± 38 *
Streptozotocin + Insulin	216 ± 35 **

* $p < 0.05$ compared to Control group, ** $p < 0.05$ compared to Streptozotocin group.

2.1. *Reduced Upregulation of Egr-1 in Growing Collaterals of Diabetic Mice*

The Egr-1 mRNA expression levels were significantly increased in growing collaterals of control mice, diabetic mice, and diabetic mice treated with insulin compared to resting collaterals isolated from the sham-operated side (Figure 1a). However, the increase in the expression levels of *Egr-1* was significantly less pronounced in diabetic mice compared to non-diabetic mice and control mice 24 h post-FAL ($2^{\wedge-ddCT}$, 3.19 ± 0.172 versus 22 ± 0.25, $p < 0.05$) (Figure 1a). Treatment of diabetic mice with insulin significantly increased *Egr-1* expression compared to the diabetic mice (3.45 ± 0.25) (Figure 1a), resulting in similar levels as in the control group. Western blot analyses revealed a significantly lower expression of Egr-1 protein in the diabetic group compared to both the non-diabetic control group and the insulin treated group (Figure 1b) 24 h after the surgical procedure.

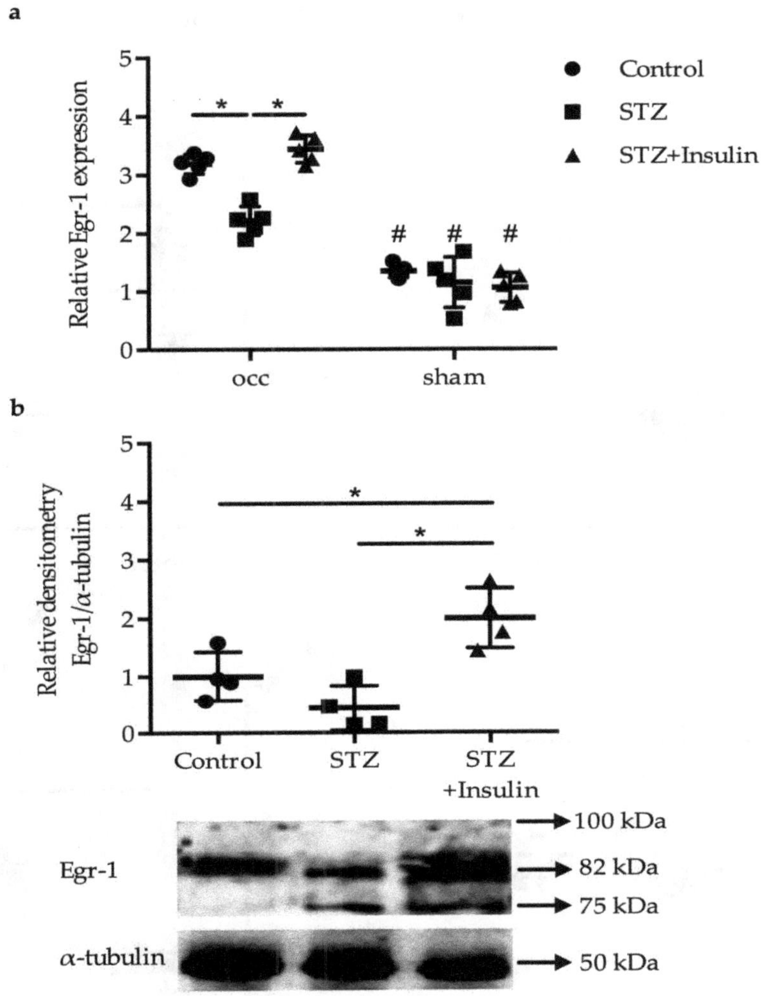

Figure 1. Gene expression studies of (**a**) mRNA levels and (**b**) protein levels of collateral arteries obtained from occluded and sham-operated mice 24 h after the surgical procedure. (**a**) Dot plots representing the results of qRT-PCR analyses ($n = 5$ per group, * $p < 0.05$ (each group compared to each other group), # $p < 0.05$ compared to corresponding occ group from one-way ANOVA with Bonferroni's multiple comparison test). Results were normalized to the expression level of the 18S rRNA. (**b**) Quantitative analyses (upper panel) and corresponding representative pictures of a Western blot (lower panel) showing the protein expression of Egr-1 as well as of α-tubulin, which was used for normalization, 24 h post-FAL ($n = 4$ per group, * $p < 0.05$ (each group compared to each other group) from one-way ANOVA with Bonferroni's multiple comparison test).

2.2. *Expression of Egr-1 Downstream Genes in Collaterals of Diabetic Mice Was Restored by Insulin Treatment*

The mRNA expression levels of Egr-1 downstream target genes, namely, Intercellular Adhesion Molecule-1 (ICAM-1), urokinase Plasminogen Activator (uPA), and Monocyte Chemoattractant Protein-1 (MCP-1) [18,23,24], were measured via qRT-PCR. Our results revealed decreased expression of ICAM-1 (Figure 2a) and uPA (Figure 2b) in the diabetic group compared to the non-diabetic control group (1.49 ± 0.49 versus 2.84 ± 0.49 and 1.53 ± 0.64 versus 3.2 ± 0.60, respectively). Mice treated with insulin showed a significant rise in ICAM-1 (2.35 ± 0.34) and uPA (3.56 ± 0.10) expression compared to the diabetic group. The expression of *MCP-1* decreased in diabetic mice (2.34 ± 0.15); however, its expression levels did not significantly rise upon treatment with insulin (2.65 ± 0.29) (Figure 2c). As previous results have shown that the transcriptional repressor Splicing Factor-1 (SF-1), which controls smooth muscle cell proliferation, is upregulated in growing collaterals during the process of arteriogenesis [22], we also investigated the expression level of the corresponding transcript. Our data showed a significant upregulation of SF-1 in the diabetic group (2.25 ± 0.36) compared to the non-diabetic group (1.15 ± 0.26), but its expression level was normalized again by insulin treatment (0.72 ± 0.04) (Figure 2d).

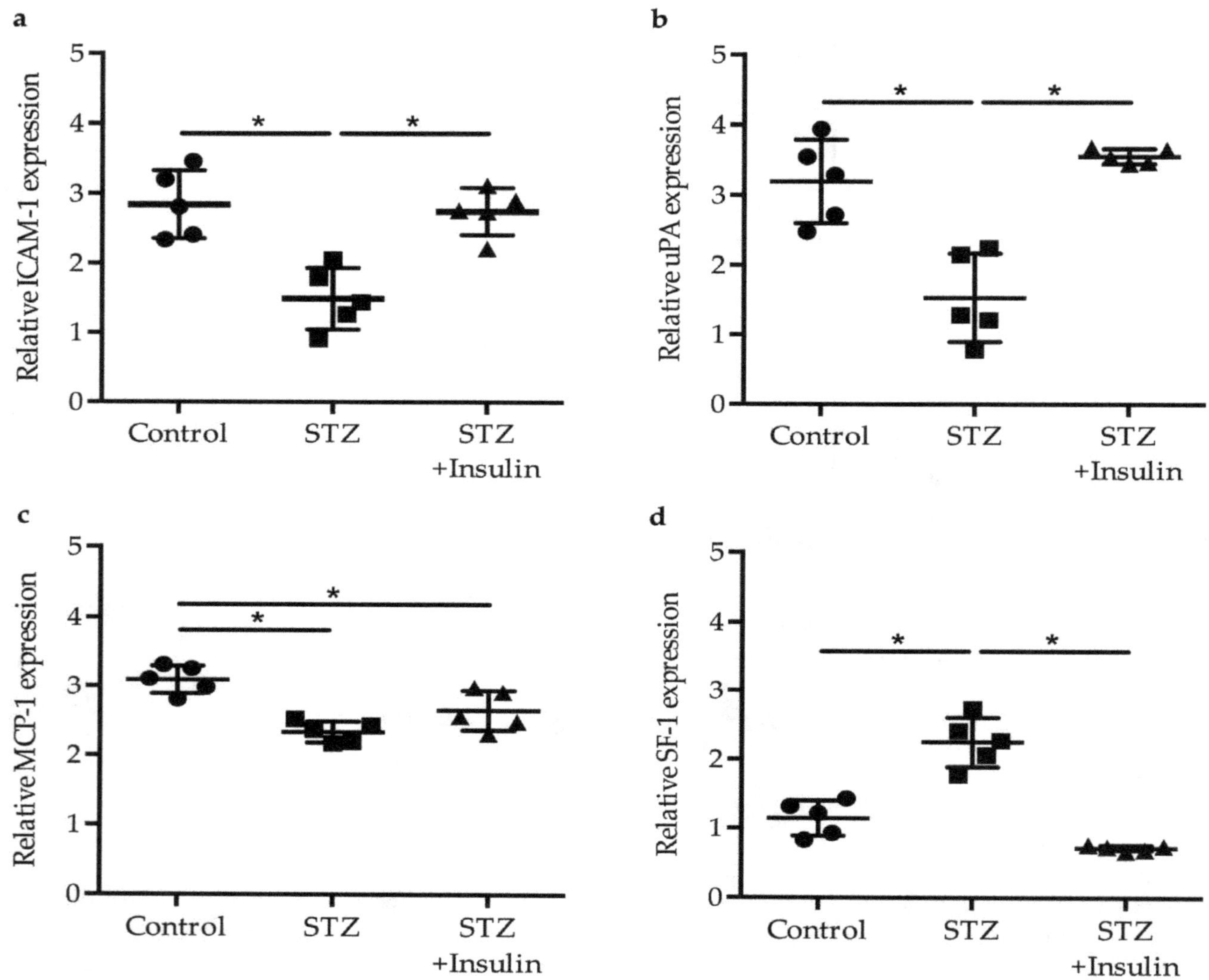

Figure 2. Gene expression of downstream targets of *Egr-1* in collateral tissues obtained from mice after induction of arteriogenesis was performed by qRT-PCR ($n = 5$ in each group, * $p < 0.05$ (each group compared to each other group) using a one-way ANOVA with Bonferroni's multiple comparison test). The relative expression is represented as $2^{\hat{}-\mathbf{ddCT}}$. The relative expressions of (**a**) *ICAM-1*, (**b**) *uPA*, (**c**) *MCP-1*, and (**d**) SF-1 were normalized to the expression level of the 18S rRNA.

2.3. Insulin Treatment Restored Vessel Growth in Diabetic Mice

The luminal collateral vessel diameter, which was measured 7 days post-FAL, was found to be significantly decreased in the diabetic group (23.61 ± 2.1 μm) compared to the control group (30.76 ± 2.5 μm); however, it was restored to control levels by insulin treatment (29.58 ± 1.8 μm) (Figure 3a). Moreover, qRT-PCR results on the cell proliferation marker Ki-67 revealed significantly reduced Ki-67 mRNA expression in the diabetic group (1.36 ± 0.37) compared to the non-diabetic control group (2.35 ± 0.50); however, Ki-67 expression levels increased when STZ mice were treated with insulin (3.02 ± 0.15) (Figure 3b).

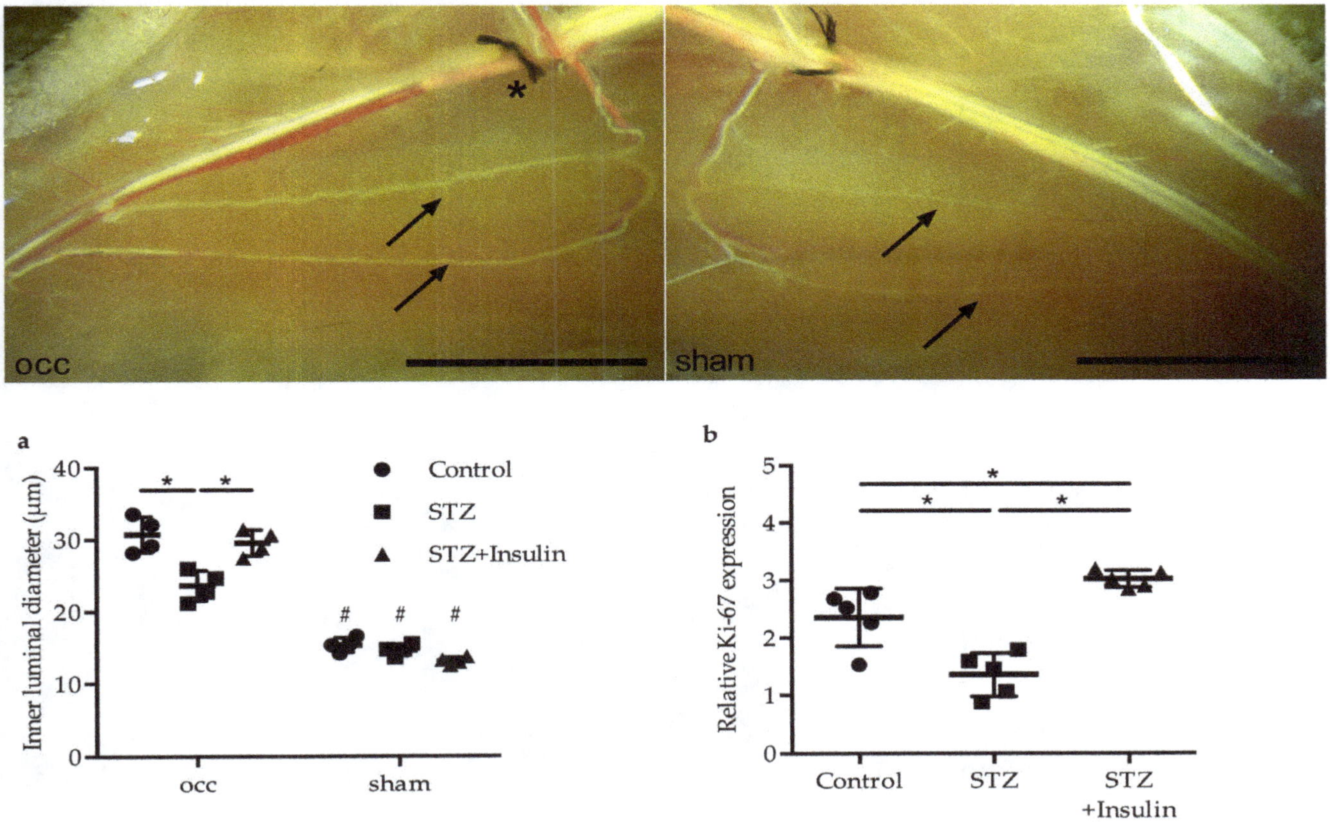

Figure 3. Upper panel: pictures of superficial collateral arteries of STZ-treated mice 7 days after femoral artery ligation (FAL, occ, left picture) or sham operation (right picture). Arrows indicate pre-existing (resting) collaterals of the sham-operated site or growth-induced collaterals of the experimental site. The ligation (*) of the femoral artery was executed downstream of the profound artery. Scale bars: 5 mm. Lower panel: (**a**) dot plots represent the inner luminal vessel diameter measured 7 days post-FAL ($n = 4$ per group, at least two collateral arteries per mouse and two sections were evaluated, * $p < 0.05$ (each group compared to each other group), # $p < 0.05$ compared to the corresponding occ group using a one-way ANOVA with Bonferroni's multiple comparison test). (**b**) Dot plots show the expression level of the proliferation marker Ki-67 in collaterals of control, STZ, and STZ + insulin-treated mice 24 h after FAL. Results were normalized to the expression level of the 18S rRNA ($n = 5$ per group, * $p < 0.05$ (each group compared to each other group) using a one-way ANOVA with Bonferroni's multiple comparison test).

2.4. Diminished Leukocyte Infiltration Was Improved in Diabetic Mice by Insulin Treatment

Fluorescent-activated cell sorting (FACS) studies from blood collected from non-ligated mice showed significantly increased levels of $CD11b^+$ cells in diabetic (55%) and insulin-treated groups (77%) compared to the non-diabetic control group (33%) with respect to $CD45^+$ cells, whereas the levels of $CD19^+$ or $CD3^+$ cells decreased in both the diabetic (10% and 14%, respectively) and the insulin-treated group (7% and 30%, respectively) (Figure 4a). There were no significant changes in leukocyte count in the adductor muscle of sham-operated mice in STZ-treated and STZ and insulin-treated mice compared to control mice (data not shown). However, in diabetic mice, there was a significant decrease in $CD11b^+$ (27% versus 13%), $CD19^+$ (45% versus 18%), and $CD3^+$ (55% versus 33%) cells three days post-ligation compared to control mice. Interestingly, insulin treatment increased the number of leukocytes in STZ-induced DM mice (Figure 4b).

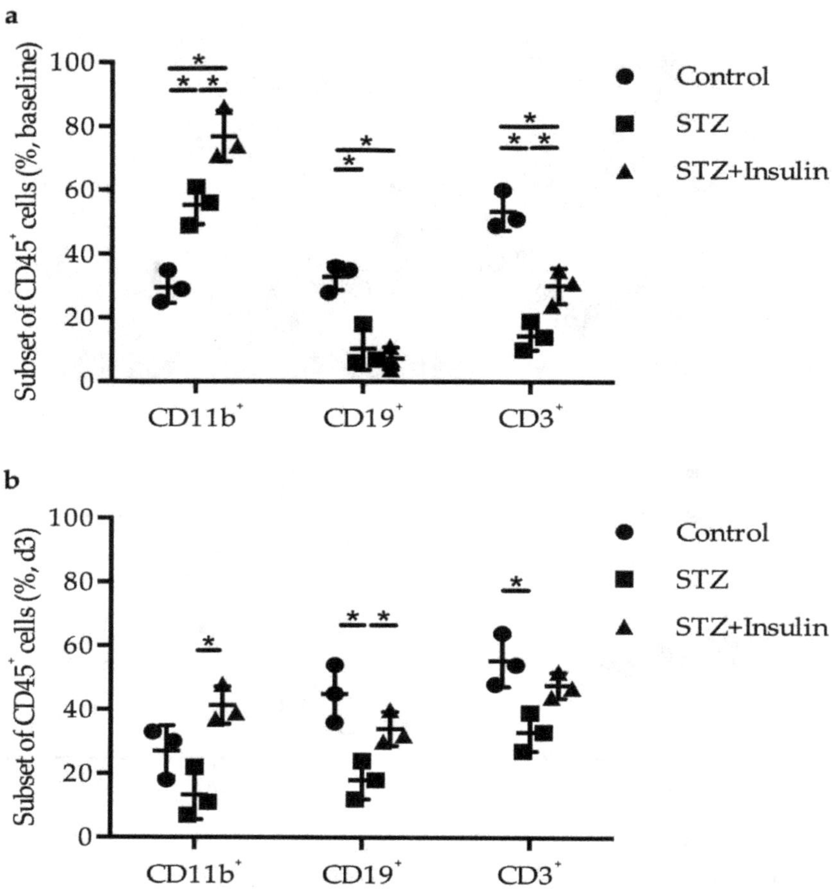

Figure 4. Dot plots represent the results of FACS analyses on CD11b$^+$, CD19$^+$, and CD3$^+$ cells performed on (**a**) whole blood of control, STZ, and STZ + insulin-treated mice without any surgical treatment and on (**b**) adductor muscles isolated from mice 3 days post-FAL (**a**,**b**: $n = 3$ per group, each group compared to each other group using a two-way ANOVA with Bonferroni's multiple comparison test).

3. Discussion

PAD is one of the common complications of DM that inflicts substantial damage to the lower limbs and has a very poor outcome. In mice, it was shown that impaired arteriogenesis is a major problem in hypercholesterolemia and DM [16]. While in the study by van Weel et al. [16], the influence of DM on perfusion recovery was less compared to that of hypercholesterolemia, our study showed a more pronounced impact of ligation on collateral vessel growth in DM. This may be due to the different experimental setup, age groups of animals under study, timepoints measured, and animal strains used. The mechanism by which impaired arteriogenesis occurs in DM is not fully understood. Earlier, Pagel et al. [22] reported the importance of *Egr-1* in promoting collateral outward remodeling through augmenting leukocyte infiltration and endothelial cell proliferation. In the present study, we report that there was a decreased expression of Egr-1 at the transcript and protein levels in collaterals of mice rendered diabetic by administration of streptozotocin. The decreased expression of *Egr-1* correlated with decreased collateral artery diameter in the diabetic mice. Important downstream targets of *Egr-1*, namely, *ICAM-1* and *uPA*, were found to be decreased, too. *ICAM-1* plays a critical role in endothelial monocyte adhesion, which is essential for arteriogenesis. An earlier study identified an upregulation of ICAM-1 mRNA in growing collateral arteries after induction of arteriogenesis by femoral artery ligation [25]. Moreover, it was shown that the process of arteriogenesis is reduced in ICAM-1 deficient mice [26]. Treatment of the diabetic mice with insulin improved the expression of *Egr-1*, increased the collateral artery diameter, and normalized the expression of downstream targets of *Egr-1*. A proposed model is shown in Figure 5.

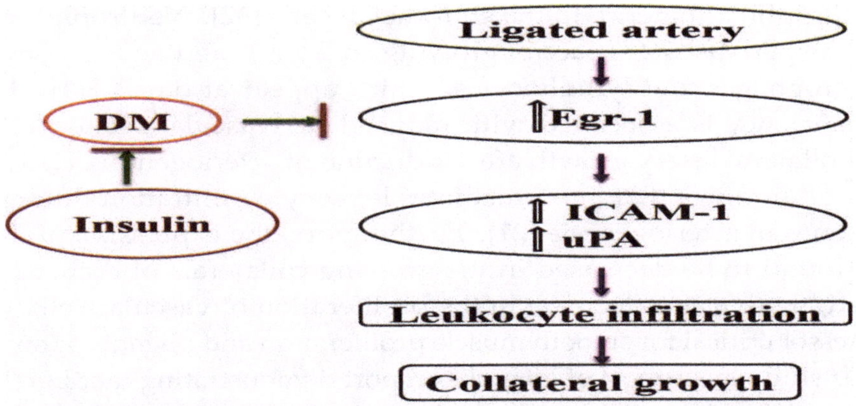

Figure 5. Graphical representation showing the mechanisms by which Egr-1 controls leukocyte recruitment, and hence, the process of collateral artery growth. While this process is impaired in DM due to the reduced *Egr-1* expression, it can be rescued by insulin treatment.

Earlier studies have clearly shown that induction of arteriogenesis in C57Bl6 mice by FAL resulted in an increased expression of *Egr-1* at the transcript and the protein levels in growing collaterals [22]. Interestingly, *Egr-1* deficient mice have been shown to have increased basal levels of $CD11b^+$ monocytes in the peripheral blood; however, levels of collateral perivascular macrophages as well as $CD3^+$ T cells and $CD19^+$ B cells in adductor muscles harvesting growing collaterals were reduced. Moreover, FAL in Egr-1−/− mice was associated with poor leukocyte recruitment and reduced collateral artery growth [22]. Our results showed that induction of DM, which was associated with reduced expression levels of *Egr-1*, also resulted in increased systemic levels of $CD11b^+$ cells, and after induction of arteriogenesis, in reduced levels of $CD11b^+$, $CD3^+$, and $CD19^+$ cells. Interestingly enough, treatment with insulin rescued perivascular leukocyte counts.

Decreased expression of *Egr-1* in DM mice in our study may support earlier findings showing that *Egr-1* is critical for collateral vessel development and that functional regulation of *Egr-1* may be compromised in DM. Evidence of induction and expression of *Egr-1* by elevated levels of glucose in murine glomerular endothelial cells and aortic smooth muscle cells have been reported. Exposure to insulin or high concentrations of D-glucose increased the expression of Egr-1 on the mRNA and protein level in glomerular endothelial cells and increased its promoter activity irrespectively of the concentration of insulin [27,28]. *TNF-α* is downstream of *Egr-1* and induces the expression of *MCP-1*. However, in arteriogenesis, increased levels of TNF-α, relevant for *MCP-1* expression, are dependent on mast cell activation [14]. Vedantham et. al. demonstrated a novel mechanism linking glucose metabolism to increased inflammatory and prothrombotic signaling in diabetic atherosclerosis via activation and post-translational modification of *Egr-1*. Hyperglycemia-induced hyper-acetylation of Egr-1 in endothelial cells was reported to be an important event linking diabetes to accelerated atherosclerosis [29]. Though acetylation of Egr-1 was not studied, it will be interesting to pursue future studies to understand the role of Egr-1 in the pathophysiology of arteriogenesis. Our observations in this study are contrary to those observed in diabetic atherosclerosis. There may be a possibility of additional regulation of Egr-1, as indicated by the shift in bands of Egr-1. Post-translational modifications of Egr-1 such as acetylation and phosphorylation have been reported to play an important role in the transcriptional activity and stability of Egr-1 [17,30]. Phosphorylation/dephosphorylation events may act as regulators for restricting the function of Egr-1. Furthermore, *SP-1* has been reported to compete for DNA binding sites of *Egr-1* [17]. Recently, a splice form of *Egr-1* was reported which lacks the N-terminal activation domain between amino acids 141 and 278 [31]. It will be interesting to further understand the mechanism through which hyperglycemia interferes with *Egr-1* upregulation during the process of arteriogenesis.

Leukocyte infiltration mediated through downstream target genes of *Egr-1*, namely, *ICAM-1*, *uPA* and *MCP-1*, was found to be decreased during collateral artery growth in diabetic mice. Endothelial uPA is vital for neutrophil adherence to the endothelial cells [32]. Neutrophils accumulate around day 1 after FAL in the perivascular space of growing collaterals and have a relevant function in the recruitment of macrophages and lymphocytes, which appear at day 3 [14]. Indeed, it has been shown that *uPA* deficiency is associated with reduced perivascular leukocyte accumulation and results in reduced collateral artery growth after induction of arteriogenesis via FAL [33]. These data comply with reported findings that *Egr-1* mediates leukocyte infiltration through activation of the abovementioned genes in arteriogenesis [21]. Furthermore, the expression of the cell proliferation marker Ki-67 was found to be decreased in the growing collaterals of diabetic mice, highlighting the fact that, indeed, there was a decrease in the proliferation of vascular cells. SF-1, an important transcriptional repressor critical for smooth muscle proliferation and phenotype switch [33], was found to be elevated in our study in support of an earlier report demonstrating that Egr-1−/− mice exhibited increased expression of SF-1 in growing collateral arteries [21]. One of the interesting findings of our study as the beneficial effect of insulin on collateral artery growth in DM mice. SF-1 regulates gene expression of pro-inflammatory cytokines in smooth muscle cells [33] and antagonizes platelet-derived growth factor BB (PDGF-BB)-induced growth and differentiation of vascular cells [34]. Several earlier reports have shown a regulation of *Egr-1* by insulin. Furthermore, Gousseva et al. [28] have reported an insulin-mediated increase in *Egr-1* promoter activity and cell proliferation in bovine aortic smooth muscle cells. Egr-1 has a role in adipocyte insulin resistance through activation of the MAPK-ERK pathway [35]. Our studies clearly show that diabetic mice treated with insulin show an increased expression of *Egr-1*, accompanied by an augmented expression of *Egr-1* downstream target genes relevant for leukocyte recruitment. Indeed, our results show that insulin treatment, moreover, goes along with increased numbers of leukocytes—relevant for the process of arteriogenesis—in collateral harboring muscles.

In summary, *Egr-1* expression decreased after induction of arteriogenesis in growing collaterals of streptozotocin-induced diabetic mice compared to control mice. Decreased *Egr-1* expression led to poor collateral growth. Insulin treatment, however, normalized the *Egr-1* expression, thereby promoting arteriogenesis. Though this was an observational study, this study assumes significance as it is the first time associating *Egr-1* with impaired arteriogenesis in DM. It will be interesting to see whether the same processes occur in patients with DM. Further investigations exploring the mechanism by which hyperglycemia suppresses *Egr-1* expression during the process of arteriogenesis will lead to better understanding of impaired arteriogenesis in DM.

4. Materials and Methods

4.1. Animal Studies

All studies with mice were performed after approval by the Institutional and Local Animal Ethics Committee (CPCSEA Approval number: H01/SASTRA/IAEC/RPP-23/12/15). Male C57B6NTac (Taconic Biosciences, USA) mice were procured through Vivo Biotech Ltd., Telangana, India and were maintained in an air-conditioned room (25 °C) with a 12 h light/12 h dark cycle. Feed and water were provided ad libitum to all the animals. Mice were rendered diabetic by treating them with STZ according to published protocols [36]. Briefly, eight-week-old male mice were made diabetic by administration of 50 mg/kg STZ dissolved in fresh citrate buffer (0.05 mol/L, pH 4.5) i.p. per day for five consecutive days. Those mice displaying blood glucose levels ≥ 250 mg/dL were considered diabetic (DM mice). The non-diabetic (NDM mice) control mice received citrate buffer alone. One group of mice received insulin after confirmation of hyperglycemia. Insulin was administered subcutaneously at a daily dose of 0.20 mL/100 g (4–5 U) until the end of the experiment.

4.2. Femoral Artery Ligation and Collection of Collaterals

Femoral artery ligation was performed as published earlier [37]. In brief, using a silk braided suture (0/7) the right femoral artery was ligated distally from the origin of the profunda femoris branching, while the left leg was sham operated. Adductor muscles and collateral arteries were collected as previously described [20]. To carry out fluorescent-activated cell sorting (FACS) analyses, adductor muscles were collected 3 days after the surgical procedure and for histological analysis, the adductor muscles were harvested 7 days after FAL. Gene expression studies on RNA and protein levels were performed with collateral arteries isolated 24 h after induction of arteriogenesis.

4.3. RNA Isolation and Quantitative Real-Time PCR Studies

Gene expression studies were performed using quantitative real time PCR (qRT-PCR). Total RNA was isolated using the RNeasy kit (TaKaRA). After DNase I (Qiagen, Hilden, Germany) digestion, one microgram of total RNA was reverse transcribed by random hexamers and Superscript RT-PCR System (Invitrogen, Carlsbad, CA, USA). After purification, the cDNA was used for qRT-PCR using specific primers for Egr-1, MCP-1, ICAM-1, SF-1, and Ki-67 [21]. Results were normalized to the expression level of the 18S rRNA.

4.4. FACS Analyses of Blood and Muscle Tissue

Whole blood withdrawn from the left ventricle 3 days post-ligation was analyzed by flow cytometry analyses (BD FACS Aria III, CA, USA) according to standard protocols. Furthermore, the adductor muscles from C57B6NTac mice were perfused with PBS (phosphate buffered saline) to eliminate the blood, harvested, and placed in small cell culture dishes. The tissue was cut into small pieces and digested 45 min at 37 °C using PBS buffer (50 mL) containing collagenase II (1 mg/mL), hyaluronidase (0.5 mg/mL) (both Sigma, St. Louis, MO, USA), dispase (1 mg/mL) (Gibco, Invitrogen, Carlsbad, CA, USA), and BSA (bovine serum albumin) (0.6 mg/mL) (Sigma). The suspension was then filtered with PBS/2%BSA through a 70 μm cell strainer (BD Falcon™), spun 10 min at 95 g, and the pellet finally resuspended in 100 μL PBS/2%BSA. The resulting cell suspension was analyzed by FACS using a panel of monoclonal antibodies against CD3 (T cells); (BioLegend Cat. No. 100201), CD11b (neutrophils, monocytes) (BioLegend Cat. No. 305902), CD19 (B cells) (BioLegend Cat. No. 115501), and CD45 (pan-leukocytes marker) (BioLegend Cat. No. 103101). Leukocyte populations were identified by fluorescence and scatter light characteristics. Cells from both peripheral blood and tissue were gated based on forward scatter (FSC-A)/side scatter (SSC-A). Leukocytes were identified by their positive staining with CD45. The final gating was based on CD45+/CD11b+, CD45+/CD19+, and CD45+/CD3+ cells (14).

4.5. Histological Analyses

Histological analyses were performed on adductor muscles (harboring collateral arteries) isolated from C57B6NTac mice as described earlier [20]. Briefly, 7 days after the surgical procedure both hind limbs were perfused with PBS containing 0.1% adenosine and 0.05% BSA (Sigma), then 4 min with fixing solution (4% buffered paraformaldehyde) via cannulation of the aorta. Thereafter, tissue samples were paraffin-embedded, cut in cross-sections, and H&E staining was performed to measure luminal collateral artery diameters.

4.6. Western Blot

Western blot analysis was performed on protein extracts, which were isolated from collaterals 24 h after femoral artery ligation or sham operation of DM and NDM mice according to standard procedures. Briefly, 30 μg of protein from all the tissue lysates was loaded onto a 10% sodium dodecyl sulfate (SDS) gel and ran at a power of 110 V. The protein in the gel was shifted to an immune-blot polyvinylidene difluoride (PVDF) membrane (1620112, Bio-Rad, USA) at 100 V for 1 h using Trans-Blot Turbo Transfer System (Bio-Rad). The blots were probed for Egr-1 protein (Egr-1 antibody (588)-Santa Cruz BioTechnology Cat.no #sc110). α-Tubulin served as a housekeeping protein (alpha tubulin antibody (B-7): Santa Cruz Biotechnology Cat.no. #sc-5286). The density of Egr-1 to α-tubulin was measured through the Quant-One software (Bio-Rad). The immunoblots are a representation of at least three independent experiments.

4.7. Statistical Analysis

All values are expressed as means ± SD unless mentioned. Statistical analyses were conducted as indicated in the figure legends using GraphPad software PRISM6 (GraphPad Software, USA). The limit of statistical significance was set at $p < 0.05$.

Author Contributions: S.V. and E.D. conceived the research idea, executed the study, and prepared the manuscript. S.T. and S.K. performed the experiments. M.L. contributed in the transfer of technology and helped in manuscript preparation. D.R.C. assisted in animal surgery.

Acknowledgments: The authors would like to acknowledge ICMR-BMBF (50/6/2013/BMS) and SASTRA Deemed to be University for supporting the research funding and facility, respectively. Moreover, we would like to thank Anna-Kristina Kluever for editing the manuscript.

Abbreviations

SF-1	Splicing Factor 1
DM	Diabetes Mellitus
NDM	Non-Diabetes Mellitus
Egr-1	Early growth response-1
uPA	urokinase Plasminogen Activator
MCP-1	Monocyte Chemoattractant Protein-1
ICAM-1	Intercellular Adhesion Molecule-1
FAL	Femoral Artery Ligation
STZ	Streptozotocin
PAD	Peripheral Artery Disease

References

1. American Diabetes Association. Peripheral Arterial Disease in People with Diabetes. *Diabetes Care* **2003**, *26*, 3333–3341. [CrossRef] [PubMed]
2. Dolan, N.C.; Liu, K.; Criqui, M.H.; Greenland, P.; Guralnik, J.M.; Chan, C.; Schneider, J.R.; Mandapat, A.L.; Martin, G.; McDermott, M.M. Peripheral artery disease, diabetes, and reduced lower extremity functioning. *Diabetes Care* **2002**, *25*, 113–120. [CrossRef] [PubMed]
3. Prompers, L.; Schaper, N.; Apelqvist, J.; Edmonds, M.; Jude, E.; Mauricio, D.; Uccioli, L.; Urbancic, V.; Bakker, K.; Holstein, P.; et al. Prediction of outcome in individuals with diabetic foot ulcers: Focus on the differences between individuals with and without peripheral arterial disease. The EURODIALE Study. *Diabetologia* **2008**, *51*, 747–755. [CrossRef] [PubMed]
4. Shu, J.; Santulli, G. Update on peripheral artery disease: Epidemiology and evidence-based facts. *Atherosclerosis* **2018**, *275*, 379–381. [CrossRef] [PubMed]
5. Beckman, J.A.; Creager, M.A.; Libby, P. Diabetes and atherosclerosis: Epidemiology, pathophysiology, and management. *JAMA* **2002**, *287*, 2570–2581. [CrossRef] [PubMed]
6. Lanzer, P. Topographic distribution of peripheral arteriopathy in non-diabetics and type 2 diabetics. *Z. Kardiol.* **2001**, *90*, 99–103. [CrossRef] [PubMed]
7. Eberhardt, R.T.; Coffman, J.D. Cardiovascular morbidity and mortality in peripheral arterial disease. *Curr. Drug Targets Cardiovasc. Haematol. Disord.* **2004**, *4*, 209–217. [CrossRef]
8. Faglia, E.; Clerici, G.; Clerissi, J.; Gabrielli, L.; Losa, S.; Mantero, M.; Caminiti, M.; Curci, V.; Quarantiello, A.; Lupattelli, T.; et al. Long-term prognosis of diabetic patients with critical limb ischemia: A population-based cohort study. *Diabetes Care* **2009**, *32*, 822–827. [CrossRef]
9. Kamalesh, M.; Shen, J. Diabetes and peripheral arterial disease in men: Trends in prevalence, mortality, and effect of concomitant coronary disease. *Clin. Cardiol.* **2009**, *32*, 442–446. [CrossRef]
10. Malmstedt, J.; Leander, K.; Wahlberg, E.; Karlstrom, L.; Alfredsson, L.; Swedenborg, J. Outcome after leg bypass surgery for critical limb ischemia is poor in patients with diabetes: A population-based cohort study. *Diabetes Care* **2008**, *31*, 887–892. [CrossRef]

11. Currie, C.J.; Morgan, C.L.; Peters, J.R. The epidemiology and cost of inpatient care for peripheral vascular disease, infection, neuropathy, and ulceration in diabetes. *Diabetes Care* **1998**, *21*, 42–48. [CrossRef] [PubMed]
12. Moraes, F.; Paye, J.; Mac Gabhann, F.; Zhuang, Z.W.; Zhang, J.; Lanahan, AA.; Simons, M. Endothelial cell-dependent regulation of arteriogenesis. *Circ. Res.* **2013**, *113*, 1076–1086. [CrossRef] [PubMed]
13. Arras, M.; Ito, W.D.; Scholz, D.; Winkler, B.; Schaper, J.; Schaper, W. Monocyte activation in angiogenesis and collateral growth in the rabbit hindlimb. *J. Clin. Invest.* **1998**, *101*, 41–50. [CrossRef] [PubMed]
14. Chillo, O.; Kleinert, E.C.; Lautz, T.; Lasch, M.; Pagel, J.I.; Heun, Y.; Troidl, K.; Fischer, S.; Caballero-Martinez, A.; Mauer, A.; et al. Perivascular Mast Cells Govern Shear Stress-Induced Arteriogenesis by Orchestrating Leukocyte Function. *Cell Rep.* **2016**, *23*, 2197–2207. [CrossRef] [PubMed]
15. De Vivo, S.; Palmer-Kazen, U.; Kalin, B.; Wahlberg, E. Risk factors for poor collateral development in claudication. *Vasc. Endovasc. Surg.* **2005**, *39*, 519–524. [CrossRef] [PubMed]
16. Van Weel, V.; de Vries, M.; Voshol, P.J.; Verloop, R.E.; Eilers, P.H.; van Hinsbergh, V.W.; van Bockel, J.H.; Quax, P.H. Hypercholesterolemia reduces collateral artery growth more dominantly than hyperglycemia or insulin resistance in mice. *Arterioscler. Thromb. Vasc. Biol.* **2006**, *26*, 1383–1390. [CrossRef] [PubMed]
17. Lambiase, P.D.; Edwards, R.J.; Anthopoulos, P.; Rahman, S.; Meng, Y.G.; Bucknall, C.A.; Redwood, S.R.; Pearson, J.D.; Marber, M.S. Circulating humoral factors and endothelial progenitor cells in patients with differing coronary collateral support. *Circulation* **2004**, *109*, 2986–2992. [CrossRef] [PubMed]
18. Gashler, A.; Sukhatme, V. Egr-1: Prototype of a zinc finger family of transcription factors. *Prog. Nucleic Acid. Res. Mol Biol.* **1995**, *50*, 191–224.
19. Yan, S.F.; Harja, E.; Andrassy, M.; Fujita, T.; Schmidt, A.M. Protein kinase C beta/early growth response-1 pathway: A key player in ischemia, atherosclerosis, and restenosis. *J. Am. Coll. Cardiol.* **2006**, *48*, A47–A55. [CrossRef]
20. Sarateanu, C.S.; Retuerto, M.A.; Beckmann, J.T.; McGregor, L.; Carbray, J.; Patejunas, G.; Nayak, L.; Milbrandt, J.; Rosengart, T.K. An Egr-1 master switch for arteriogenesis: Studies in Egr-1 homozygous negative and wild-type animals. *J. Thorac. Cardiovasc. Surg.* **2006**, *131*, 138–145. [CrossRef]
21. Lee, J.S.; Lee, J.Y.; Li Kim, K.; Shin, I.S.; Suh, W.; Choi, J.H.; Jeon, E.S.; Byun, J.; Kim, D.K. Adenoviral-mediated delivery of early growth response factor-1 gene increases tissue perfusion in a murine model of hindlimb ischemia. *Mol. Ther.* **2005**, *12*, 328–336. [CrossRef] [PubMed]
22. Pagel, J.I.; Ziegelhoeffer, T.; Heil, M.; Fischer, S.; Fernández, B.; Schaper, W.; Preissner, K.T.; Deindl, E. Role of early growth response 1 in arteriogenesis: Impact on vascular cell proliferation and leukocyte recruitment in vivo. *Thromb. Haemost.* **2012**, *107*, 562–574. [PubMed]
23. McMahon, S.B.; Monroe, J.G. The role of early growth response gene 1 (egr-1) in regulation of the immune response. *J. Leukoc. Biol.* **1996**, *60*, 159–166. [CrossRef] [PubMed]
24. Yan, SF.; Fujita, T.; Lu, J.; Okada, K.; Shan Zou, Y.; Mackman, N.; Pinsky, DJ.; Stern, DM. Egr-1, a master switch coordinating upregulation of divergent gene families underlying ischemic stress. *Nat. Med.* **2000**, *6*, 1355–1361. [CrossRef] [PubMed]
25. Scholz, D.; Ito, W.; Fleming, I.; Deindl, E.; Sauer, A.; Babiak, A.; Bühler, A.; Wiesnet, M.; Busse, R.; Schaper, J.; et al. Ultrastructure and molecular histology of rabbit hindlimb collateral artery growth (arteriogenesis). *Virchows. Arch.* **2000**, *436*, 257–270. [CrossRef] [PubMed]
26. Hoefer, I.E.; van Royen, N.; Rectenwald, J.E.; Deindl, E.; Hua, J.; Jost, M.; Grundmann, S.; Voskuil, M.; Ozaki, C.K.; et al. Arteriogenesis proceeds via ICAM-1/Mac-1- mediated mechanisms. *Circ. Res.* **2004**, *94*, 1179–1185. [CrossRef] [PubMed]
27. Hasan, R.N.; Phukan, S.; Harada, S. Differential regulation of early growth response gene-1 expression by insulin and glucose in vascular endothelial cells. *Arterioscler. Thromb. Vasc. Biol.* **2003**, *23*, 988–993. [CrossRef] [PubMed]
28. Gousseva, N.; Kugathasan, K.; Chesterman, C.N.; Khachigian, L.M. Early growth response factor-1 mediates insulin-inducible vascular endothelial cell proliferation and regrowth after injury. *J. Cell. Biochem.* **2001**, *81*, 523–534. [CrossRef]
29. Vedantham, S.; Thiagarajan, D.; Ananthakrishnan, R.; Wang, L.; Rosario, R.; Zou, S.; Goldberg, I.J.; Yan, S.F.; Schmidt, A.M.; Ramasamy, R. Aldose Reductase drives hyperacetylation of Egr-1 in hyperglycemia and consequent upregulation of proinflammatory and prothrombotic signals. *Diabetes* **2014**, *63*, 761–774. [CrossRef]

30. Aliperti, V.; Sgueglia, G.; Aniello, F.; Vitale, E.; Fucci, L.; Donizetti, A. Identification, Characterization, and Regulatory Mechanisms of a Novel EGR-1 Splicing Isoform. *Int. J. Mol. Sci.* **2019**, *20*, 1548. [CrossRef]
31. Reichel, C.A.; Uhl, B.; Lerchenberger, M.; Puhr-Westerheide, D.; Rehberg, M.; Liebl, J.; Khandoga, A.; Schmalix, W.; Zahler, S.; Deindl, E.; et al. Urokinase-type plasminogen activator promotes paracellular transmigration of neutrophils via Mac-1, but independently of urokinase-type plasminogen activator receptor. *Circulation* **2011**, *124*, 1848–1859. [CrossRef] [PubMed]
32. Deindl, E.; Ziegelhöffer, T.; Kanse, S.M.; Fernandez, B.; Neubauer, E.; Carmeliet, P.; Preissner, K.T.; Schaper, W. Receptor-independent role of the urokinase-type plasminogen activator during arteriogenesis. *FASEB J.* **2003**, *17*, 1174–1176. [CrossRef] [PubMed]
33. Cattaruzza, M.; Schafer, K.; Hecker, M. Cytokine-induced down-regulation of zfm1/splicing factor-1 promotes smooth muscle cell proliferation. *J. Biol. Chem.* **2002**, *277*, 6582–6589. [CrossRef]
34. Cattaruzza, M.; Nogoy, N.; Wojtowicz, A.; Hecker, M. Zinc finger motif-1 antagonizes PDGF-BB-induced growth and dedifferentiation of vascular smooth muscle cells. *FASEB J.* **2012**, *26*, 4864–4875. [CrossRef] [PubMed]
35. Yu, X.; Shen, N.; Zhang, M.L.; Pan, F.Y.; Wang, C.; Jia, W.P.; Liu, C.; Gao, Q.; Gao, X.; Xue, B.; et al. Egr-1 decreases adipocyte insulin sensitivity by tilting PI3K/Akt and MAPK signal balance in mice. *EMBO J.* **2011**, *30*, 3754–3765. [CrossRef] [PubMed]
36. Jawerbaum, A.; White, V. Animal models in diabetes and pregnancy. *Endocr. Rev.* **2010**, *31*, 680–701. [CrossRef]
37. Limbourg, A.; Korff, T.; Napp, L.C.; Schaper, W.; Drexler, H.; Limbourg, F.P. Evaluation of postnatal arteriogenesis and angiogenesis in a mouse model of hind-limb ischemia. *Nat. Protoc.* **2009**, *4*, 1737–1746. [CrossRef]

5

Atherosclerosis and the Capillary Network; Pathophysiology and Potential Therapeutic Strategies

Tilman Ziegler [1,2], Farah Abdel Rahman [1], Victoria Jurisch [1] and Christian Kupatt [1,2,*]

1. Klinik & Poliklinik für Innere Medizin I, Klinikum rechts der Isar, Technical University of Munich, 81675 Munich, Germany; tilman.ziegler@tum.de (T.Z.); farah.abdel-rahman@tum.de (F.A.R.); victoria.jurisch@googlemail.com (V.J.)
2. DZHK (German Center for Cardiovascular Research), Partner Site Munich Heart Alliance, 80802 Munich, Germany

* Correspondence: christian.kupatt@tum.de

Abstract: Atherosclerosis and associated ischemic organ dysfunction represent the number one cause of mortality worldwide. While the key drivers of atherosclerosis, arterial hypertension, hypercholesterolemia and diabetes mellitus, are well known disease entities and their contribution to the formation of atherosclerotic plaques are intensively studied and well understood, less effort is put on the effect of these disease states on microvascular structure an integrity. In this review we summarize the pathological changes occurring in the vascular system in response to prolonged exposure to these major risk factors, with a particular focus on the differences between these pathological alterations of the vessel wall in larger arteries as compared to the microcirculation. Furthermore, we intend to highlight potential therapeutic strategies to improve microvascular function during atherosclerotic vessel disease.

Keywords: atherosclerosis; pericyte; rAAV; capillary; endothelial cells

---

1. Introduction

Atherosclerosis remains an entity with continually growing incidence associated with a variety of disease states, which include ischemic stroke, peripheral artery disease and coronary artery disease. Taken together, cardiovascular disease, which can be seen as an expression of advanced atherosclerosis, account for 17.9 million deaths or 31% of all deaths per year globally, thus ranking it the number one cause of mortality today [1]. Multiple risk factors contributing to atherosclerosis have been identified and well-studied, mainly arterial hypertension, hypercholesterolemia, nicotine abuse and diabetes.

Atherosclerosis describes a pathological remodeling of the arterial wall initiated by the accumulation of lipids in the sub-endothelial layer of arteries. The retention of lipids triggers an inflammatory reaction leading to the invasion of multiple classes of leukocytes. This inflammatory state facilitates further endothelial dysfunction and remodeling of the extracellular matrix (ECM), ultimately leading to the formation of calcified, vulnerable plaques prone to rupture, which can lead to complete vessel occlusion via platelet activation and thrombosis.

This process of increasing vascular remodeling manifests initially as diffuse thickening of the Tunica intima, the innermost vascular layer, and an increase of intima thickness relative to the underlying Tunica media. Interestingly, these early stages in remodeling have been observed already at early ages, starting in the second decade of life [2]. The diffuse intimal thickening is mainly driven by the accumulation of lipids [3]. As proposed by Williams and Tabas in their response-to-retention hypothesis in 1995 [4,5], this accumulation of ECM-associated lipoproteins constitutes the initial step in the formation of an atherosclerotic lesion. The ECM-protein class of proteoglycans in particular has been identified as a key binding partner for lipid-complexes owing to their high affinity for lipoproteins [6,7].

Subsequently, the lipoprotein-proteoglycan complexes, which are prone to oxidation and aggregation, represent a source of oxidative stress on the surrounding endothelial cells and vascular smooth muscle cells (vSMC). This process induces the recruitment of macrophages, in part due to the increase in SMC-derived Monocyte chemoattractant protein-1 [8], which phagocytose the lipoprotein-proteoglycan complexes, leading to the accumulation of foam cells in the atherosclerotic plaque [9,10]. Owing to the increased number of macrophages and the subsequent release of inflammatory cytokines, vascular smooth muscle cells change from their resting state into a more fibroproliferative condition, e.g. they display a drastic increase in activation and expansion. They simultaneously demonstrate a heightened susceptibility to apoptosis, mediated by the induced expression of the pro-apoptotic regulator BAX (Bcl-2-associated X protein) [11]. In addition, activated vSMCs produce transforming growth factor β (TGF-β), tissue factor (TF) and further proteoglycans, thus attracting more lipoproteins and additional macrophages, which further worsens the progression of the atherosclerotic lesion [12–14]. In the later stages of atherosclerotic plaque formation, atherosclerotic lesions can transform into thin cap fibroatheromas, characterized by a thin fibrous cap containing calcifications covering a necrotic lipid core. These atherosclerotic lesions are prone to rupture, exposing the blood stream to the underlying extracellular matrix, containing Von Willebrand factor, collagen and fibrin. These ECM-proteins subsequently bind to platelets and lead to their activation and subsequent organization into a thrombus, resulting in the occlusion of the vessel [15–17].

In clinical practice, strategies for the treatment of atherosclerosis focus on the reduction of the risk factors of this pathological condition and on interventional or surgical revascularization. However, atherosclerosis is generally seen as a predominant problem of the macrocirculation with a focus on the formation of atherosclerotic plaques, rather than a disease affecting the whole circulatory system. In this review we discuss the impact of the known predominant risk factors—arterial hypertension, hypercholesterolemia and diabetes—on the development and progression of atherosclerosis with a focus on their influence on the microcirculation, e.g., arterioles, capillaries and venules. Furthermore, we highlight potential therapeutic strategies that might improve overall vascular function in atherosclerotic patients.

2. Cardiovascular Risk Factors Contributing to Atherosclerosis: The Macro

Arterial Hypertension represents a key driver in the development of atherosclerosis, and thus, cardiovascular disease. The prevalence of hypertension in ischemic stroke, coronary or peripheral artery disease lies reportedly around 60–90% depending on the localization of the atherosclerotic lesion [18,19]. Arterial hypertension can be divided into two classes: primary or essential hypertension, triggered by an interplay of underlying causes as well as secondary hypertension, caused by either endocrinological disorders or stenosis of the renal arteries. While the causes of arterial hypertension vary, the effect on the vascular system remains the same. It is currently unclear whether arterial hypertension represents the cause of vascular dysfunction or the result of it; however, a bidirectional interaction between hypertension and atherosclerosis appears the most likely explanation. Initial evidence that endothelial dysfunction causes hypertension stems from early observations that the inhibition of the endothelial nitric oxide synthase, which produces the potent vasodilator NO, leads to hypertension in human subjects [20]. One key regulator of arterial blood pressure is identified in the Renin-Angiotensin-Aldosterone system (RAAS), also regulating fluid and electrolyte homeostasis. Here, Angiotensin II, the main effector peptide of this system, has been demonstrated to directly induce endothelial dysfunction via the recruitment of macrophages to the vascular wall in a CCR2/MCP-1 dependent manner. Angiotensin II furthermore increases endothelial oxidative stress via NADPH oxidase–derived superoxide anion production, predominantly by interacting with the endothelial AT_{1A} receptor [21–23].

Hypercholesterolemia represents an additional risk factor with increasing prevalence in the development of cardiovascular disease [24,25]. Particularly, western style diets (high-fat and cholesterol, high-protein, high-sugar) lead to an increase in cholesterol, LDL-levels and LDL/HDL ratios [26].

Low density lipoproteins enter the vascular wall at predilection sites characterized by disturbed blood flow and preexisting endothelial dysfunction [27]. Once LDLs enter the vascular wall, they form complexes with proteoglycans (with versican, decorin, syndecan-4, biglycan and perlecan being the predominant proteoglycans in the vascular wall [28]) via the interaction of the LDL-component Apolipoprotein B [29]. This interaction facilitates changes to the lipid composition and the configuration of Apolipoprotein B [30], which enhances the oxidation of LDL to oxidized LDL (oxLDL) via reactive oxygen species generated by the activated endothelium and vascular smooth muscle cells [31]. This oxidation step represents a prerequisite for the detection and phagocytosis of LDL-particles by macrophages [32], leading to the formation of foam cells. This transformation increases the expression of inflammatory cytokines and oxidative stress markers in those macrophages [33]. Furthermore, oxLDL facilitates endothelial expression of leucocyte adhesion molecules (vacular cell adhesion protein 1, P-Selectin [34,35]) and cytokines [36], attracting additional macrophages, thus, enhancing the inflammatory state of the atherosclerotic lesion.

The last main contributor to the development of atherosclerosis can be identified in diabetes mellitus (DM). The hallmark feature of diabetes is the elevation of blood glucose levels (hyperglycemia). One key effect of hyperglycemia lies in the increased formation of superoxides, which enhances the oxidative stress of the vascular wall further. This process is partly mediated by the increased formation of advanced glycation end products (AGEs). Advanced glycation end products occur when excess glucose forms dicarbonyl compounds, which react spontaneously with amino groups of proteins [37]. These AGEs then bind to their respective receptor (RAGE), expressed on endothelial cells, macrophages and vascular smooth muscle cells. Particularly in endothelial cells, AGEs induce the activation of the NAD(P)H-oxidase [38] and also the expression of adhesion proteins and cytokines via the nuclear translocation of NFκB [39,40]. In macrophages, AGE-signaling enhances oxLDL uptake via an upregulation of CD36 and Macrophage Scavenger Receptor Class A [41]. Additionally, RAGE itself acts as an endothelial adhesion protein in concert with ICAM-1 [42], necessary for the adhesion of leukocytes. Further mechanisms enhancing ROS production upon hyperglycemic conditions are to be found in the Lipoxygenase pathway [43] and the Polypol pathway, respectively [44].

As discussed in the previous paragraphs, the formation of atherosclerotic lesions can be driven by multiple interdependent risk factors. However, arterial hypertension, diabetes mellitus and hypercholesterolemia also drastically change the functionality of the microcirculatory vessels, a fact rarely pointed out as compared to classical large-vessel pathologies. Therefore, in the following paragraphs we focus on the pathologies elicited by these risk factors in small vessels.

3. Hypertension, Hypercholesterolemia and Diabetes Mellitus in Capillaries: The Micro

Unlike larger vessels (arteries and veins), the smaller units of the vascular system lose their classical three layered structure consisting of Tunica intima, Tunica media and Tunica adventitia. While arterioles still contain a covering sheet of vascular smooth muscle cells throughout, capillaries are only sporadically covered in pericytes, a sort of mural cell closely related to vascular smooth muscle cells, but often lacking their contractile phenotype [45–47]. Venules on the other hand generally lack a complete cover of vSMCs. In their biological function, pericytes further differ from vascular smooth muscle cell layers due to their close interaction with endothelial cells. In the microcirculation, pericytes represent key regulators of endothelial quiescence, predominantly by secreting the growth factor Angiopoietin-1, which binds to the endothelial Tie-2 receptor [48]. Activation of this receptor tyrosine kinase facilitates the expression of survival factors, such as Survivin, and suppressing the expression of pro-apoptotic signaling molecules, like procaspase-9 and BAD (BCL2 Associated Agonist Of Cell Death) in endothelial cells [49,50]. Furthermore, Angiopoietin-1 enhances the recruitment of additional pericytes to the endothelial monolayer in a HB-EGF (heparin binding EGF like growth factor) and HGF (hepatocyte growth factor) dependent positive feedback loop [51,52]. In addition to Ang-1, pericytes regulate endothelial proliferation rates via TGF-β (transforming growth factor β) [53,54], bFGF (basic fibroblast growth factor) [55] and VEGF (vascular endothelial growth factor) [56]. Of note, pathological stimuli such as inflammation, hypoxia and neoplasia generally do not manifest themselves in a proliferation of mural cells in the microcirculation but, rather, a decrease in endothelial pericyte coverage. While this loss in pericytes has been widely reported, their fate remains unknown. Speculations range from de-differentiation to migration or apoptosis, depending on the particular vascular bed and stimulus [57–60]. Furthermore, the influx of macrophages into the vessel wall and subsequent transition into foam cells, one key driver in the development of atherosclerosis, does not occur in the same way in capillaries, since there is no comparable structure – e.g., tunica media – in these smallest vessels. These differences in morphology and in the reaction of pericytes to pathological stimuli also have an impact on the functional and morphological changes of capillaries exposed to those stimuli. However, while some reactions of the vascular system to the exposure to risk factors still remain in effect in capillaries (increased expression of endothelial adhesion molecules and of reactive oxygen species leading to a state of endothelial dysfunction), the following paragraphs will focus on the specific differences between the microcirculation and larger vessels in response to pro-atherosclerotic stimuli.

Arterial hypertension leads to an increase in the vascular pericyte coverage. Apart from this enhancement of the number of pericytes, this cell type also undergoes a transformation into a more vascular smooth muscle cell like phenotype, indicated by an increase in the expression of contractile proteins [61,62]. This effect is in part mediated by an upregulation of the endothelial-derived growth factor FGF-2 and interleukin-6 [63]. Interestingly, this increase is not accompanied by a gain in capillary density, but rather the opposite. Capillary rarefication is routinely seen both in human as well as in animal studies during arterial hypertension [64,65]. The growing number of pericytes and endothelial coverage with pericytes during arterial hypertension however appears to be unique to the hypertensive stimulus, since hypercholesterolemia, hyperglycemia and the subsequent inflammation elicited generally leads to a drastic decrease in pericyte coverage. To this end, hypercholesterolemia leads to a decrease in endothelial pericyte coverage in part via the downregulation of the endothelial NO synthase, a potent driver of microvascular mural cell recruitment [66–68]. In addition, hypercholesterolemia facilitates the above mentioned accumulation of reactive oxygen species and the increased recruitment of leukocytes [69]. Other effects seen during states of increased lipid deposition are the reduction of angiogenic sprouting via a downregulation of vascular endothelial growth factor (VEGF-A) and an additional reduction of endothelial N-Cadherin, the key anchoring protein with which endothelial cells and pericytes interact [70,71]. Diabetes as well seems to be associated with a drastic loss in pericytes. In this context, pericyte loss represents a key feature in the case of diabetic retinopathy. This complication of end-stage diabetes constitutes a well-studied phenomenon, due to the accessibility of the vascular bed to investigation both in human specimens as well as animal models. In both, capillary rarefication as well as a loss in pericytes is observed during diabetic retinopathy [72,73], while this process has also been demonstrated in additional vascular beds [74], mediated in part by advanced glycation end product accumulation [75].

4. Current and Future Treatment Strategies

Multiple therapies have been in clinical use to treat atherosclerotic lesions and the underlying cardiovascular risk factors. Two treatment options can be destinguished: firstly, the treatment of the predisposing factors causing atherosclerosis in order to reduce the progression of the disease once diagnosed. For primary arterial hypertension a host of antihypertensive drugs are available with varying efficacies and substance-class specific secondary effects. Notably, ACE-inhibitors and angiotensin 2 receptor antagonists not only lower the blood pressure but also reduce the degree of endothelial dysfunction by reducing leukocyte recruitment and the production of reactive oxygen species [76], an effect also demonstrated for calcium channel blockers [77]. Antidiabetic drugs too display pleiotropic effects beneficial for cardiovascular mortality. To this end, metformin and the novel class of PCSK9 inhibitors additionally reduce reactive oxygen species production [78,79]. Lastly, the pleiotropic effects of statins, the first line treatment option for hypercholesterolemia, have been well documented throughout the last decades. These drugs reduce endothelial cytokine production [80], production of reactive oxygen species [81] and vascular smooth muscle cell proliferation [82].

Mechanical revascularization, either via bypass surgery or percutaneous angioplasty, represents the second category in the treatment of atherosclerosis. These methods have demonstrated their merit over time for both coronary as well as peripheral artery disease. However, while extensive research has been undertaken to optimize surgery procedures and percutaneous vascular intervention strategies, no-reflow phenomena routinely occur in patients undergoing revascularization both in acute ischemic events as well as chronic vascular occlusion with rates varying from 2% up to 25%, depending on the vascular bed and the abruptness of occlusion [83,84]. In the case of acute myocardial or limb ischemia, these events can be attributed to a high thrombotic burden in the occluded vessel. However, the predominant vascular risk factors for the development of atherosclerotic lesions can have additional effects in the microcirculation as described above. In particular, the rarefication of capillaries and the dysfunctionality of the remaining capillaries, leading to a dysfunctional downstream vessels system, resulting in a drastic decrease in overall capillary diameter. This reduction in available runoff contributes to low-flow phenomena through recently implanted stents and increase the risk of stent thrombosis (see Figure 1).

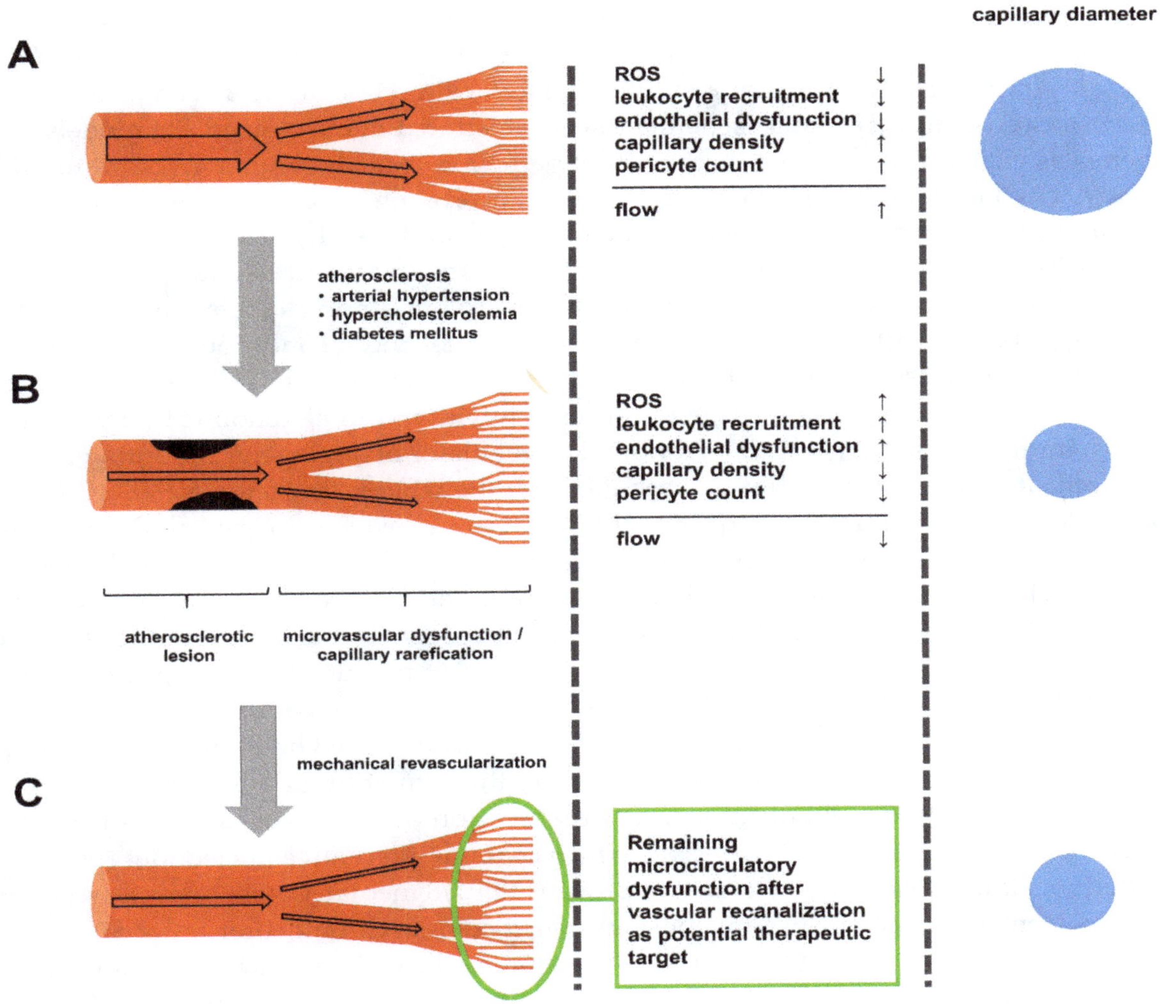

Figure 1. (**A**) The healthy circulatory system is characterized by minimal lipid accumulation in larger arteries and an overall low state of endothelial activation, leading to low levels of ROS production and leukocyte recruitment. (**B**) Upon prolonged exposure to the atherosclerotic risk factors arterial hypertension, hypercholesterolemia and diabetes, endothelial cells experience constant activation enhancing leukocyte recruitment, oxidative stress and loss of pericytes in the microcirculation, leading

to capillary rarefication, limiting the potential blood flow through the now sparse capillary network. (**C**) Even after mechanical revascularization, via bypass operations or percutaneous angioplasty, the capillary rarefication remains, continuously limiting blood flow, thus hindering the recovery of the ischemic tissue and leaving newly opened vessels susceptible for restenosis and stent thrombosis. Here, strategies to improve capillary density, and thus, microcirculatory flow, appear to be worthwhile therapeutic targets in the treatment of atherosclerosis currently not yet addresses.

Consequently, therapeutic strategies to ameliorate capillary rarefication and improve the functionality of the downstream capillary network need to be established. Since capillary stability crucially relies on proper pericyte adhesion to the endothelial tube, factors increasing pericyte abundance, as well as promoting angiogenic sprouting appear to be among the most promising targets to reduce the loss in capillaries during chronic.

One such agent can be found in the small peptide Thymosin β4. Thymosin β4 was first identified as an actin sequestering peptide binding G-actin in competition with Myocardin-related transcription factor A (MRTF-A) [85]. MRTF-A in its unbound form, i.e., free of G-actin binding, is capable to translocate into the nucleus, where it regulates the expression of SRF (serum response factor) target genes, in particular *CCN1* and *CCN2* [86]. CCN1 and CCN2 have been shown to promote angiogenic sprouting and vascular maturation via the recruitment of pericytes to newly formed vessels [87,88]. Increasing either the availability of Thymosin β4 or MRTF-A can promote MRTF-A nuclear translocation during chronic ischemia, as demonstrated in mouse and pig models of chronic limb ischemia as well as myocardial ischemia and reperfusion and hibernating myocardium [74,86,89]. Interestingly, Thymosin β4 has proven successful in improving myocardial perfusion in a model of chronic myocardial ischemia in otherwise healthy pigs and also hypercholesterolemic pigs and transgenic diabetic pigs [74,89], indicating its potential in the treatment of patients with underlying risk factors. Since arterial hypertension, hypercholesterolemia and diabetes mellitus are chronic disease states, a long term treatment seems preferable under these conditions. Thus, recombinant adeno-associated viral vectors (rAAV), as used in these studies, appear a favorable option, given their ability to facilitate long-term transgene expression with minimal genomic integration and low levels of host immune responses [90,91]. Another key regulator of angiogenic sprouting ameliorating capillary rarefication can be identified in vascular endothelial growth factor A (VEGF-A). VEGF-A promotes endothelial proliferation and tip-cell formation. However, long-term overexpression of VEGF-A leads to the formation of hemangioma-like structures with poor perfusion [92]. This effect can be prevented, when VEGF-A is administered as a combination treatment with a pericyte recruiting agent, such as PDGF-B, which stabilize newly formed vessels via the integration of pericytes into the sprouting vascular network [93]. Thus, a cotransfection of rabbits undergoing chronic hind limb ischemia with both rAAV.PDGF-B as well as rAAV. VEGF-A can induce collateral growth, increases capillary density and enhances the perfusion of the chronically occluded hind limb. Seeing as increased VEGF-A levels over prolonged periods of time lead to the formation of dysfunctional vessel, other modes of delivery might be advantageous. Overexpression of target genes in short bursts can be achieved via the transfection of modified RNA, which contains alternative nucleotides (pseudouridine, methylpseudouridine or 5-methyl-cytosine) to prevent TLR7/8 mediated host immune responses [94]. Using modRNA encoding for VEGF-A in mouse and pig models of chronic coronary occlusion, Carlsson et al. demonstrated a robust and short term VEGF-A expression, leading to an increase in both capillary and arteriole density. After proving the efficacy of an intramyocardial injection of VEGF-A modRNA, Gan et al. demonstrated in a recent phase Ia/b clinical study in diabetic patients, that localized injection of VEGF-A modRNA leads to a robust short term transgene expression without the induction of a significant immunresponse while locally improving perfusion [95]. Thus, capillary rarefication and loss of pericytes are treatment targets accessible for gene therapy approaches in vascular disease. However, other disease states accompanied by capillary rarefication might profit from similar gene therapy approaches, such as Duchenne muscular dystrophy (DMD). DMD is caused by mutations in the dystrophin gene, leading to the production of unstable, truncated and dysfunctional proteins [96,97]. While Duchenne muscular dystrophy is mostly recognized as a disease of the peripheral muscle and myocardium, it is also accompanied by capillary rarefication. This process contributes to the dire health status of patients afflicted by this genetic disorder by aggravating tissue ischemia [98]. In this context, our group was able to demonstrate that pigs lacking the exon 52 of the dystrophin gene (DMDΔ52), which leads to the expression of a similarly shortened and unstable dystrophin protein [99], also display a decrease in tissue capillary density and pericyte coverage. Once treated with rAAV containing a split Cas9 protein and guide RNAs targeting Exon 51, these animals not only regained expression of a functional dystrophin gene, but also showed a drastic improvement of tissue capillarization, a process accompanied by a reduction in CD68 positive macrophages (Figure 2, Moretti et al., Nature Medicine, accepted for publishing).

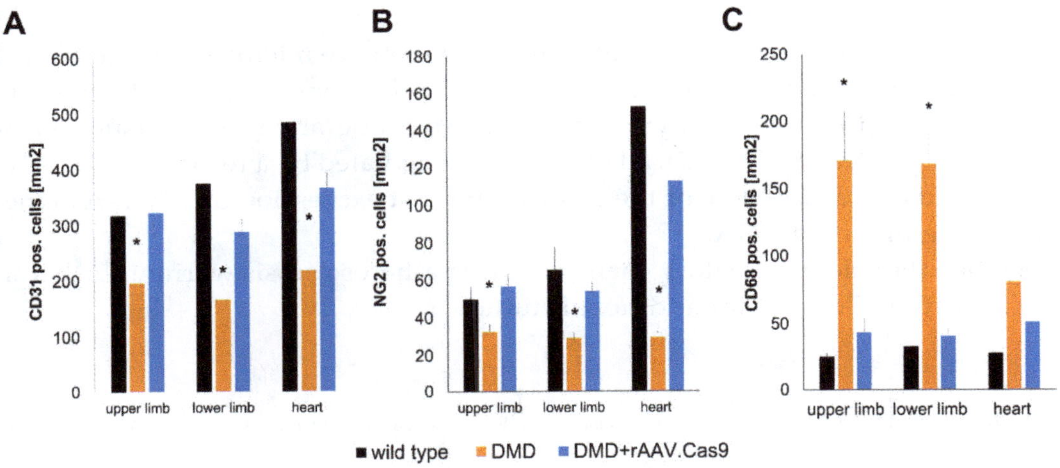

Figure 2. Effect of in vivo genome editing via rAAV and Cas9 mediated deletion of exon 51 of Duchenne muscular dystrophy on the vascularization and macrophage recruitment in the heart and upper and lower hind limb in DMDΔ52 pigs. (**A**) staining for CD31 positive endothelial cells highlights a significant decrease in capillary density in pigs suffering from Duchenne muscular dystrophy which ins ameliorated in pigs receiving Cas9 mediated Exon 51 deletion thus restoring dystrophin expression. (**B**) Similarly, edited DMD pigs display an amelioration of pericyte loss seen in dystrophin deficient pigs. (**C**) Lastly, the reduction in both endothelial cells as well as pericytes in dystrophin deficient pigs is accompanied by an increased recruitment of CD68 positive macrophages into the tissue, similarly to the recruitment seen in atherosclerotic states, which is again reversed upon normalization of dystrophin expression (*$p < 0.05$ versus wild type and DMD+rAAV.Cas9, error bars are given as SEM).

Interestingly, these findings combined highlight potential therapeutic strategies to target the rather neglected pathophysiological changes mediated by atherosclerotic risk factors in the microcirculation and represent a potential addition to the classical treatment strategies to ameliorate the disease burden of vascular occlusive disease.

5. Conclusions

Atherosclerosis represents a multifactorial disease mainly driven by arterial hypertension, hypercholesterolemia and diabetes mellitus, which, through the stenosis and occlusion of arteries, leads to organ ischemia and thus constitutes a main driver of mortality worldwide. The three main contributors to the development of atherosclerosis can originate from similar sources, such as sedentary lifestyle, western diet and obesity and exerted damage to the vessel wall via distinct but overlapping pathomechanisms. The hallmark of vascular alterations elicited by all three disease entities lies in the endothelial dysfunction seen in atherosclerosis, which is largely driven by an increase in endothelial activation with an elevated uptake of lipids, namely low-density lipoproteins, into the vascular wall.

This process triggers the production of reactive oxygen species as well as the attraction of macrophages to the site of plaque formation, leading to their transformation into foam cells. All of those pathological alterations can enter into a positive feedback loop aggravating the development of plaque formation. One additional component in this disease progression is the proliferation of vascular smooth muscle cells, which can participate in the uptake of oxidized LDL and can also transform into foam cells, which serve as a source for inflammatory cytokines, attracting more macrophages. Herein lies one key difference between the macrocirculation (e.g., larger arteries) and the microcirculation exemplified by capillaries. Capillaries are surrounded not by vascular smooth muscle cells but by pericytes, a cell type related to vascular smooth muscle cells but with distinct functions in the vascular unit. Unlike vSMCs, pericytes react to the pathological stimuli elicited by hyperglycemia and hypercholesterolemia with a detachment from the underlying endothelium, resulting in further endothelial activation and apoptosis. This leads to capillary rarefication and reduced blood flow due to a decrease in capillary surface area.

Here, we highlighted potential therapeutic targets to improve microvascular dysfunction, namely by expressing proangiogenic growth factors and pericyte chemoattractants, either combined in one signaling molecule (as is the case for Thymosin β4) or in a cooperative fashion (such as the combined overexpression of VEGF-A and PDGF-B), all of which are mediated by a recombinant adeno-associated viral vector mediated overexpression, or the short-term burst expression of VEGF-A alone in the form of VEGF-A encoding modified RNA.

Taken together, the microcirculatory changes during atherosclerosis warrant further investigation and represent a worthwhile topic for additional studies.

References

1. World Health Organization. *Cardiovascular Disease (CVDs)*; World Health Organization: Geneva, Switzerland, 2017.
2. Nakashima, Y.; Chen, Y.X.; Kinukawa, N.; Sueishi, K. Distributions of diffuse intimal thickening in human arteries: Preferential expression in atherosclerosis-prone arteries from an early age. *Virchows Arch.* **2002**, *441*, 279–288. [CrossRef]
3. Guyton, J.R.; Bocan, T.M.; Schifani, T.A. Quantitative ultrastructural analysis of perifibrous lipid and its association with elastin in nonatherosclerotic human aorta. *Arteriosclerosis* **1985**, *5*, 644–652. [CrossRef]
4. Tabas, I.; Williams, K.J.; Boren, J. Subendothelial lipoprotein retention as the initiating process in atherosclerosis: Update and therapeutic implications. *Circulation* **2007**, *116*, 1832–1844. [CrossRef]
5. Williams, K.J.; Tabas, I. The response-to-retention hypothesis of early atherogenesis. *Arterioscler. Thromb. Vasc. Biol.* **1995**, *15*, 551–561. [CrossRef]
6. Lee, R.T.; Yamamoto, C.; Feng, Y.; Potter-Perigo, S.; Briggs, W.H.; Landschulz, K.T.; Turi, T.G.; Thompson, J.F.; Libby, P.; Wight, T.N. Mechanical strain induces specific changes in the synthesis and organization of proteoglycans by vascular smooth muscle cells. *J. Biol. Chem.* **2001**, *276*, 13847–13851. [CrossRef]
7. Little, P.J.; Tannock, L.; Olin, K.L.; Chait, A.; Wight, T.N. Proteoglycans synthesized by arterial smooth muscle cells in the presence of transforming growth factor-beta1 exhibit increased binding to LDLs. *Arterioscler. Thromb. Vasc. Biol.* **2002**, *22*, 55–60. [CrossRef]
8. Cushing, S.D.; Berliner, J.A.; Valente, A.J.; Territo, M.C.; Navab, M.; Parhami, F.; Gerrity, R.; Schwartz, C.J.; Fogelman, A.M. Minimally modified low density lipoprotein induces monocyte chemotactic protein 1 in human endothelial cells and smooth muscle cells. *Proc. Natl. Acad. Sci. USA* **1990**, *87*, 5134–5138. [CrossRef]
9. Hurt-Camejo, E.; Camejo, G.; Rosengren, B.; Lopez, F.; Ahlstrom, C.; Fager, G.; Bondjers, G. Effect of arterial proteoglycans and glycosaminoglycans on low density lipoprotein oxidation and its uptake by human macrophages and arterial smooth muscle cells. *Arterioscler. Thromb.* **1992**, *12*, 569–583. [CrossRef]
10. Karakikes, I.; Chaanine, A.H.; Kang, S.; Mukete, B.N.; Jeong, D.; Zhang, S.; Hajjar, R.J.; Lebeche, D. Therapeutic cardiac-targeted delivery of miR-1 reverses pressure overload-induced cardiac hypertrophy and attenuates pathological remodeling. *J. Am. Heart Assoc.* **2013**, *2*, e000078. [CrossRef]
11. Kockx, M.M.; De Meyer, G.R.; Muhring, J.; Jacob, W.; Bult, H.; Herman, A.G. Apoptosis and related proteins in different stages of human atherosclerotic plaques. *Circulation* **1998**, *97*, 2307–2315. [CrossRef]

12. Merrilees, M.J.; Beaumont, B. Structural heterogeneity of the diffuse intimal thickening and correlation with distribution of TGF-beta 1. *J. Vasc. Res.* **1993**, *30*, 293–302. [CrossRef]
13. Murry, C.E.; Gipaya, C.T.; Bartosek, T.; Benditt, E.P.; Schwartz, S.M. Monoclonality of smooth muscle cells in human atherosclerosis. *Am. J. Pathol.* **1997**, *151*, 697–705.
14. Nakata, A.; Miyagawa, J.; Yamashita, S.; Nishida, M.; Tamura, R.; Yamamori, K.; Nakamura, T.; Nozaki, S.; Kameda-Takemura, K.; Kawata, S.; et al. Localization of heparin-binding epidermal growth factor-like growth factor in human coronary arteries. Possible roles of HB-EGF in the formation of coronary atherosclerosis. *Circulation* **1996**, *94*, 2778–2786. [CrossRef]
15. Alshehri, O.M.; Hughes, C.E.; Montague, S.; Watson, S.K.; Frampton, J.; Bender, M.; Watson, S.P. Fibrin activates GPVI in human and mouse platelets. *Blood* **2015**, *126*, 1601–1608. [CrossRef]
16. Naimushin, Y.A.; Mazurov, A.V. Von Willebrand factor can support platelet aggregation via interaction with activated GPIIb-IIIa and GPIb. *Platelets* **2004**, *15*, 419–425. [CrossRef]
17. Sarratt, K.L.; Chen, H.; Zutter, M.M.; Santoro, S.A.; Hammer, D.A.; Kahn, M.L. GPVI and alpha2beta1 play independent critical roles during platelet adhesion and aggregate formation to collagen under flow. *Blood* **2005**, *106*, 1268–1277. [CrossRef]
18. Cassese, S.; Byrne, R.A.; Tada, T.; Pinieck, S.; Joner, M.; Ibrahim, T.; King, L.A.; Fusaro, M.; Laugwitz, K.L.; Kastrati, A. Incidence and predictors of restenosis after coronary stenting in 10 004 patients with surveillance angiography. *Heart* **2014**, *100*, 153–159. [CrossRef]
19. Gray, W.A.; Keirse, K.; Soga, Y.; Benko, A.; Babaev, A.; Yokoi, Y.; Schroeder, H.; Prem, J.T.; Holden, A.; Popma, J.; et al. A polymer-coated, paclitaxel-eluting stent (Eluvia) versus a polymer-free, paclitaxel-coated stent (Zilver PTX) for endovascular femoropopliteal intervention (IMPERIAL): A randomised, non-inferiority trial. *Lancet* **2018**, *392*, 1541–1551. [CrossRef]
20. Sander, M.; Chavoshan, B.; Victor, R.G. A large blood pressure-raising effect of nitric oxide synthase inhibition in humans. *Hypertension* **1999**, *33*, 937–942. [CrossRef]
21. Bush, E.; Maeda, N.; Kuziel, W.A.; Dawson, T.C.; Wilcox, J.N.; DeLeon, H.; Taylor, W.R. CC chemokine receptor 2 is required for macrophage infiltration and vascular hypertrophy in angiotensin II-induced hypertension. *Hypertension* **2000**, *36*, 360–363. [CrossRef]
22. Ryan, M.J.; Didion, S.P.; Mathur, S.; Faraci, F.M.; Sigmund, C.D. Angiotensin II-induced vascular dysfunction is mediated by the AT1A receptor in mice. *Hypertension* **2004**, *43*, 1074–1079. [CrossRef]
23. Wang, H.D.; Xu, S.; Johns, D.G.; Du, Y.; Quinn, M.T.; Cayatte, A.J.; Cohen, R.A. Role of NADPH oxidase in the vascular hypertrophic and oxidative stress response to angiotensin II in mice. *Circ. Res.* **2001**, *88*, 947–953. [CrossRef]
24. World Health Organization. *Global Health Observatory*; World Health Organization: Geneva, Switzerland, 2018.
25. Landsberg, L.; Aronne, L.J.; Beilin, L.J.; Burke, V.; Igel, L.I.; Lloyd-Jones, D.; Sowers, J. Obesity-related hypertension: Pathogenesis, cardiovascular risk, and treatment—A position paper of the The Obesity Society and The American Society of Hypertension. *Obesity* **2013**, *21*, 8–24. [CrossRef]
26. Nahrendorf, M.; Swirski, F.K. Lifestyle effects on hematopoiesis and atherosclerosis. *Circ. Res.* **2015**, *116*, 884–894. [CrossRef]
27. Gimbrone, M.A., Jr.; Garcia-Cardena, G. Vascular endothelium, hemodynamics, and the pathobiology of atherosclerosis. *Cardiovasc. Pathol.* **2013**, *22*, 9–15. [CrossRef]
28. Fogelstrand, P.; Boren, J. Retention of atherogenic lipoproteins in the artery wall and its role in atherogenesis. *Nutr. Metab. Cardiovasc. Dis.* **2012**, *22*, 1–7. [CrossRef]
29. Iverius, P.H. The interaction between human plasma lipoproteins and connective tissue glycosaminoglycans. *J. Biol. Chem.* **1972**, *247*, 2607–2613.
30. Flood, C.; Gustafsson, M.; Pitas, R.E.; Arnaboldi, L.; Walzem, R.L.; Boren, J. Molecular mechanism for changes in proteoglycan binding on compositional changes of the core and the surface of low-density lipoprotein-containing human apolipoprotein B100. *Arterioscler. Thromb. Vasc. Biol.* **2004**, *24*, 564–570. [CrossRef]
31. Ungvari, Z.; Wolin, M.S.; Csiszar, A. Mechanosensitive production of reactive oxygen species in endothelial and smooth muscle cells: Role in microvascular remodeling? *Antioxid. Redox Signal.* **2006**, *8*, 1121–1129. [CrossRef]
32. Krieger, M. Scavenger receptor class B type I is a multiligand HDL receptor that influences diverse physiologic systems. *J. Clin. Investig.* **2001**, *108*, 793–797. [CrossRef]

33. Lara-Guzman, O.J.; Gil-Izquierdo, A.; Medina, S.; Osorio, E.; Alvarez-Quintero, R.; Zuluaga, N.; Oger, C.; Galano, J.M.; Durand, T.; Munoz-Durango, K. Oxidized LDL triggers changes in oxidative stress and inflammatory biomarkers in human macrophages. *Redox Biol.* **2018**, *15*, 1–11. [CrossRef]
34. Khan, B.V.; Parthasarathy, S.S.; Alexander, R.W.; Medford, R.M. Modified low density lipoprotein and its constituents augment cytokine-activated vascular cell adhesion molecule-1 gene expression in human vascular endothelial cells. *J. Clin. Investig.* **1995**, *95*, 1262–1270. [CrossRef]
35. Vora, D.K.; Fang, Z.T.; Liva, S.M.; Tyner, T.R.; Parhami, F.; Watson, A.D.; Drake, T.A.; Territo, M.C.; Berliner, J.A. Induction of P-selectin by oxidized lipoproteins. Separate effects on synthesis and surface expression. *Circ. Res.* **1997**, *80*, 810–818. [CrossRef]
36. Berliner, J.A.; Schwartz, D.S.; Territo, M.C.; Andalibi, A.; Almada, L.; Lusis, A.J.; Quismorio, D.; Fang, Z.P.; Fogelman, A.M. Induction of chemotactic cytokines by minimally oxidized LDL. *Adv. Exp. Med. Biol.* **1993**, *351*, 13–18. [CrossRef]
37. Brownlee, M. Biochemistry and molecular cell biology of diabetic complications. *Nature* **2001**, *414*, 813–820. [CrossRef]
38. Wautier, M.P.; Chappey, O.; Corda, S.; Stern, D.M.; Schmidt, A.M.; Wautier, J.L. Activation of NADPH oxidase by AGE links oxidant stress to altered gene expression via RAGE. *Am. J. Physiol. Endocrinol. Metab.* **2001**, *280*, E685–E694. [CrossRef]
39. Basta, G.; Schmidt, A.M.; De Caterina, R. Advanced glycation end products and vascular inflammation: Implications for accelerated atherosclerosis in diabetes. *Cardiovasc. Res.* **2004**, *63*, 582–592. [CrossRef]
40. Neumann, A.; Schinzel, R.; Palm, D.; Riederer, P.; Munch, G. High molecular weight hyaluronic acid inhibits advanced glycation endproduct-induced NF-kappaB activation and cytokine expression. *FEBS Lett.* **1999**, *453*, 283–287. [CrossRef]
41. Iwashima, Y.; Eto, M.; Hata, A.; Kaku, K.; Horiuchi, S.; Ushikubi, F.; Sano, H. Advanced glycation end products-induced gene expression of scavenger receptors in cultured human monocyte-derived macrophages. *Biochem. Biophys. Res. Commun.* **2000**, *277*, 368–380. [CrossRef]
42. Ziegler, T.; Horstkotte, M.; Lange, P.; Ng, J.; Bongiovanni, D.; Hinkel, R.; Laugwitz, K.L.; Sperandio, M.; Horstkotte, J.; Kupatt, C. Endothelial RAGE exacerbates acute postischaemic cardiac inflammation. *Thromb. Haemost.* **2016**, *116*, 300–308. [CrossRef]
43. Natarajan, R.; Gerrity, R.G.; Gu, J.L.; Lanting, L.; Thomas, L.; Nadler, J.L. Role of 12-lipoxygenase and oxidant stress in hyperglycaemia-induced acceleration of atherosclerosis in a diabetic pig model. *Diabetologia* **2002**, *45*, 125–133. [CrossRef]
44. Wu, L.; Vikramadithyan, R.; Yu, S.; Pau, C.; Hu, Y.; Goldberg, I.J.; Dansky, H.M. Addition of dietary fat to cholesterol in the diets of LDL receptor knockout mice: Effects on plasma insulin, lipoproteins, and atherosclerosis. *J. Lipid Res.* **2006**, *47*, 2215–2222. [CrossRef]
45. Ho, K.L. Ultrastructure of cerebellar capillary hemangioblastoma. IV. Pericytes and their relationship to endothelial cells. *Acta Neuropathol.* **1985**, *67*, 254–264. [CrossRef]
46. Larson, D.M.; Carson, M.P.; Haudenschild, C.C. Junctional transfer of small molecules in cultured bovine brain microvascular endothelial cells and pericytes. *Microvasc. Res.* **1987**, *34*, 184–199. [CrossRef]
47. Rucker, H.K.; Wynder, H.J.; Thomas, W.E. Cellular mechanisms of CNS pericytes. *Brain Res. Bull.* **2000**, *51*, 363–369. [CrossRef]
48. Davis, S.; Aldrich, T.H.; Jones, P.F.; Acheson, A.; Compton, D.L.; Jain, V.; Ryan, T.E.; Bruno, J.; Radziejewski, C.; Maisonpierre, P.C.; et al. Isolation of angiopoietin-1, a ligand for the TIE2 receptor, by secretion-trap expression cloning. *Cell* **1996**, *87*, 1161–1169. [CrossRef]
49. Cardone, M.H.; Roy, N.; Stennicke, H.R.; Salvesen, G.S.; Franke, T.F.; Stanbridge, E.; Frisch, S.; Reed, J.C. Regulation of cell death protease caspase-9 by phosphorylation. *Science* **1998**, *282*, 1318–1321. [CrossRef]
50. Papapetropoulos, A.; Fulton, D.; Mahboubi, K.; Kalb, R.G.; O'Connor, D.S.; Li, F.; Altieri, D.C.; Sessa, W.C. Angiopoietin-1 inhibits endothelial cell apoptosis via the Akt/survivin pathway. *J. Biol. Chem.* **2000**, *275*, 9102–9105. [CrossRef]
51. Kobayashi, H.; DeBusk, L.M.; Babichev, Y.O.; Dumont, D.J.; Lin, P.C. Hepatocyte growth factor mediates angiopoietin-induced smooth muscle cell recruitment. *Blood* **2006**, *108*, 1260–1266. [CrossRef]
52. Iivanainen, E.; Nelimarkka, L.; Elenius, V.; Heikkinen, S.M.; Junttila, T.T.; Sihombing, L.; Sundvall, M.; Maatta, J.A.; Laine, V.J.; Yla-Herttuala, S.; et al. Angiopoietin-regulated recruitment of vascular smooth muscle cells by endothelial-derived heparin binding EGF-like growth factor. *FASEB J. Off. Publ. Fed. Am. Soc. Exp. Biol.* **2003**, *17*, 1609–1621. [CrossRef]

53. Orlidge, A.; D'Amore, P.A. Inhibition of capillary endothelial cell growth by pericytes and smooth muscle cells. *J. Cell Biol.* **1987**, *105*, 1455–1462. [CrossRef] [PubMed]
54. Marra, F.; Bonewald, L.F.; Park-Snyder, S.; Park, I.S.; Woodruff, K.A.; Abboud, H.E. Characterization and regulation of the latent transforming growth factor-beta complex secreted by vascular pericytes. *J. Cell. Physiol.* **1996**, *166*, 537–546. [CrossRef]
55. Watanabe, S.; Morisaki, N.; Tezuka, M.; Fukuda, K.; Ueda, S.; Koyama, N.; Yokote, K.; Kanzaki, T.; Yoshida, S.; Saito, Y. Cultured retinal pericytes stimulate in vitro angiogenesis of endothelial cells through secretion of a fibroblast growth factor-like molecule. *Atherosclerosis* **1997**, *130*, 101–107. [CrossRef]
56. Takagi, H.; King, G.L.; Robinson, G.S.; Ferrara, N.; Aiello, L.P. Adenosine mediates hypoxic induction of vascular endothelial growth factor in retinal pericytes and endothelial cells. *Investig. Ophthalmol. Vis. Sci.* **1996**, *37*, 2165–2176.
57. Austin, K.M.; Nguyen, N.; Javid, G.; Covic, L.; Kuliopulos, A. Noncanonical matrix metalloprotease-1-protease-activated receptor-1 signaling triggers vascular smooth muscle cell dedifferentiation and arterial stenosis. *J. Biol. Chem.* **2013**, *288*, 23105–23115. [CrossRef] [PubMed]
58. Pfister, F.; Feng, Y.; vom Hagen, F.; Hoffmann, S.; Molema, G.; Hillebrands, J.L.; Shani, M.; Deutsch, U.; Hammes, H.P. Pericyte migration: A novel mechanism of pericyte loss in experimental diabetic retinopathy. *Diabetes* **2008**, *57*, 2495–2502. [CrossRef]
59. Zehendner, C.M.; Wedler, H.E.; Luhmann, H.J. A novel in vitro model to study pericytes in the neurovascular unit of the developing cortex. *PLoS ONE* **2013**, *8*, e81637. [CrossRef]
60. Ziegler, T.; Horstkotte, J.; Schwab, C.; Pfetsch, V.; Weinmann, K.; Dietzel, S.; Rohwedder, I.; Hinkel, R.; Gross, L.; Lee, S.; et al. Angiopoietin 2 mediates microvascular and hemodynamic alterations in sepsis. *J. Clin. Investig.* **2013**, *123*, 3436–3445. [CrossRef]
61. Herman, I.M.; Jacobson, S. In situ analysis of microvascular pericytes in hypertensive rat brains. *Tissue Cell* **1988**, *20*, 1–12. [CrossRef]
62. Wallow, I.H.; Bindley, C.D.; Reboussin, D.M.; Gange, S.J.; Fisher, M.R. Systemic hypertension produces pericyte changes in retinal capillaries. *Investig. Ophthalmol. Vis. Sci.* **1993**, *34*, 420–430.
63. Ricard, N.; Tu, L.; Le Hiress, M.; Huertas, A.; Phan, C.; Thuillet, R.; Sattler, C.; Fadel, E.; Seferian, A.; Montani, D.; et al. Increased pericyte coverage mediated by endothelial-derived fibroblast growth factor-2 and interleukin-6 is a source of smooth muscle-like cells in pulmonary hypertension. *Circulation* **2014**, *129*, 1586–1597. [CrossRef] [PubMed]
64. Chen, I.I.; Prewitt, R.L.; Dowell, R.F. Microvascular rarefaction in spontaneously hypertensive rat cremaster muscle. *Am. J. Physiol.* **1981**, *241*, H306–H310. [CrossRef] [PubMed]
65. Cheng, C.; Daskalakis, C.; Falkner, B. Capillary rarefaction in treated and untreated hypertensive subjects. *Ther. Adv. Cardiovasc. Dis.* **2008**, *2*, 79–88. [CrossRef] [PubMed]
66. Wolfle, S.E.; de Wit, C. Intact endothelium-dependent dilation and conducted responses in resistance vessels of hypercholesterolemic mice in vivo. *J. Vasc. Res.* **2005**, *42*, 475–482. [CrossRef]
67. Steinberg, H.O.; Bayazeed, B.; Hook, G.; Johnson, A.; Cronin, J.; Baron, A.D. Endothelial dysfunction is associated with cholesterol levels in the high normal range in humans. *Circulation* **1997**, *96*, 3287–3293. [CrossRef]
68. Ha, J.M.; Jin, S.Y.; Lee, H.S.; Shin, H.K.; Lee, D.H.; Song, S.H.; Kim, C.D.; Bae, S.S. Regulation of retinal angiogenesis by endothelial nitric oxide synthase signaling pathway. *Korean J. Physiol. Pharmacol.* **2016**, *20*, 533–538. [CrossRef]
69. Garcia-Quintans, N.; Sanchez-Ramos, C.; Prieto, I.; Tierrez, A.; Arza, E.; Alfranca, A.; Redondo, J.M.; Monsalve, M. Oxidative stress induces loss of pericyte coverage and vascular instability in PGC-1alpha-deficient mice. *Angiogenesis* **2016**, *19*, 217–228. [CrossRef]
70. Radice, G.L. N-cadherin-mediated adhesion and signaling from development to disease: Lessons from mice. *Prog. Mol. Biol. Transl. Sci.* **2013**, *116*, 263–289. [CrossRef]
71. Zechariah, A.; ElAli, A.; Hagemann, N.; Jin, F.; Doeppner, T.R.; Helfrich, I.; Mies, G.; Hermann, D.M. Hyperlipidemia attenuates vascular endothelial growth factor-induced angiogenesis, impairs cerebral blood flow, and disturbs stroke recovery via decreased pericyte coverage of brain endothelial cells. *Arterioscler. Thromb. Vasc. Biol.* **2013**, *33*, 1561–1567. [CrossRef]

72. Beltramo, E.; Porta, M. Pericyte loss in diabetic retinopathy: Mechanisms and consequences. *Curr. Med. Chem.* **2013**, *20*, 3218–3225. [CrossRef]
73. Kim, Y.H.; Park, S.Y.; Park, J.; Kim, Y.S.; Hwang, E.M.; Park, J.Y.; Roh, G.S.; Kim, H.J.; Kang, S.S.; Cho, G.J.; et al. Reduction of experimental diabetic vascular leakage and pericyte apoptosis in mice by delivery of alphaA-crystallin with a recombinant adenovirus. *Diabetologia* **2012**, *55*, 2835–2844. [CrossRef] [PubMed]
74. Hinkel, R.; Howe, A.; Renner, S.; Ng, J.; Lee, S.; Klett, K.; Kaczmarek, V.; Moretti, A.; Laugwitz, K.L.; Skroblin, P.; et al. Diabetes Mellitus-Induced Microvascular Destabilization in the Myocardium. *J. Am. Coll. Cardiol.* **2017**, *69*, 131–143. [CrossRef] [PubMed]
75. Yamagishi, S.; Takeuchi, M.; Matsui, T.; Nakamura, K.; Imaizumi, T.; Inoue, H. Angiotensin II augments advanced glycation end product-induced pericyte apoptosis through RAGE overexpression. *FEBS Lett.* **2005**, *579*, 4265–4270. [CrossRef] [PubMed]
76. Fiordaliso, F.; Cuccovillo, I.; Bianchi, R.; Bai, A.; Doni, M.; Salio, M.; De Angelis, N.; Ghezzi, P.; Latini, R.; Masson, S. Cardiovascular oxidative stress is reduced by an ACE inhibitor in a rat model of streptozotocin-induced diabetes. *Life Sci.* **2006**, *79*, 121–129. [CrossRef]
77. Lupo, E.; Locher, R.; Weisser, B.; Vetter, W. In vitro antioxidant activity of calcium antagonists against LDL oxidation compared with alpha-tocopherol. *Biochem. Biophys. Res. Commun.* **1994**, *203*, 1803–1808. [CrossRef]
78. Algire, C.; Moiseeva, O.; Deschenes-Simard, X.; Amrein, L.; Petruccelli, L.; Birman, E.; Viollet, B.; Ferbeyre, G.; Pollak, M.N. Metformin reduces endogenous reactive oxygen species and associated DNA damage. *Cancer Prev. Res.* **2012**, *5*, 536–543. [CrossRef]
79. Sabatine, M.S.; Leiter, L.A.; Wiviott, S.D.; Giugliano, R.P.; Deedwania, P.; De Ferrari, G.M.; Murphy, S.A.; Kuder, J.F.; Gouni-Berthold, I.; Lewis, B.S.; et al. Cardiovascular safety and efficacy of the PCSK9 inhibitor evolocumab in patients with and without diabetes and the effect of evolocumab on glycaemia and risk of new-onset diabetes: A prespecified analysis of the FOURIER randomised controlled trial. *Lancet Diabetes Endocrinol.* **2017**, *5*, 941–950. [CrossRef]
80. Inoue, I.; Goto, S.; Mizotani, K.; Awata, T.; Mastunaga, T.; Kawai, S.; Nakajima, T.; Hokari, S.; Komoda, T.; Katayama, S. Lipophilic HMG-CoA reductase inhibitor has an anti-inflammatory effect: Reduction of MRNA levels for interleukin-1beta, interleukin-6, cyclooxygenase-2, and p22phox by regulation of peroxisome proliferator-activated receptor alpha (PPARalpha) in primary endothelial cells. *Life Sci.* **2000**, *67*, 863–876. [CrossRef]
81. Bouitbir, J.; Charles, A.L.; Echaniz-Laguna, A.; Kindo, M.; Daussin, F.; Auwerx, J.; Piquard, F.; Geny, B.; Zoll, J. Opposite effects of statins on mitochondria of cardiac and skeletal muscles: A 'mitohormesis' mechanism involving reactive oxygen species and PGC-1. *Eur. Heart J.* **2012**, *33*, 1397–1407. [CrossRef]
82. Raiteri, M.; Arnaboldi, L.; McGeady, P.; Gelb, M.H.; Verri, D.; Tagliabue, C.; Quarato, P.; Ferraboschi, P.; Santaniello, E.; Paoletti, R.; et al. Pharmacological control of the mevalonate pathway: Effect on arterial smooth muscle cell proliferation. *J. Pharmcol. Exp. Ther.* **1997**, *281*, 1144–1153.
83. Tokuda, T.; Hirano, K.; Sakamoto, Y.; Takimura, H.; Kobayashi, N.; Araki, M.; Yamawaki, M.; Ito, Y. Incidence and clinical outcomes of the slow-flow phenomenon after infrapopliteal balloon angioplasty. *J. Vasc. Surg.* **2017**, *65*, 1047–1054. [CrossRef] [PubMed]
84. Harrison, R.W.; Aggarwal, A.; Ou, F.S.; Klein, L.W.; Rumsfeld, J.S.; Roe, M.T.; Wang, T.Y.; American College of Cardiology National Cardiovascular Data, Registry. Incidence and outcomes of no-reflow phenomenon during percutaneous coronary intervention among patients with acute myocardial infarction. *Am. J. Cardiol.* **2013**, *111*, 178–184. [CrossRef] [PubMed]
85. Morita, T.; Hayashi, K. G-actin sequestering protein thymosin-beta4 regulates the activity of myocardin-related transcription factor. *Biochem. Biophys. Res. Commun.* **2013**, *437*, 331–335. [CrossRef] [PubMed]
86. Hinkel, R.; Trenkwalder, T.; Petersen, B.; Husada, W.; Gesenhues, F.; Lee, S.; Hannappel, E.; Bock-Marquette, I.; Theisen, D.; Leitner, L.; et al. MRTF-A controls vessel growth and maturation by increasing the expression of CCN1 and CCN2. *Nat. Commun.* **2014**, *5*, 3970. [CrossRef]
87. Hall-Glenn, F.; De Young, R.A.; Huang, B.L.; van Handel, B.; Hofmann, J.J.; Chen, T.T.; Choi, A.; Ong, J.R.; Benya, P.D.; Mikkola, H.; et al. CCN2/connective tissue growth factor is essential for pericyte adhesion and endothelial basement membrane formation during angiogenesis. *PLoS ONE* **2012**, *7*, e30562. [CrossRef]

88. Hanna, M.; Liu, H.; Amir, J.; Sun, Y.; Morris, S.W.; Siddiqui, M.A.; Lau, L.F.; Chaqour, B. Mechanical regulation of the proangiogenic factor CCN1/CYR61 gene requires the combined activities of MRTF-A and CREB-binding protein histone acetyltransferase. *J. Biol. Chem.* **2009**, *284*, 23125–23136. [CrossRef]
89. Ziegler, T.; Bahr, A.; Howe, A.; Klett, K.; Husada, W.; Weber, C.; Laugwitz, K.L.; Kupatt, C.; Hinkel, R. Tbeta4 Increases Neovascularization and Cardiac Function in Chronic Myocardial Ischemia of Normo- and Hypercholesterolemic Pigs. *Mol. Ther.* **2018**, *26*, 1706–1714. [CrossRef]
90. Chirmule, N.; Propert, K.; Magosin, S.; Qian, Y.; Qian, R.; Wilson, J. Immune responses to adenovirus and adeno-associated virus in humans. *Gene Ther.* **1999**, *6*, 1574–1583. [CrossRef]
91. Nowrouzi, A.; Penaud-Budloo, M.; Kaeppel, C.; Appelt, U.; Le Guiner, C.; Moullier, P.; von Kalle, C.; Snyder, R.O.; Schmidt, M. Integration frequency and intermolecular recombination of rAAV vectors in non-human primate skeletal muscle and liver. *Mol. Ther.* **2012**, *20*, 1177–1186. [CrossRef]
92. Yla-Herttuala, S.; Rissanen, T.T.; Vajanto, I.; Hartikainen, J. Vascular endothelial growth factors: Biology and current status of clinical applications in cardiovascular medicine. *J. Am. Coll. Cardiol.* **2007**, *49*, 1015–1026. [CrossRef]
93. Hellstrom, M.; Kalen, M.; Lindahl, P.; Abramsson, A.; Betsholtz, C. Role of PDGF-B and PDGFR-beta in recruitment of vascular smooth muscle cells and pericytes during embryonic blood vessel formation in the mouse. *Development* **1999**, *126*, 3047–3055. [PubMed]
94. Kariko, K.; Buckstein, M.; Ni, H.; Weissman, D. Suppression of RNA recognition by Toll-like receptors: The impact of nucleoside modification and the evolutionary origin of RNA. *Immunity* **2005**, *23*, 165–175. [CrossRef] [PubMed]
95. Gan, L.M.; Lagerstrom-Fermer, M.; Carlsson, L.G.; Arfvidsson, C.; Egnell, A.C.; Rudvik, A.; Kjaer, M.; Collen, A.; Thompson, J.D.; Joyal, J.; et al. Intradermal delivery of modified mRNA encoding VEGF-A in patients with type 2 diabetes. *Nat. Commun.* **2019**, *10*, 871. [CrossRef] [PubMed]
96. Aartsma-Rus, A.; Van Deutekom, J.C.; Fokkema, I.F.; Van Ommen, G.J.; Den Dunnen, J.T. Entries in the Leiden Duchenne muscular dystrophy mutation database: An overview of mutation types and paradoxical cases that confirm the reading-frame rule. *Muscle Nerve* **2006**, *34*, 135–144. [CrossRef] [PubMed]
97. White, S.; Kalf, M.; Liu, Q.; Villerius, M.; Engelsma, D.; Kriek, M.; Vollebregt, E.; Bakker, B.; van Ommen, G.J.; Breuning, M.H.; et al. Comprehensive detection of genomic duplications and deletions in the DMD gene, by use of multiplex amplifiable probe hybridization. *Am. J. Hum. Genet.* **2002**, *71*, 365–374. [CrossRef] [PubMed]
98. Shimizu-Motohashi, Y.; Asakura, A. Angiogenesis as a novel therapeutic strategy for Duchenne muscular dystrophy through decreased ischemia and increased satellite cells. *Front. Physiol.* **2014**, *5*, 50. [CrossRef]
99. Klymiuk, N.; Blutke, A.; Graf, A.; Krause, S.; Burkhardt, K.; Wuensch, A.; Krebs, S.; Kessler, B.; Zakhartchenko, V.; Kurome, M.; et al. Dystrophin-deficient pigs provide new insights into the hierarchy of physiological derangements of dystrophic muscle. *Hum. Mol. Genet.* **2013**, *22*, 4368–4382. [CrossRef]

6

Collateral Vessels have Unique Endothelial and Smooth Muscle Cell Phenotypes

Hua Zhang, Dan Chalothorn and James E Faber *

Department of Cell Biology and Physiology, Curriculum in Neuroscience, McAllister Heart Institute, University of North Carolina, Chapel Hill, NC 27599-7545, USA

* Correspondence: jefaber@med.unc.edu

Abstract: Collaterals are unique blood vessels present in the microcirculation of most tissues that, by cross-connecting a small fraction of the outer branches of adjacent arterial trees, provide alternate routes of perfusion. However, collaterals are especially susceptible to rarefaction caused by aging, other vascular risk factors, and mouse models of Alzheimer's disease—a vulnerability attributed to the disturbed hemodynamic environment in the watershed regions where they reside. We examined the hypothesis that endothelial and smooth muscle cells (ECs and SMCs, respectively) of collaterals have specializations, distinct from those of similarly-sized nearby distal-most arterioles (DMAs) that maintain collateral integrity despite their continuous exposure to low and oscillatory/disturbed shear stress, high wall stress, and low blood oxygen. Examination of mouse brain revealed the following: Unlike the pro-inflammatory cobble-stoned morphology of ECs exposed to low/oscillatory shear stress elsewhere in the vasculature, collateral ECs are aligned with the vessel axis. Primary cilia, which sense shear stress, are present, unexpectedly, on ECs of collaterals and DMAs but are less abundant on collaterals. Unlike DMAs, collaterals are continuously invested with SMCs, have increased expression of *Pycard, Ki67, Pdgfb, Angpt2, Dll4, Ephrinb2*, and eNOS, and maintain expression of *Klf2/4*. Collaterals lack tortuosity when first formed during development, but tortuosity becomes evident within days after birth, progresses through middle age, and then declines—results consistent with the concept that collateral wall cells have a higher turnover rate than DMAs that favors proliferative senescence and collateral rarefaction. In conclusion, endothelial and SMCs of collaterals have morphologic and functional differences from those of nearby similarly sized arterioles. Future studies are required to determine if they represent specializations that counterbalance the disturbed hemodynamic, pro-inflammatory, and pro-proliferative environment in which collaterals reside and thus mitigate their risk factor-induced rarefaction.

Keywords: collateral circulation; cerebral collaterals; endothelial cells; ischemic stroke; primary cilia

---

1. Introduction

Obstructive disease, i.e., stroke and atherosclerosis of the coronary and peripheral arteries, is the leading cause of morbidity and mortality. Collateral circulation, which is composed of anastomotic vessels called collaterals, is the most important system capable of mitigating the effects of obstructive disease [1–5]. However, the number and diameter of collaterals in tissues vary greatly among individuals for reasons that are only beginning to be understood [1]. Moreover, little is known about the basic biology of collaterals, in part because of their small diameter and low density in tissues, difficulty in distinguishing them from other vessels, and lack of methodologies allowing study of their endothelial cells (ECs) and smooth muscle cells (SMCs) in cell culture. It is known, however, that collaterals are unique with regard to their: mechanism of formation during development (collaterogenesis) and its high sensitivity to genetic background-dependent variation, anatomic location in the circulation, hemodynamic forces acting on their ECs and SMCs, hallmark tortuosity, high susceptibility to risk factor-induced rarefaction, robust shear stress-dependent outward remodeling, and protective function in ischemic disease [1–5].

In mice, collaterals form late during gestation by the sprouting of ephrin-B2$^+$ ECs off of a small number of distal arterioles that subsequently undergo a tip cell-led proliferation, migration, and lumenization process to establish anastomoses between adjacent arterial trees [6–8]. This process varies greatly due to naturally-occurring polymorphisms in certain genes in the collaterogenesis pathway, resulting in wide differences in collateral extent and thus collateral-dependent blood flow and tissue injury in experimental models of occlusive arterial disease [9–11]. Collateral blood flow also varies widely in humans suffering stroke [3,4], coronary, and peripheral artery diseases [12,13], with recent evidence supporting involvement of the same key variant gene identified in the mouse [14]. Since collaterals interconnect adjacent arterial trees, there is little or no pressure drop across them in the absence of obstructive disease. Thus, blood flow within collaterals is near zero, oscillating slowly toward one or the other tree that they anastomose [6,15]. Endothelial cells and SMCs that compose the collateral wall are therefore continuously exposed to low and disturbed shear stress, high circumferential wall stress, and low blood oxygen content. Accompanying this adverse hemodynamic environment, which favors vascular inflammation and endothelial dysfunction elsewhere in the circulation, collaterals in mice undergo a progressive decline in number and a loss of diameter with aging, presence of vascular risk factors, and in models of Alzheimer's disease [16–21]. Supportive evidence, based on measurement of collateral-dependent flow induced by acute ischemic stroke, has been reported in humans with aging and presence of vascular risk factors [22–24]. This so call "collateral rarefaction" has been linked in mice to chronic low-level inflammation, endothelial dysfunction, and increased proliferation of collateral ECs and SMCs [16–20,25]. Collaterals are also capable of undergoing robust anatomic outward remodeling in steno-occlusive disease, compared to similarly sized arterioles [2,5,9,10]. Additionally, different from arterioles in the trees that they interconnect, collaterals lack myogenic responsiveness and have less SMC tone at baseline [26,27].

Despite these important unique features of collaterals, no studies have examined cellular and molecular aspects of their endothelial and smooth muscle cells to determine whether they differ from those of similarly sized arterioles. For example, blood flow in arteries and arterioles of healthy tissues, and thus fluid shear stress experienced by their ECs, is laminar, orthograde, and high velocity, with the exception of the inner curvature of the aortic arch and sites immediately downstream of arterial bifurcations where flow varies from high-velocity and orthograde to low-velocity with transient flow reversals in a fraction of the fluid laminae during each cardiac cycle (i.e., "disturbed" flow) [28–31]. Endothelial cells at these sites of disturbed shear stress are cobblestone in shape, as opposed to elsewhere where they are elongated and aligned with the vessel axis. They also evidence higher levels of proliferation, apoptosis, permeability, lipid uptake, oxidative stress, and markers of inflammation and aging, i.e., displaying the well-known pro-atherogenic EC phenotype specific to these sites. Flow and shear stress in collaterals in the absence of obstruction share similarly disturbed conditions [6,15]. Yet this is the normal environment in which collateral ECs and SMCs reside.

The purpose of this study was to examine the hypothesis that collateral ECs and SMCs express unique morphological and functional phenotypes that serve as adaptations or specializations to maintain the integrity of the collateral wall and balance against collateral rarefaction favored by the low and disturbed shear stress, high wall stress, and low blood oxygen levels—the latter caused by low flow-induced hemoglobin unloading to tissue. Such differences, if present, could offer insights into how collaterals are able to persist in healthy individuals but also why they are so susceptible to rarefaction with aging and other vascular risk factors. In addition, knowledge concerning the molecular features of collateral wall cells is fundamental to better understand how collaterals form during development, remodel in obstructive disease, and undergo risk factor-induced rarefaction, and to investigate possible treatments to augment or intervene with these processes.

2. Results

2.1. Collateral Endothelial Cells Are Aligned with the Vessel Axis Despite their Chronic Exposure to Low and Oscillatory Shear Stress

As a first-test of the hypothesis that collateral wall cells have unique phenotypes, we assessed the orientation of collateral ECs using scanning electron microscopy (SEM) and staining of the junctional protein zona occludens-1 (ZO-1). Despite the unique low and disturbed shear stress present in collaterals, ECs of collaterals were aligned with the vessel axis to the same extent, i.e., ~4 degrees off the longitudinal axis, which was present in nearby distal-most arterioles (DMAs) and in the descending thoracic aorta where blood flow is high-velocity and laminar (Figures 1 and 2). The area, perimeter, length, and width of collateral ECs were also comparable to ECs lining DMAs (Figure S1).

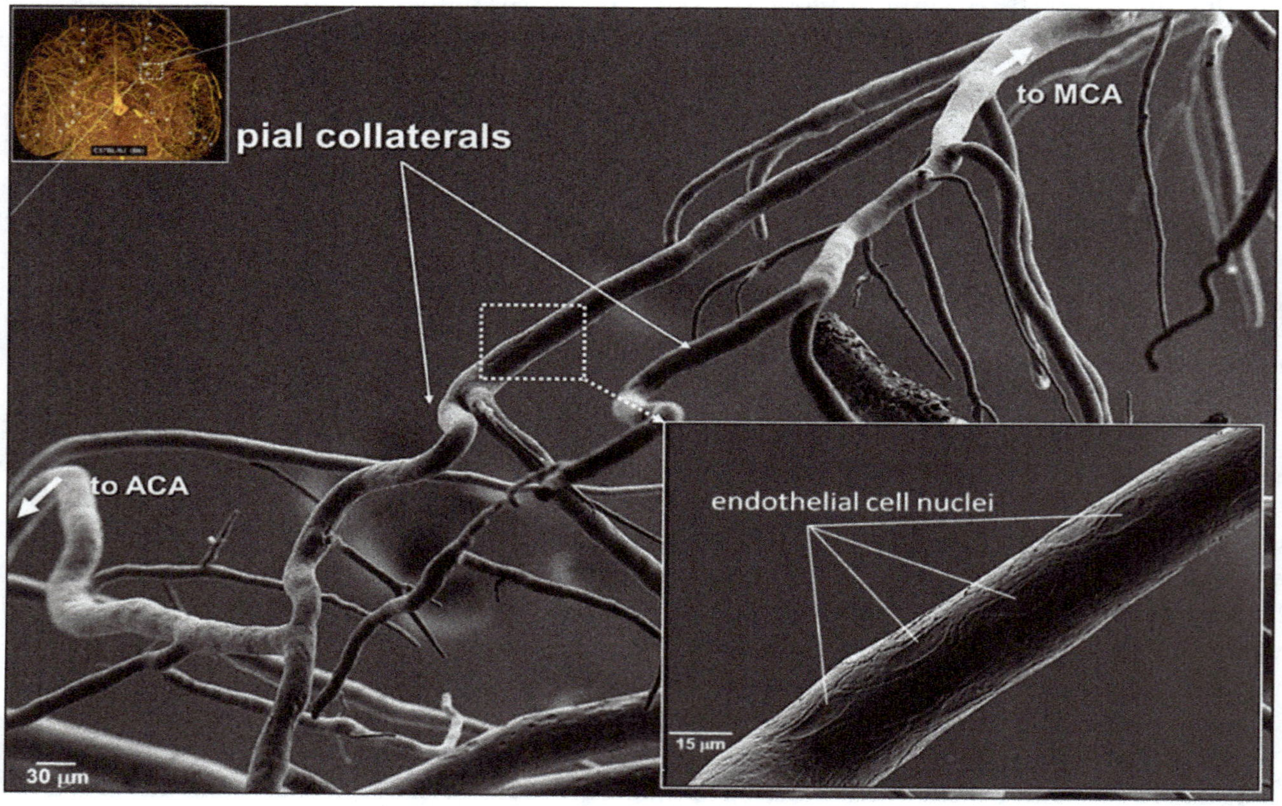

Figure 1. Pial collateral endothelial cells are aligned with the vessel axis. Scanning electron micrograph (SEM) of a corrosion cast of Batson's #17-filled cerebral pial arterial vessels and 2 collaterals, fixed after maximal dilation, which overlie the watershed zone between the anterior (ACA) and middle (MCA) cerebral artery trees. Upper inset, Microfil® cast of arterial vessels and collaterals (stars) in optically cleared brain. SEMs were obtained from six mice (see also Figure S1). Penetrating arterioles are evident branching from collaterals and pial arterioles.

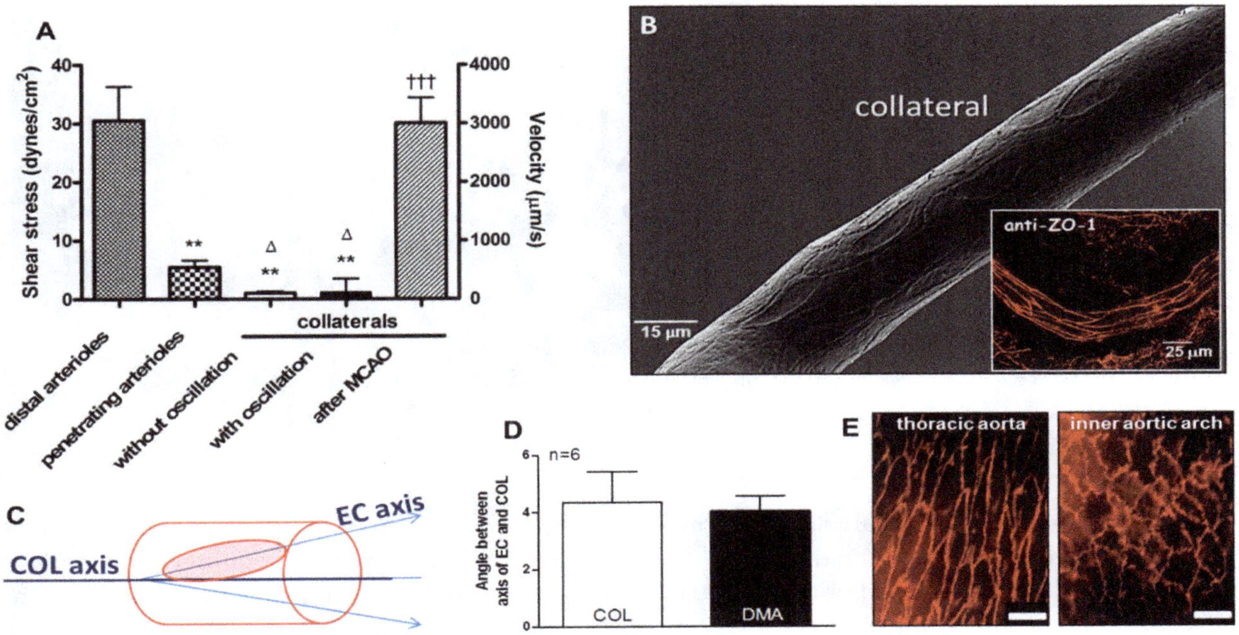

Figure 2. Collateral endothelial cells are aligned with the vessel axis despite having low and oscillatory flow/shear stress in the absence of arterial obstruction. (**A**) Data were obtained in anesthetized mice via cranial window and previously published in reference [6]; unlike distal-most arterioles (DMAs) with diameters comparable to collaterals (COLs) and penetrating arterioles, COLs examined over 30 s intervals have either no flow or slowly oscillating, low velocity, to-and-fro flow with ~zero net-direction. After ligation of the MCA trunk (MCAO), flow to its territory reaches that evident in DMAs within 10–30 s. (**B**–**E**) Collateral endothelial cells (ECs) have the same "anti-inflammatory" alignment (~4 degrees from horizontal) as ECs of DMAs and the descending thoracic aorta, despite having low/disturbed shear stress at baseline. This is in contrast to the "pro-inflammatory" non-alignment present in the inner curvature of the aortic arch. In this and subsequent figures, data are means ± SE for "n" number of mice. Data in D determined from SEM images, $n = 6$ mice. Panel E magnification bar is 25 μm. Panel A 2-sided t-tests for shear stress followed by Bonferroni correction for ** $p < 0.01$ vs distal arterioles; Δ $p < 0.05$ vs penetrating arterioles; 2-sided t-test for ttt $p < 0.001$ vs before MCAO. ZO-1, zona occludens-1 immunohistochemistry.

2.2. *Endothelial Cells of Collaterals and Distal-Most Arterioles Have Primary Cilia; Collaterals Have Fewer*

While examining EC orientation using SEM we noticed the presence of casts of channels penetrating into a fraction of the ECs lining collaterals (Figure 3). Based on studies in other cell types including bovine aorta and human umbilical vein ECs [32–34], these are invaginations of the plasmalemma that abut the ciliary membrane to form the ciliary pocket, which houses the proximal end of luminal primary cilia (PrC) that were removed by shearing forces ("depilated/de-ciliated") during infusion of Batson's #17. The Batson's-filled ciliary pockets (i.e., PrC) were commonly located near the nucleus, in accordance with the base of the cilium being associated with the basal body [34–40]. Distal arterioles also have cilia (Figure S1). One, two, or rarely three cilia were present in ECs that expressed them (Figure 3, Figure S2). More than one cilium per EC has not been found in previous studies, to our knowledge; however, previous reports have only examined large conduit vessels. The above method, which serendipitously identified PrC, is indirect since ciliary pockets were what were detected. We therefore confirmed their presence using immunofluorescence (Figure 4). Eighteen percent of collateral ECs expressed PrC, as compared to 28% of DMAs; thus ECs lining collaterals had 34% fewer cilia. We have not found other reports that ECs within vessels of the microcirculation express primary cilia.

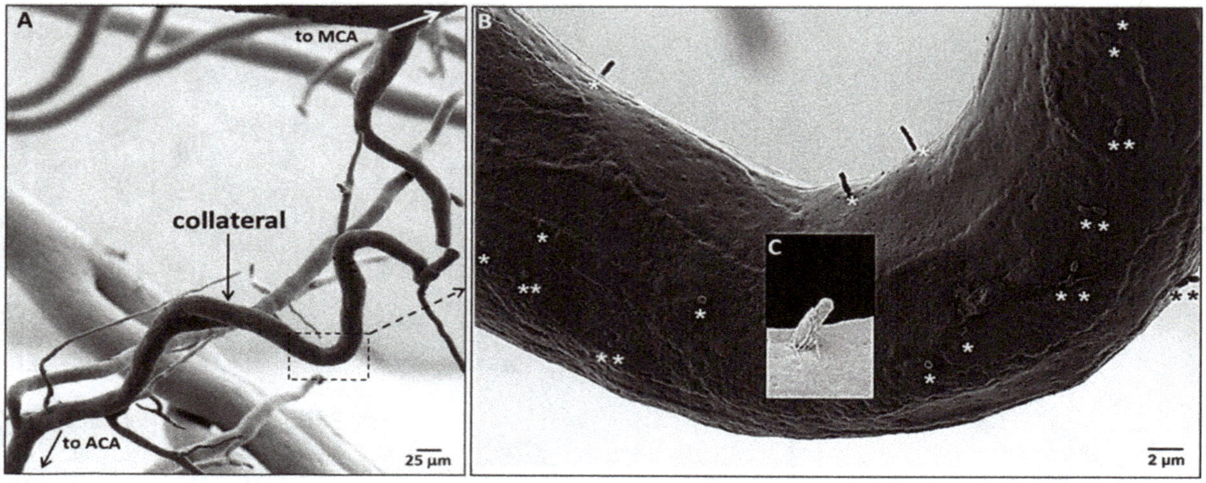

Figure 3. Collateral endothelial cells have primary cilia. (**A**) SEM of a corrosion cast of pial arterial vessels and a collateral, fixed at maximal dilation. (**B**) Stars identify casts of plasmalemmmal invaginations that contain the proximal end of the primary cilia (PrC) filled with Batson's #17 after removal of the PrC by shearing during infusion of the casting agent; each EC has 0–3 PrC. (**C**) Higher magnification SEM of a ~2 µm long PrC invagination.

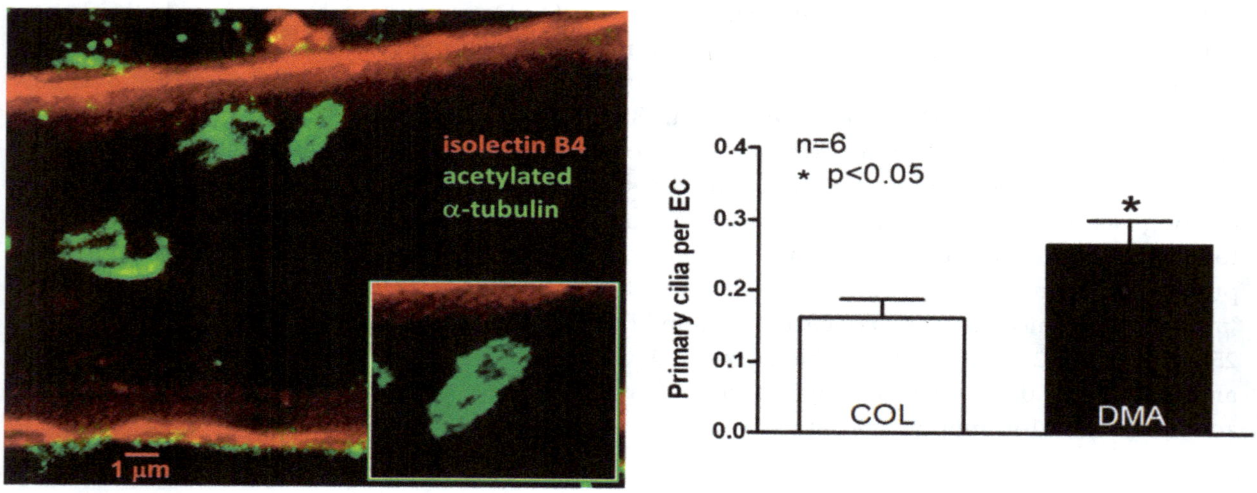

Figure 4. Collateral endothelial cells have fewer primary cilia than distal-most arterioles (DMA). Immunofluorescent-stained collaterals (COL) with focal plane set within the lumen above the far-wall, showing primary cilia. Figure S2 shows cilia on DMAs. Inset, higher magnification. Right panel, $n = 6$ mice, 2-sided t-test.

2.3. Collaterals Are Invested with a Continuous Layer of Smooth Muscle Cells, unlike Distal-Most Arterioles Whose Smooth Muscle Cells Are Discontinuous

Smooth muscle cells (SMCs) become sparse and discontinuous on distal arterioles in many tissue types [41–43]. Unlike arterioles that have orthograde flow, collateral blood flow converges from opposite directions, resulting in an average flow of near or at zero in the center-most segment of the collateral in the absence of occlusion (Figure 2A). The kinetic energy of flow is therefore converted to potential energy, which increases the circumferential wall stress of collaterals. Accordingly, we reasoned that SMC investment of collaterals might be greater than that present on DMAs to balance this increased wall stress. Figure 5 supports this hypothesis.

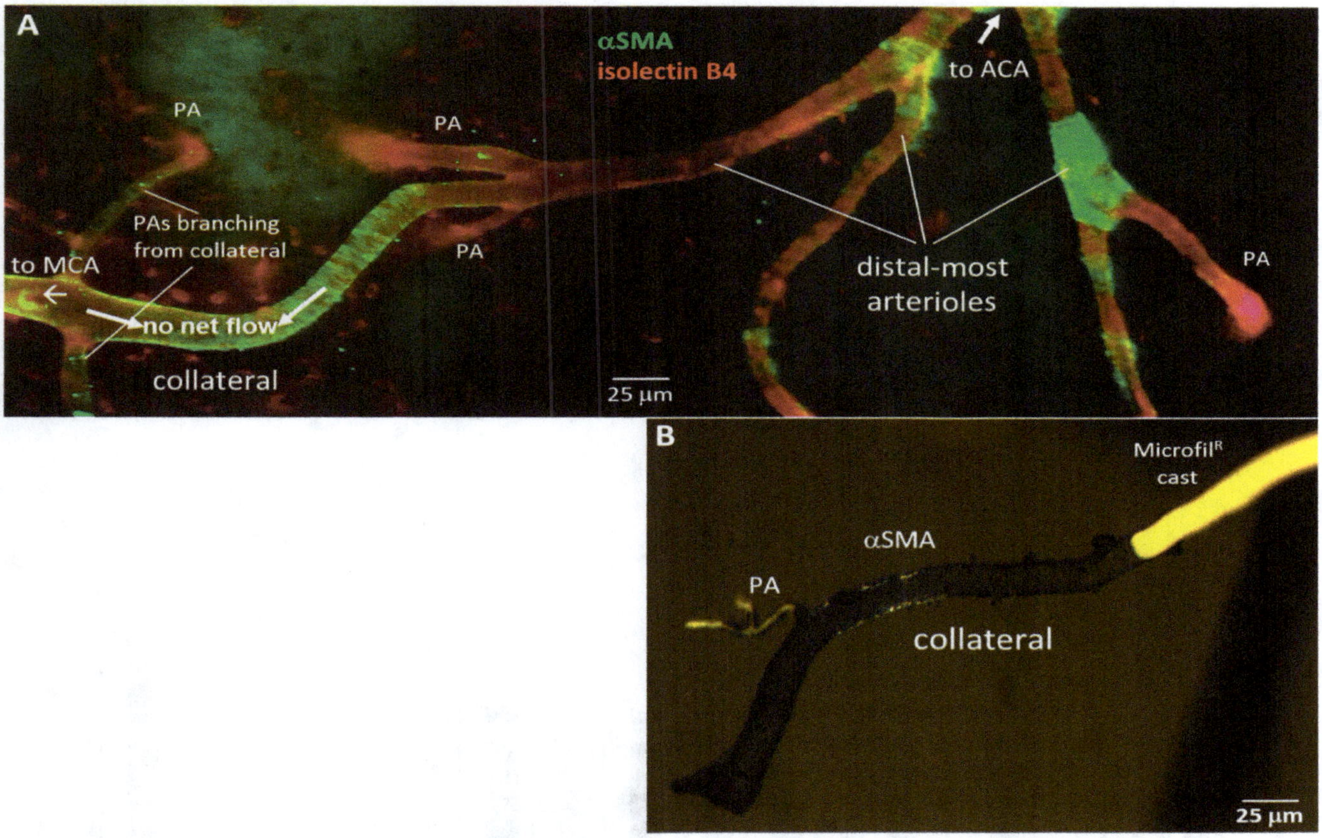

Figure 5. Collaterals are invested with a continuous layer of smooth muscle cells (SMCs), unlike distal-most arterioles (DMAs) that lack or have discontinuous SMCs. (**A**), Immuno-fluorescent staining of SMCs (αSM-actin) and ECs (IB4-lectin). Representative image of pial collaterals, DMAs and penetrating arterioles (PA). (**B**), Brightfield image of αSMA-stained collateral and PA filled with yellow Microfil®, then freed from surrounding pial membrane.

2.4. Gene Expression Differs for Collaterals Versus Distal-Most Arterioles

Given the disturbed hemodynamic, pro-oxidative stress (i.e., low blood oxygen content) environment in which collateral mural cells reside, plus the high susceptibility of collaterals to undergo rarefaction with aging, vascular risk factor presence, and eNOS/NO deficiency [16–21,25] compared to nearby DMAs [17], we postulated that expression of genes involved with inflammation, cell proliferation, aging, and angiogenesis differ for collaterals and DMAs. To test this hypothesis, we measured transcript levels of 22 such genes (Figure 6), as well as eNOS immunofluorescence (Figure 7). Collaterals had increased expression of *Pycard, Ki67, Pdgfb, Angpt2, Dll4, Ephrinb2,* and eNOS, whereas 16 other genes were not significantly different. Of note, expression of the EC shear stress-sensitive transcription factors Klf2 and Klf4, which promote anti-proliferative, -inflammatory, and -angiogenic processes, upregulate eNOS, and are sharply downregulated at vascular sites of low and disturbed shear stress [35–37,44,45], were, in contrast, not downregulated in collaterals compared to DMAs with laminar high-velocity flow.

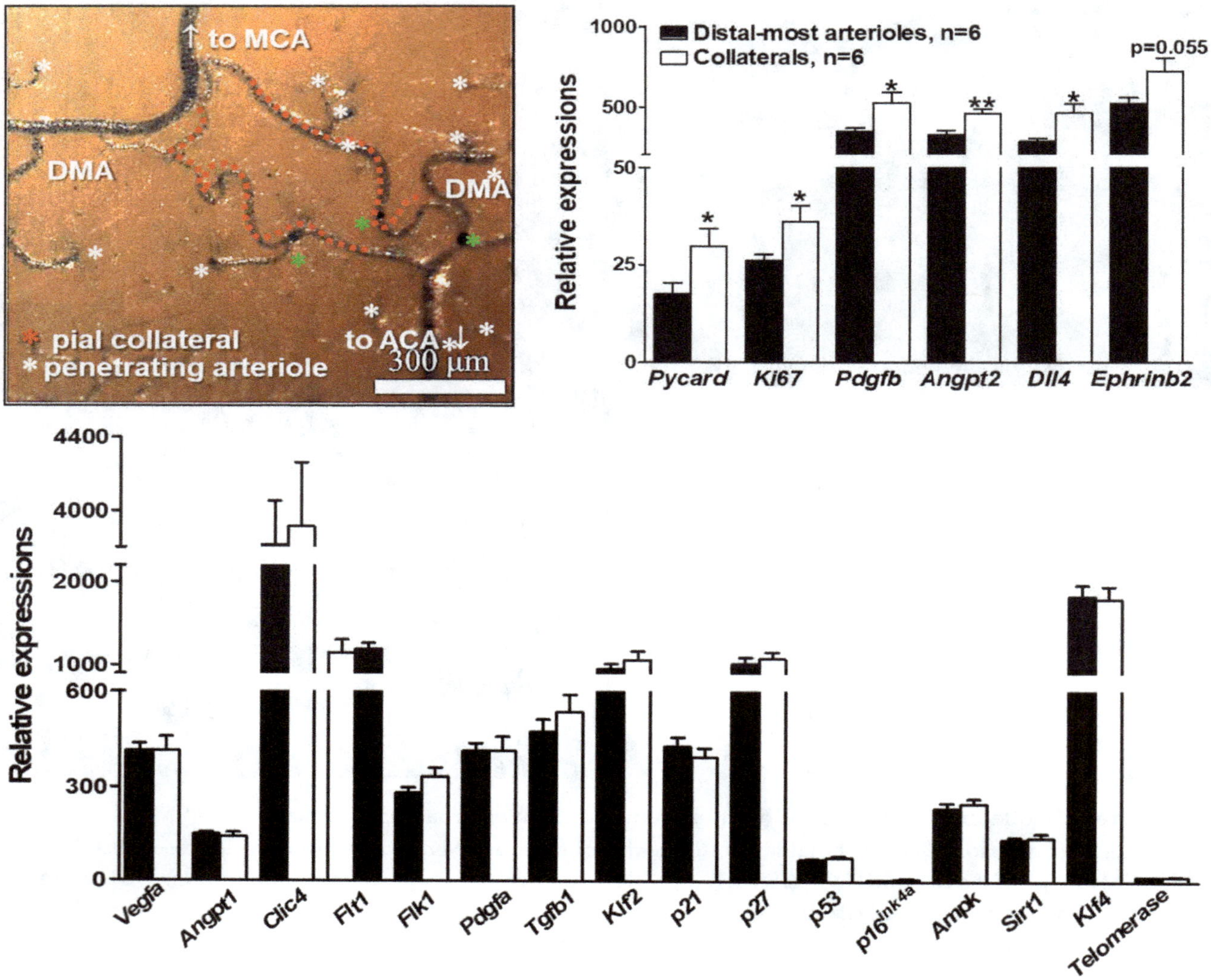

Figure 6. Gene expression differs for collaterals versus distal-most arterioles. Upper left panel, pial arterial vasculature perfusion-fixed at maximal dilation then filled with PU4ii polyurethane. Stars identify penetrating arterioles, including three that bifurcate and descend into the cortex immediately below the arteriole or collateral (green stars). Ten collaterals and 10 nearby similarly-sized distal-most arterioles DMAs were dissected from each of 36 mice and pooled into six samples for extraction of RNA. Transcript abundance was determined by Nanostring n-Counter® for 22 genes, each normalized to one of six housekeeping genes (*Gapdh, βactin, Tubb5, Hprt1, Ppia, Tbp*) selected for comparable level of expression [46]. * $p < 0.05$, ** $p < 0.01$ by 2-sided t-test for collaterals versus DMAs.

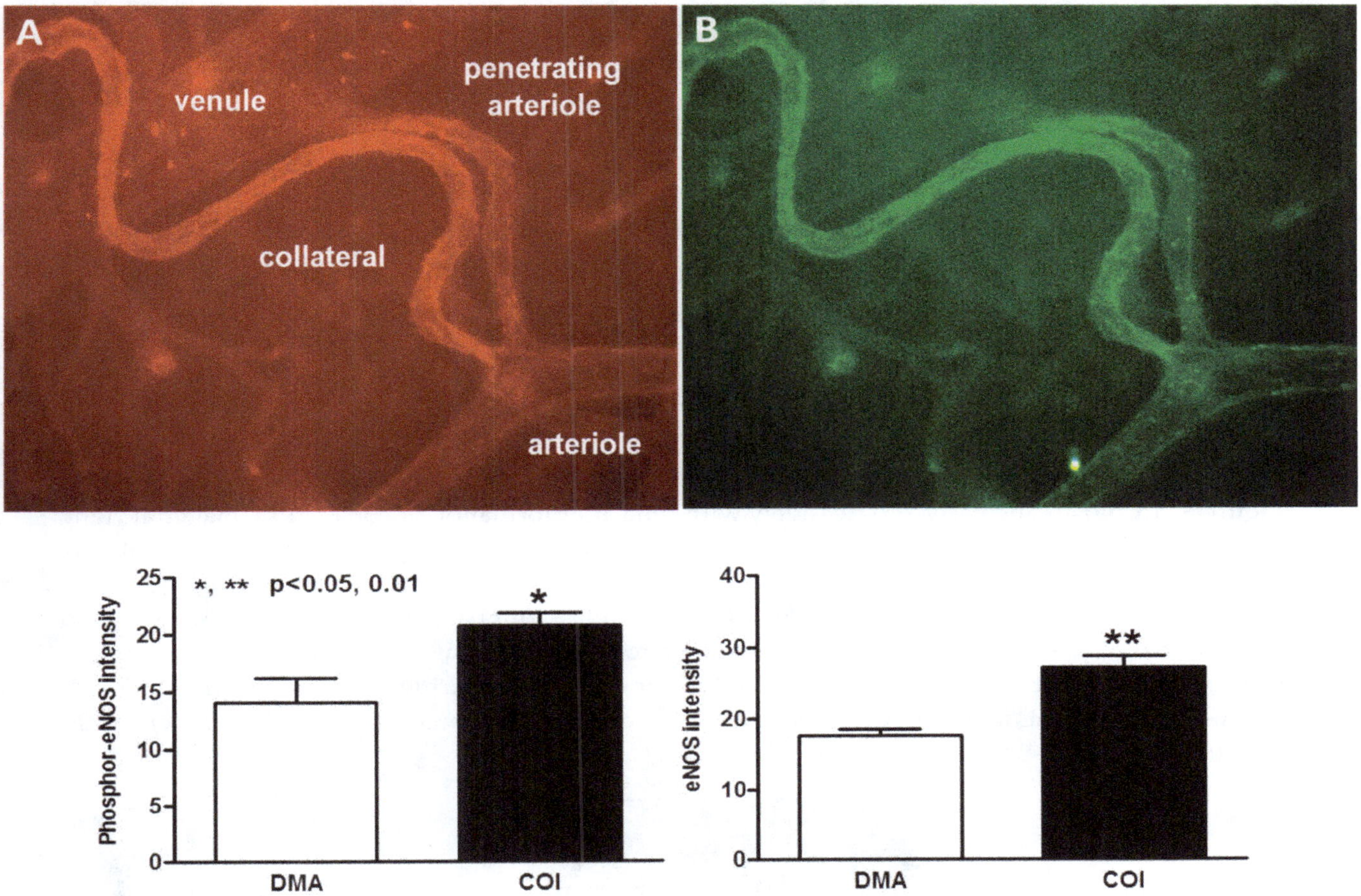

Figure 7. Collaterals express increased levels of phospho- and total eNOS compared to arterioles. Top panels, immunohistochemistry for phospho- (**A**, red) and total (**B**, green) eNOS, $n = 4$ mice, 1-sided t-tests, 163x magnification. * $p < 0.05$, ** $p < 0.01$.

2.5. Changes in Tortuosity over a Collateral's "Lifetime" Suggests Accelerated Proliferative Senescence of their Mural Cells

We previously reported that aging, hypertension, and other vascular risk factors cause a loss of collateral number and a smaller diameter in those that remain [17–19,25]. Aging-induced rarefaction becomes evident in late middle-age in mice (16 months of age), is not seen in DMAs, is accelerated in onset by the presence of other vascular risk factors, and is associated with increased cellular markers of oxidative stress, inflammation, proliferation, and aging, as well as increased vessel tortuosity [17–19,25]. Tortuosity is a hallmark of collaterals. We postulated that it arises from a persistently increased rate of proliferation of collateral wall cells (confirmed in [18]) that is driven by the disturbed hemodynamic conditions present in collaterals. The above studies did not examine tortuosity at time points earlier than 3 months of age. To determine whether collaterals begin to acquire tortuosity from formation onward, we examined mice on embryonic day E15.5 (collaterals form between E15.5 and E18.5 [6,7]) and on post-natal day-1 and day-21. Tortuosity was absent at E15.5 but became evident by P1 and was significant by P21 (Figure 8). When viewed in context with our previous data for tortuosity at later ages (Figure 9; human year-equivalents for the latter five bars are approximately 13, 19, 49, 69, 84 years [47]), these findings support the hypothesis that collateral rarefaction, which becomes evident in late middle-age in mice [17], is caused by proliferative senescence of collateral ECs and SMCs due to a lifetime elevation in proliferation in excess of apoptosis that is caused by the disturbed hemodynamic conditions in which collaterals reside.

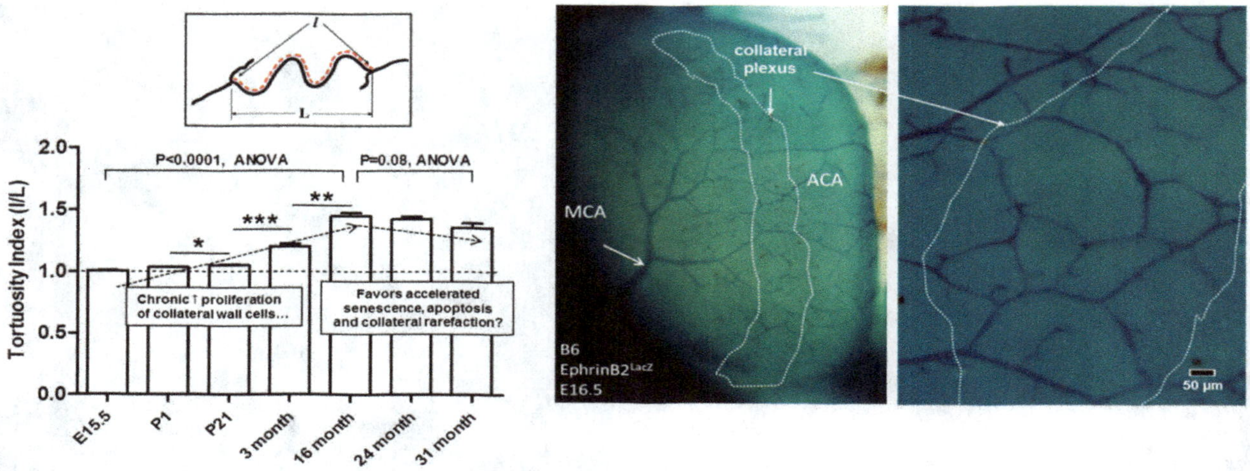

Figure 8. Tortuosity increases progressively with time after formation of collaterals. Images at right, ephrin-B2^{LacZ} reporter mouse (construction of mutant described in [6]) showing embryonic collaterals. Bar graph, tortuosity index = l/L (axial length of collateral ÷ scalar length connecting collateral endpoints). E, embryonic day, P, post-natal day. Data for last four bars from Faber et al. [17] who also showed that collateral diameter and number begin to decline at or after 16 months of age. Number of mice (C57BL/6, B6) for bars 1–7: 8,9,8,9,10,7,8. For each mouse tortuosity, was determined for all MCA–ACA collaterals and averaged. ANOVA followed by 1-sided Bonferroni t-tests, *, **, ***, $p < 0.05$, 0.01, 0.001, respectively.

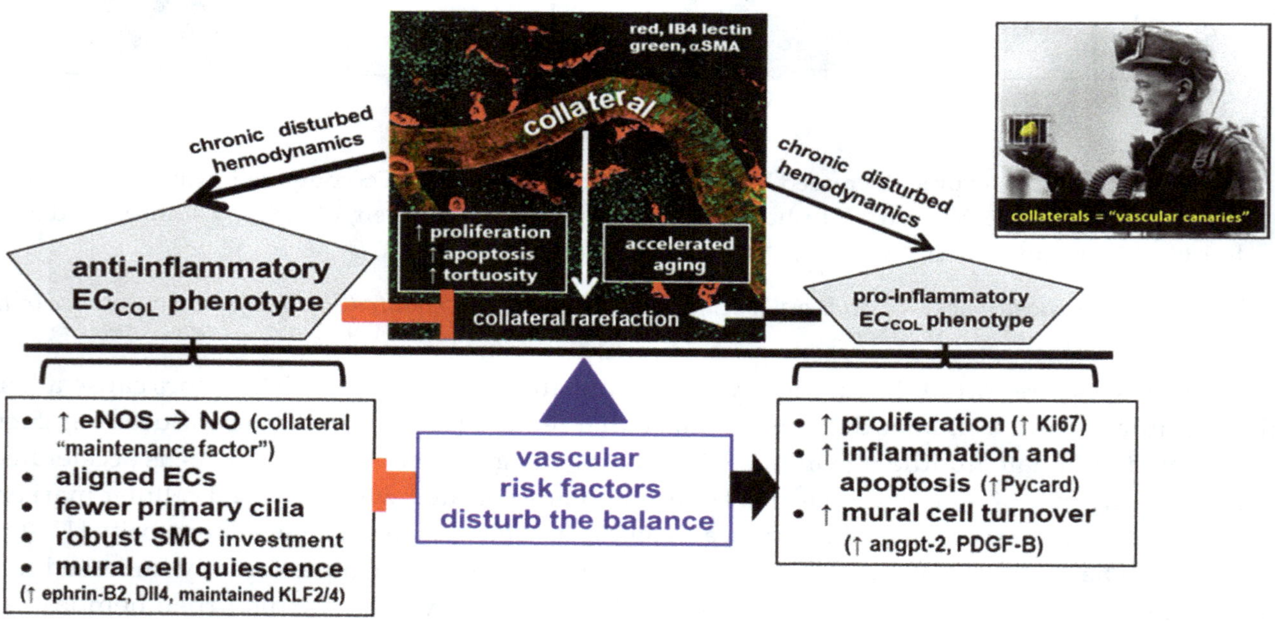

Figure 9. Persistence/maintenance versus rarefaction/pruning of collaterals "hangs in the balance". Proposed model whereby collateral (COL) mural cells reside in an environment of low/disturbed shear stress, high circumferential wall stress, and low blood oxygen content. This favors a pro-inflammatory, pro-proliferative, pro-apoptotic, and accelerated aging EC phenotype, leading to loss of collateral number and diameter (rarefaction). Compared to distal arterioles, collaterals have specializations and differential gene expression (left box) that provide adaptations that mitigate against factors that promote collateral rarefaction (right box). Vascular risk factors, e.g., aging, hypertension, EC dysfunction, and oxidative stress, disturb the balance. Collaterals are more sensitive than other vessels to these environmental risk factors, like "canaries in a mine-shaft".

3. Discussion

The present study identified a number of distinct features of collateral ECs and SMCs that may underlie or contribute to the unique characteristics of collaterals outlined in the Introduction. We found that despite the low and oscillatory shear stress present in collaterals at baseline in the absence of obstruction, their ECs are aligned with the vessel axis to the same degree present in distal-most arterioles and the descending aorta—vessels with high-velocity orthograde laminar flow. Endothelial cells of both collaterals and arterioles have primary cilia, and collaterals possess fewer of them. Smooth muscle cells of collaterals are continuous, unlike those of DMAs. Collaterals have higher levels of expression of genes associated with both pro- and anti-inflammatory and pro- and anti-proliferation pathways, compared to DMAs. A bias towards a higher rate of cell proliferation in collateral mural cells [18] is supported by the observation that collaterals begin to acquire tortuosity shortly after their formation in the embryo that increases through middle age (16 months, 49 human year-equivalents [47]). The above findings provide insights into structural and molecular specializations that may underlie the unique features and functions of collateral vessels.

Convergence of blood flow in collaterals at baseline imposes low and "disturbed" flow/shear stress forces on their mural cells, i.e., either absence of flow or very low flow that oscillates to-and-fro (~1–10 times per minute) and averages zero [6,15]. This results in increased wall stress according to the Bernoulli relationship. When present elsewhere in the arterial circulation, e.g., at bifurcations, the inner arch of the aorta or downstream of plaques, low and disturbed shear stress favors a non-aligned cobblestoned EC morphology that is associated with increased oxidative stress, inflammation, markers of aging, and low eNOS/NO activity (i.e., endothelial dysfunction) [28–31,44,45]. Surprisingly, however, we found that collateral ECs have the same alignment (and cell dimensions) as ECs in DMAs and the descending aorta. We did not investigate how this anti-inflammatory structural phenotype is specified. It is possible that one or more of the other unique features that we identified are involved (see below). On the other hand, the data in Figure 2 for flow and shear stress were obtained in anesthetized animals. During awake behaviors, collaterals may have periods of sustained flow in one or the other direction induced by changes in regional metabolic activity in the territory supplied by the arterial trees that they cross-connect. It is not known if collaterals contribute in this way to physiological metabolic regulation of blood flow and oxygen delivery, i.e., neurovascular coupling in brain and functional hyperemia elsewhere. However, such periods of sustained unidirectional flow could promote the EC orientation we observed. Irrespective of underlying cause, we speculate that the aligned phenotype of collateral ECs is part (or a marker) of a group of protective mechanisms that favor maintenance of collaterals and mitigate their rarefaction (Figure 9).

To our knowledge, this is the first report showing that ECs lining collaterals and arterioles have primary cilia. They are much more abundant than reported previously for conduit vessels from healthy individuals (i.e., absent or present on less than 1% of ECs [32,34]): 18% of collateral ECs have PrC compared to 28% for DMAs. Primary cilia on ECs were described in 1984 by Haust in aorta of rabbits and humans with atherosclerosis [48]. Subsequent reports described ciliated ECs in capillaries of the pineal gland of a 20 week-old human fetus [49], developing heart and aortic valve leaflets [33,50,51], and references therein], surrounding atheromas [52], ectopically in the common carotid artery of *ApoE*$^{-/-}$ mice, and in healthy individuals at bifurcations of conduit arteries and the inner curvature of the aortic arch; by contrast cilia are absent or nearly so in regions of arteries where shear stress is laminar [33,40,50]. Most other cell types express PrC during development, under certain conditions of cell culture [53], and in adults [35–37]. Depending on cell type, PrC participate in specification of embryo asymmetry, centriole disposition, proliferation/cell cycle regulation, autophagy, flow-sensing mechanotransduction, chemoception, and compartmentalization and trafficking of signaling proteins among the cilioplasm, cytoplasm, and nucleoplasm (e.g., for Gli and PDGFRα) [35–37]. When present, cilia are most abundant in non-proliferating cells, with the proximal end anchored in an invagination of the plasmalemma (ciliary pocket) in ECs and other but not all cell types [33,34,36]. Primary cilia are complexed with the mother centriole of the basal body that links to the microtubule-organizing center

(MTOC) [32,35–37,54]. Disassembly/resorption of the cilium during S-phase and centriole liberation are essential for cell division [36,37,54]. Since PrC are linked to the cytoskeleton via the MTOC, flow-induced ciliary bending in ECs [55] is capable of being transmitted throughout the cell, including to cell–cell and cell–matrix junctions [33,37]. Primary cilia transduce fluid shear stress in renal tubular epithelial cells and ECs through a pathway that that is exceptionally sensitive to shear stress and involves polycystin-1 and polycystin-2, which are encoded by *Pkd1* and *Pkd2* [35–37]. Polycystin-1 has mechanosensitive properties while polycystin-2 is a TRP calcium channel. Both proteins are required to sense shear stress and in turn release nitric oxide [33,37]. Defects in PrC are associated with many abnormalities. For example, mutations of *PKD1* and *PKD2* are causal for autosomal dominant polycystic kidney disease, with kidney ECs and tubular cells of patients evidencing deficient calcium and NO responses and increased proliferation [33,35–37].

Primary cilia are absent in human umbilical vein ECs maintained under laminar shear stress and proliferative quiescence in cell culture. In human umbilical veins less than one percent of ECs have cilia that protrude into the lumen, while in a larger fraction the cilia are located intracellularly [34,55]. Embryonic aorta and ECs cultured from it have a single cilium that projects into the lumen [38–40]. Endothelial cilia are present in regions of high shear stress during embryonic development, along with expression of the shear stress-sensitive transcription factor, KLF2, which transactivates *eNOS* and other anti-inflammatory and anti-proliferative genes [44,45]. In regions with low or disturbed shear stress PrC are disassembled/absent and expression of *Klf2* and *eNOS* are abolished and reduced, respectively [33,56]. Expression of *Klf2* is also inhibited in non-ciliated ECs isolated from embryonic arteries, and chemical removal of PrC from ECs in culture has a similar effect, i.e., abolishing *Klf2* expression [57]. Interestingly, in ECs of adult $ApoE^{-/-}$ mice, which have endothelial dysfunction but do not develop plaques, cilia are expressed ectopically in the common carotid artery despite the presence of laminar flow, compared to wildtype mice that are devoid of cilia [33]. Cilia were lost when high shear stress was induced via implantation of a flow-restricting cast around the vessel. Casting of common carotids in wildtype mice induced ciliogenesis only in regions of low and disturbed shear stress. These findings suggest that expression of PrC on ECs in vivo in adults is limited to regions of low/disturbed shear stress but can occur ectopically in arteries with laminar flow in the presence of endothelial dysfunction caused by hyperlipidemia [33] and possibly other vascular risk factors. Of note, in highly ciliated, disturbed-flow areas such as the inner curvature of the aortic arch or downstream of plaques, approximately 25% of ECs have a single cilium while the rest are devoid [33], a percentage similar to what we observed in arterioles and collaterals.

Our findings that PrC are also present on arterioles and collaterals in healthy young adult mice highlight the need for studies examining cilia function in these vessel types. This includes determining whether our observation of fewer cilia on collateral ECs than arterioles has functional significance. Endothelial cells are coupled mechanically, electrically, and diffusionally to adjacent ECs and SMCs [58], thus only a fraction of ECs may need to express cilia for transduction of mechano-sensitive or other signals. High shear stress causes disassembly of cilia in cultured ECs, while oscillatory flow reversal induces their expression [33]. We speculate that cilia on arteriole and collateral ECs may reflect the lower flow/shear stress in arterioles and very low and disturbed flow in collaterals and that fewer PrC on collateral ECs may serve to reduce their sensitivity to the prevailing disturbed shear stress environment. In other words, fewer cilia on collateral ECs may be part of a repertoire of adaptations that balance against or oppose—through maintained or increased expression of KLF2/4, eNOS, and other anti-inflammatory/anti-proliferative factors—the low-grade inflammatory, oxidative, proliferative, and apoptotic signals promoted by the disturbed hemodynamic environment present in collaterals (Figure 9). Egorova et al. [36] proposed something similar, i.e., that since presence of PrC on ECs is associated with KLF2 expression, endothelial cilia may signal a brake on EC activation in regions of low and disturbed flow. A protective role for cilia in these regions [36,37] is supported by the recent report that removal of endothelial cilia using conditional deletion of *Ift88* increased atherosclerosis and inflammatory gene expression, and decreased eNOS activity in $Apoe^{-/-}$ mice fed a high-fat diet [59], and that the endothelium becomes sensitized in athero-prone regions to undergo osteogenic differentiation in Tg737 (*orpk/orpk*) cilium-defective mice [60]. It is also possible that if PrC are protective, fewer of them in collaterals could contribute to the high susceptibility of these vessels to rarefaction from aging and other vascular risk factors. However, fewer cilia on collaterals might simply reflect a secondary or bystander effect, being a consequence, for example, of a higher inherent proliferation rate of collateral ECs as evidenced by the progressive increase in collateral tortuosity (discussed below), since presence of PrC and their association with the basal body is believed to favor removal of cells from the cell cycle [35–37]. Future studies will be required to determine if our finding of multiple cilia on ECs reflects ECs that have undergone proliferative senescence and associated failed cytokinesis and nuclear polyploidy [39].

It has recently been shown that ECs in the developing mouse retina rely on PrC to stabilize vessel connections during remodeling of the vascular plexus in regions with low to intermediate shear stress [61]. Endothelial cilia sense flow in zebrafish embryos, participate in recruitment of mural cells to arterial fated vessels, and are required for normal vascular morphogenesis [62,63]. The number and diameter of collaterals declines beginning in middle age [17]. This age-induced rarefaction is strongly accelerated by genetic or pharmacologically induced eNOS/NO deficiency or the presence of vascular risk factors [16,19]. Increased shear stress induces collateral outward remodeling following acute or slowly developing arterial obstruction [1,2,5]. *Pkd1*$^{+/-}$ mice and patients with autosomal dominant polycystic kidney disease have endothelial eNOS/NO dysfunction [64]. It will be important to examine in future studies whether collateral PrC participate in one or more of the above functions using EC-specific knockdown of polycystin-1, since: 1) deficiency in it leads to altered ciliary function, 2) polycystin-1 together with polycystin-2 participate in flow-sensing by PrC, 3) mutant forms of either protein cause polycystic kidney disease [35–37], 4) there is evidence that VHL, independent of its role in the degradation of Hif1α, together with GSK3β are required for structural maintenance of the cilium [65], and 5) the protein Rabep2, which is required for collaterogenesis [11], is a novel substrate of GSK3β [66], localizes at the cilium–basal body complex, and knockdown of it leads to defective ciliogenesis [67]. Other approaches to interfere with cilia presence and function, e.g., with knockdown of other ciliary proteins such as *Pkd2* and *Ift88*, also will need to be examined.

In contrast to distal arterioles, which have sparse and discontinuous SMCs in various tissues including retina (we were unable to identify studies in brain) [41–43], SMCs were continuous on collaterals. We speculate this may be an adaptive increase in wall thickness to balance the increase in circumferential wall stress caused by the Bernoulli-specified conversion of kinetic energy of flow to increased potential energy (transmural pressure) as a consequence of flow-convergence in collaterals. It would be interesting to examine whether the composition and amount of extracellular matrix, which could assist SMCs in balancing the increased wall stress in collaterals, differs in collaterals versus arterioles. Of note, despite their increased SMC coverage, collaterals have less rather than more tone compared to similarly-sized arterioles, and lack myogenic responsiveness—additional unique features of collateral vessels [26,27].

The disturbed hemodynamic, pro-oxidative environment in which collateral mural cells reside led us to examine whether expression of genes involved in inflammation, cell proliferation, aging, and angiogenesis differ for collaterals versus distal arterioles. Collaterals displayed increased mRNA levels for the pro-inflammatory, pro-apoptosis inflammasome gene, *Pycard*, the pro-proliferative genes, *Ki67*, *Pdgfb*, and *Angpt2*, the anti-proliferative gene, *Dll4*, and the differentiated arterial-type EC marker gene, *Ephrinb2*. However, expression of cell cycle inhibitor genes, *p21*, *p27*, and *p53*, were not different, nor were other genes associated with proliferation, cell cycle arrest, and aging (*p16*^{Ink4a}, *Ampk*, *Sirt1*, *telomerase*). Neither were there differences in expression of other genes associated with EC and/or SMC proliferation (*Vegfa*, *Flk1*, *Clic4*, *Pdgfa*, *Flt1*) and that are required (in the case of the first three genes [7,8]) for formation of collaterals during development or involved with specifying EC and SMC differentiation and quiescence (*Tgfb*, *Angpt1*). Increased expression by collaterals of the above pro-proliferation genes is consistent with our tortuosity measurements, which suggest that collateral mural cells have a higher proliferation rate, compared to other arterial vessels: collateral tortuosity was evident by the first day after birth, continued to increase through middle age, and then declined. The latter occurred at the same time that collaterals experience a decline in number and diameter with advanced aging [17]. These findings support the hypothesis that age-associated collateral rarefaction is caused by proliferative senescence and subsequent apoptosis of collateral ECs and SMCs due to a lifetime elevation in proliferation rate caused by the disturbed hemodynamic and low blood oxygen content environment in which collaterals reside (Figure 9).

Collaterals also displayed increased activity of eNOS, which previous studies have shown opposes rarefaction of collaterals caused by aging and other vascular risk factors [16,18,19]. eNOS-derived NO inhibits oxidative stress, inflammation, proliferation, leukocyte adhesion, platelet aggregation, and cellular aging and promotes SMC relaxation [58,68]. Since shear stress is a proximate stimulus for eNOS-derived NO, increased eNOS/NO in collaterals with their low and disturbed shear stress environment may lessen the effect of factors promoting collateral rarefaction (Figure 9). Likewise, maintained expression of the EC shear stress-sensitive transcription factors, *Klf2* and *Klf4*, in collaterals despite their low and oscillatory flow, which inhibits expression of these factors elsewhere in the arterial vasculature with disturbed flow [44], may act as additional "balancing" factors or collateral specializations, along with increased eNOS, aligned ECs, fewer cilia, robust SMC coverage, and increased ephrin-B2 and Dll4. Expression of KLF2 and KLF4, which negatively regulate proliferation, inflammation, and angiogenesis, upregulate eNOS, and are sharply downregulated at sites of low and disturbed shear stress, were not different in collaterals versus DMAs. Interestingly, PrC promote *Klf2*, *Klf4*, and *eNOS* expression [35–37,44,69,70].

A limitation of the above studies is that RNA was obtained from dissected vessels, which are composed of ECs, SMCs, and, although less so, pericytes, fibroblasts, and resident myeloid cells. Studies are needed that employ separation of cell types and examination of a wider array of genes and their respective protein levels. However, the difficulty in manually dissecting collaterals and distal arterioles in the required numbers, the effect of cell dissociation techniques on baseline levels of RNA and protein, the absence of cell culture models of "collateral" ECs and SMCs, and the as of yet lack of any collateral-specific marker gene, preclude the use of these approaches. Of note, however, expression of several of the genes examined are specific or enriched for ECs, e.g., *Flk1*, *Angpt1*, *Angpt2*, *Ephrinb2*, *DLL4*, *eNOS*, *Clic4*, *Klf2*, and *Klf4*. However, analysis of gene transcription does not always reflect changes in protein level or function; thus the investigation of oxidative stress, inflammatory, proliferation, or senescence markers at the protein level may better reflect differences in cellular characteristics.

4. Materials and Methods

Three to 4 month-old male C57BL/6 (B6) wildtype (lab colony, Jackson Laboratories breeders, Bar Harbor, ME, USA) or genetically modified mice were studied. Scanning electron microscopy was performed on the cerebral arterial vasculature that was filled with Batson's #17. Angiography and morphometry were performed after filling with yellow Microfil® [18]. Prior to infusion of the casting agents, and also for immunohistochemistry, the vasculature was cleared of blood and perfusion-fixed after maximal dilation with 10^{-4} M nitroprusside. Filling was confined to the pre-capillary vessels by adjusting the viscosity and input pressure of the casting material. All pial collaterals between the anterior cerebral artery (ACA) and middle (MCA) trees of both hemispheres were identified; tortuosity (axial length of the collateral ÷ scalar length connecting the collateral's endpoints [17]) and lumen diameter, EC orientation, and other morphometrics were obtained at midpoint for each collateral and an average value obtained for each animal unless indicated otherwise in the figure legends. Permanent MCA occlusion was by electro-cautery occlusion of the M1-MCA just distal to the lenticulostriate branches [18]. Right femoral artery (FA) occlusion was achieved by ligating the superficial FA immediately proximal and distal to the superior epigastric artery, which was also ligated [18]. Hindlimb perfusion was measured by laser Doppler perfusion imaging of the plantar foot and the adductor thigh regions. Values reported are means ± SE, with significance at $p < 0.05$; n-sizes (number of animals studied) and statistical tests are given in the figure legends.

All applicable international, national, and/or institutional guidelines for the care and use of animals were followed, including the National Institutes of Health Guide for the Care and Use of Laboratory Animals (UNC IACUC #18-123.0-A, 1 April 2019). This article does not contain any studies with human participants performed by any of the authors.

4.1. *Angiography and Morphometry*

As previously described in detail [20] animals were anesthetized deeply with ketamine and xylazine and heparinized. The distal thoracic aorta was cannulated, right atrium perforated, and the mouse was perfused with PBS containing freshly prepared sodium nitroprusside (10^{-4} M, for maximal dilation) and Evans blue dye (for light staining of brain and the endothelial surface) at ~100 mmHg. One ml of yellow Microfil (Flowtech Inc, Carver, MA, USA) was infused at a viscosity adjusted to fill the entire pial arterial and collateral circulations with sufficient pressure (~100 mmHg) and duration to cause limited capillary transit and venous filling to assure complete filling of all precapillary vessels and collaterals. After the Microfil had set for 20 min, brains were kept in 4% PFA and collaterals were imaged the next day using a Leica fluorescent stereomicroscope. All collaterals between the anterior cerebral artery (ACA) and middle cerebral artery (MCA) trees of both hemispheres were counted and divided by 2 to give the average number per hemisphere. Images were subsequently analyzed (ImageJ, NIH, Bethesday, MD, USA): Collateral lumen diameter was determined at midpoint at 50X for all ACA-MCA collaterals and averaged for each mouse.

4.2. *Permanent Middle Cerebral Artery Occlusion (pMCAO)*

As previously described [20], mice were anesthetized with ketamine and xylazine (100 and 10 mg/kg, ip, respectively) and rectal temperature was maintained at 37 ± 0.5 °C. The temporalis muscle between the eye and ear on one side was retracted after a 4 mm incision. After a 2 mm craniotomy (18000-17 drill, FST, Foster City, CA, USA), the dura was incised with a 27 gauge needle tip and reflected to reveal the main trunk of the MCA which was cauterized (18010-00, FST, modified) distal to the lenticulostriate branches. The incision was closed with suture and Vetbond (3M, Minneapolis, MN, USA), intramuscular cefazolin 50 mg/kg and buprenorphine were administered, and the animal was monitored in a warmed cage during recovery from anesthesia to maintain the above rectal temperature. Mice were euthanized 4 days after pMCAO. Pial collateral morphometry was then performed as described above.

4.3. *Laser Doppler Perfusion Imaging and Hindlimb Ischemia Model*

Femoral artery ligation (FAL) was performed and hindlimb perfusion was measured using a laser Doppler perfusion imager (Model LDI2-IR, Moor Instruments, Wilmington, DE, USA, ~2 mm penetration and high resolution) as described previously [71]. Briefly, the anterior thigh and adductor regions were depilated followed by 24 h to recover from any erythema. Mice were then anesthetized with 1.25% isoflurane/O_2, rectal temperature was maintained at 37 ± 0.5 °C. A 3 mm incision was made overlying the femoral vessels 5 mm proximal to the knee. The femoral artery was gently isolated and ligated twice with 7-0 suture immediately distal to the lateral caudal femoral artery and 1 mm further distally, followed by transection between the ligatures. The superficial epigastric artery was also ligated. The skin was closed using 5-0 silk. Mice were placed in a heated chamber to block ambient light, and rectal temperature was maintained at 37 ± 0.5 °C. Less than 5 min after ligation, the plantar and adductor regions of both legs were laser-scanned. Average perfusion within the region of interest, drawn to outline the plantar surface of the paws, was calculated using Moor LDI Image Processing V5.0 software and reported as the ratio of ligated to the non-ligated hindlimb, where the region of interest was defined according to anatomic landmarks as described previously [71].

4.4. *Quantitative NanoString Expression Analysis*

As described previously [46], mice placed under deep anesthesia (ketamine and xylazine, 100 and 10 mg/kg, ip, respectively) were perfused with 1 ml RNAlater®(Sigma-Aldrich Corp, St. Louis, MO, USA) premixed with 10% Evans blue dye through the thoracic aorta. The brain was then removed and immersed in RNAlater®. Approximately 10 pial collaterals and 10 nearby similarly sized distal-most arterioles per mouse (total 36 mice) were micro-dissected and pooled in RNAlater®as 6 samples. Samples were homogenized (TH, Omni International, Marietta, GA, USA) in Trizol Reagent (Invitrogen, Carlsbad, CA, USA). Total RNA was purified using the RNeasy Micro Kit according to the manufacturer (Qiagen, Valencia, CA, USA). RNA concentration and quality were determined by NanoDrop 1000 (Thermo Scientific, Wilmington, DE, USA) and Bioanalyzer 2100 (Agilent, Foster City, CA, USA), respectively. Measurement of transcript number was conducted for 22 selected genes by the genomics facility at UNC using NanoString custom-synthesized probes (NanoString, Seattle, WA, USA). Transcript number for each gene was normalized to one of the following 6 housekeeping genes selected to be in range of the target gene under analysis: *Gapdh*, *βactin*, *Tubb5*, *Hprt1*, *Ppia* and *Tbp*.

4.5. *Immunohistochemistry*

Mice under deep anesthesia (ketamine and xylazine, 100 and 10 mg/kg, ip, respectively) were perfused with nitroprusside (10^{-4} M) in PBS at ~100 mmHg with a reservoir for 3 minutes for maximal dilation and then with 2% PFA for 15 min for fixation. Brains were blocked with 10% goat serum in 0.3% PBS-triton 1 hr at room temperature. Then the cortex area were incubated with 1:50 anti-eNOS rabbit IgG (sc-654, Santa Cruz Biotechnology, Santa Cruz, CA, USA); 1:100 anti-phospho eNOS rabbit IgG (ab75639, Abcam, Cambridge, MA, USA), 1:100 anti-acetylated-tubulin (T7451, Sigma), 1:100 anti-ZO1 (ab96587, Abcam), 1;400 anti-aSMA (Abcam, 32575, clone E184), overnight, 4 °C in a shaker, followed by incubation of 1:200 goat anti rabbit-fluorescent conjugated with Alexa fluor®568 (A10042, ThermoFisher Scientific, Grand Island, NY, USA) or Alexa fluor®488 (A21208). Images of eNOS and phorpho-eNOS for pial collaterals and DMAs were taken using a Leica fluorescent stereomicroscope (Richmond, IL, USA), and the signal strength was measured using ImageJ (Bethesda, MD, USA). Endothelial cells were probed with Isolectin-GS-IB4-Alexa568 (I121415, ThermoFisher Scientific). Primary cilia (probed with anti-acetylated-tubulin antibody) in the lumen of pial collaterals were observed with a Zeiss 710 confocal microscope (Thornwood, NT, USA), with z stack scanning from the top of cortex down to a depth of ~30 um. Endothelial junctions (probed with ZO-1) were visualized with a Zeiss 710 confocal microscope.

4.6. *Collateral Primary Cilia and Endothelial Orientation Assessed by Scanning Electron Microscopy*

Mice were perfused with maximal vessel dilation as described above. Brain arterial vasculature was then casted using a Batson's No 17 Plastic Replica and Corrosion Kit (Polysciences, Inc, Warrington, PA, USA). Briefly, 1 ml of Batson's 17 was infused through the thoracic aorta. After fully curing, the brain tissue was removed using maceration solution, and the cerebral vasculature including the pial collateral regions were carefully persevered for emission scanning electron microscopy. The vasculature was observed under a Zeiss Supra 25 Field emission scanning electron microscope. Images of pial collateral and DMAs were saved for analysis of primary cilia and endothelial cell morphology. To measure the orientation of collateral endothelial cells, we use Photoshop to draw a line coordinate with the collateral axis and a second line coordinate with the endothelial cell axis (see Figure 2, panel C), and the angle formed was measured.

4.7. *Statistics*

Experiments were performed in accordance with the University of North Carolina's Institutional Animal Care and Use Committee, the NIH Guide for the Care and Use of Laboratory Animals, the ARRIVE guidelines, and the following suggested STAIR criteria [72]: investigators were blinded during data analysis where possible; no data points were identified as outliers by statistical test and none were excluded; all results were fully disclosed including negative results; the review, discussion and citation of the literature was unbiased; pMCAO was used to permanently recruit blood flow across pial collaterals. Values are mean ± SEM. Statistical analysis ($p < 0.05$ = significant) is described in the figure legends.

5. Conclusions

In conclusion, collaterals are unique among blood vessel types with regard to their formation, structure, function, prevailing shear stress, and susceptibility to variation in their extent caused primarily by differences in genetic background but also by environmental factors such as aging and risk factors. The present study provides our first look into how differences in collateral endothelial and smooth muscle cells may accommodate and contribute to these unique features. Moreover, the model/hypothesis shown in Figure 9, if correct, may begin to provide answers to two perplexing questions: Why do collaterals undergo rarefaction with aging and other vascular risk factors? They are chronically exposed to adverse hemodynamic conditions. How do they resist more extensive pruning away? Their mural cells have specializations or adaptations in structure and expression of factors that mitigate the effects of these conditions.

Author Contributions: H.Z. performed angiography, morphometry, in vivo experiments, immunostaining, expression analysis, animal husbandry, and statistical analysis; D.C. performed SEM and determined collateral tortuosity in perinatal mice; J.E.F. designed the experiments, data analysis, and figures and wrote the manuscript.

Acknowledgments: We thank Kirk McNaughton for histological tissue sectioning and Katy Liu for assistance in preparation of the SEM samples.

Abbreviations

ACA	anterior cerebral artery
B6	C57BL/6 mouse strain
COL	collateral
DMA	distal-most arteriole
EC	endothelial cell
eNOS	endothelial nitric oxide synthase
Flt 1	VEGF receptor 1
Flk1	VEGF receptor 2
MCA	middle cerebral artery
NO	nitric oxide
PA	penetrating arteriole
Pkd1	gene that encodes polycystin-1
PrC	primary cilia
SMC	smooth muscle cell
VECAD	vascular endothelial cell adhesion protein, selectively expressed by ECs
WT	wildtype littermate controls

References

1. Faber, J.E.; Chilian, W.M.; Deindl, E.; van Royen, N.; Simons, M. A brief etymology of the collateral circulation. *Atherioscler. Thromb. Vasc. Biol.* **2014**, *34*, 1854–1859. [CrossRef] [PubMed]
2. Nishijima, Y.; Akamatsu, Y.; Weinstein, P.R.; Liu, J. Collaterals: Implications in cerebral ischemic diseases and therapeutic interventions. *Brain Res.* **2015**, *1623*, 18–29. [CrossRef] [PubMed]
3. Bang, O.Y.; Goyal, M.; Liebeskind, D.S. Collateral circulation in ischemic stroke: Assessment tools and therapeutic strategies. *Stroke* **2015**, *46*, 3302–3309. [CrossRef]

4. Ginsberg, M.D. The cerebral collateral circulation: Relevance to pathophysiology and treatment of stroke. *Neuropharmacology* **2018**, *134*, 280–292. [CrossRef] [PubMed]
5. Schaper, W. Collateral circulation: Past and present. *Basic Res. Cardiol.* **2009**, *104*, 5–21. [CrossRef] [PubMed]
6. Chalothorn, D.; Faber, J.E. Formation and maturation or the murine native cerebral collateral circulation. *J. Mol. Cell. Cardiol.* **2010**, *49*, 251–259. [CrossRef] [PubMed]
7. Lucitti, J.L.; Mackey, J.K.; Morrison, J.C.; Haigh, J.J.; Adams, R.H.; Faber, J.E. Formation of the collateral circulation is regulated by vascular endothelial growth factor-A and A disintegrin and metalloprotease family members 10 and 17. *Circ. Res.* **2012**, *111*, 1539–1550. [CrossRef] [PubMed]
8. Lucitti, J.L.; Tarte, N.J.; Faber, J.E. Chloride intracellular channel 4 is required for maturation of the cerebral collateral circulation. *Am. J. Physiol. Heart Circ. Physiol.* **2015**, *309*, H1141–H1150. [CrossRef] [PubMed]
9. Zhang, H.; Prabhakar, P.; Sealock, R.; Faber, J.E. Wide genetic variation in the native pial collateral circulation is a major determinant of variation in severity of stroke. *J. Cereb. Blood Flow Metab.* **2010**, *30*, 923–934. [CrossRef]
10. Chalothorn, D.; Faber, J.E. Strain-dependent variation in native collateral function in mouse hindlimb. *Physiol. Genom.* **2010**, *42*, 469–479. [CrossRef]
11. Lucitti, J.L.; Sealock, R.; Buckley, B.K.; Zhang, H.; Xiao, L.; Dudley, A.C.; Faber, J.E. Variants of Rab GTPase-effector binding protein-2 cause variation in the collateral circulation and severity of stroke. *Stroke* **2016**, *47*, 3022–3031. [CrossRef] [PubMed]
12. Seiler, C.; Stoller, M.; Pitt, B.; Meier, P. The human coronary collateral circulation: Development and clinical importance. *Eur. Heart J.* **2013**, *34*, 2674–2682. [CrossRef] [PubMed]
13. Traupe, T.; Ortmann, J.; Stoller, M.; Baumgartner, I.; de Marchi, S.F.; Seiler, C. Direct quantitative assessment of the peripheral artery collateral circulation in patients undergoing angiography. *Circulation* **2013**, *128*, 737–744. [CrossRef] [PubMed]
14. Rost, N.S.; Giese, A.K.; Worrall, B.B.; Williams, S.; Malik, R.; Cloonan, L.; Furie, K.L.; Lindgren, A.; Frid, P.; Wasselius, J.; et al. *RABEP2* (Rab GTPase-effector binding protein-2) is associated with ischemic stroke phenotypes: a translational replication study. *Eur. Stroke J.* **2018**, *3*, 42–43.
15. Toriumi, H.; Tatarishvili, J.; Tomita, M.; Tomita, Y.; Unekawa, M.; Suzuki, N. Dually supplied T-junctions in arteriolo-arteriolar anastomosis in mice: Key to local hemodynamic homeostasis in normal and ischemic states? *Stroke* **2009**, *40*, 3378–3383. [CrossRef] [PubMed]
16. Dai, X.; Faber, J.E. eNOS deficiency causes collateral vessel rarefaction and impairs activation of a cell cycle gene network during arteriogenesis. *Circ. Res.* **2010**, *106*, 1870–1881. [CrossRef] [PubMed]
17. Faber, J.E.; Zhang, H.; Lassance-Soares, R.M.; Prabhakar, P.; Najafi, A.H.; Burnett, M.S.; Epstein, S.E. Aging causes collateral rarefaction and increased severity of ischemic injury in multiple tissues. *Arterioscler. Thromb. Vasc. Biol.* **2011**, *31*, 1748–1756. [CrossRef] [PubMed]
18. Moore, S.M.; Zhang, H.; Maeda, N.; Doerschuk, C.; Faber, J.E. Cardiovascular risk factors cause premature rarefaction of the collateral circulation and greater ischemic tissue injury. *Angiogenesis* **2015**, *18*, 265–281. [CrossRef]
19. Rzechorzek, W.; Zhang, H.; Buckley, B.K.; Hua, H.; Pomp, D.; Faber, J.E. Exercise training prevents rarefaction of pial collaterals and increased severity of stroke with aging. *J. Cereb. Blood Flow Metab.* **2017**, *37*, 3544–3555. [CrossRef]
20. Zhang, H.; Jin, B.; Faber, J.E. Mouse models of Alzheimer's disease cause loss of pial collaterals and increased severity of ischemic stroke. *Angiogenesis* **2018**, *22*, 263–279. [CrossRef]
21. Hecht, N.; He, J.; Kremenetskaia, I.; Nieminen, M.; Vajkoczy, P.; Woitzik, J. Cerebral hemodynamic reserve and vascular remodeling in C57/BL6 mice are influenced by age. *Stroke* **2012**, *43*, 3052–3062. [CrossRef] [PubMed]
22. Menon, B.K.; Smith, E.E.; Coutts, S.B.; Welsh, D.G.; Faber, J.E.; Damani, Z.; Goyal, M.; Hill, M.D.; Demchuk, A.M.; Hee Cho, K.H.; et al. Leptomeningeal collaterals are associated with modifiable metabolic risk factors. *Ann. Neurol.* **2013**, *74*, 241–248. [CrossRef] [PubMed]
23. Malik, N.; Hou, Q.; Vagal, A.; Patrie, J.; Xin, W.; Michel, P.; Eskandari, A.; Jovin, T.; Wintermark, M. Demographic and clinical predictors of leptomeningeal collaterals in stroke patients. *J. Stroke Cerebrovasc. Dis.* **2014**, *23*, 2018–2022. [CrossRef] [PubMed]
24. Arsava, E.M.; Vural, A.; Akpinar, E.; Gocmen, R.; Akcalar, S.; Oguz, K.K.; Topcuoglu, M.A. The detrimental effect of aging on leptomeningeal collaterals in ischemic stroke. *J. Stroke Cerebrovasc. Dis.* **2014**, *23*, 421–426. [CrossRef] [PubMed]

25. Wang, J.; Peng, X.; Lassance-Soares, R.M.; Najafi, A.H.; Alderman, L.O.; Sood, S.; Xue, Z.; Chan, R.; Faber, J.E.; Epstein, S.E.; et al. Aging-induced collateral dysfunction: Impaired responsiveness of collaterals and susceptibility to apoptosis via dysfunctional eNOS signaling. *J. Cardiovasc. Transl. Res.* **2011**, *4*, 779–789. [CrossRef] [PubMed]
26. Chan, S.L.; Sweet, J.G.; Bishop, N.; Cipolla, M.J. Pial collateral reactivity during hypertension and aging: Understanding the function of collaterals for stroke therapy. *Stroke* **2016**, *47*, 1618–1625. [CrossRef] [PubMed]
27. Beard, D.J.; Murtha, L.A.; McLeod, D.D.; Spratt, N.J. Intracranial pressure and collateral blood flow. *Stroke* **2016**, *47*, 1695–1700. [CrossRef] [PubMed]
28. Davies, P.F.; Civelek, M.; Fang, Y.; Fleming, I. The atherosusceptible endothelium: Endothelial phenotypes in complex haemodynamic shear stress regions in vivo. *Cardiovasc. Res.* **2013**, *99*, 315–327. [CrossRef]
29. Abe, J.; Berk, B.C. Novel mechanisms of endothelial mechanotransduction. *Arterioscler. Thromb. Vasc. Biol.* **2014**, *34*, 2378–2386. [CrossRef]
30. Zhou, J.; Li, Y.S.; Chien, S. Shear stress-initiated signaling and its regulation of endothelial function. *Arterioscler. Thromb. Vasc. Biol.* **2014**, *34*, 2191–2198. [CrossRef]
31. Zakkar, M.; Angelini, G.D.; Emanueli, C. Regulation of vascular endothelium inflammatory signaling by shear stress. *Curr. Vasc. Pharmacol.* **2016**, *14*, 181–186. [CrossRef]
32. Briffeuil, P.; Thibaut-Vercruyssen, R.; Ronveaux-Dupal, M.F. Ciliation of bovine aortic endothelial cells in culture. *Atherosclerosis* **1994**, *106*, 75–81. [CrossRef]
33. Van der Heiden, K.; Hierck, B.P.; Krams, R.; de Crom, R.; Cheng, C.; Baiker, M.; Pourquie, J.; Alkemade, F.E.; DeRuiter, M.C.; Gittenberger-de Groot, A.C.; et al. Endothelial primary cilia in areas of disturbed flow are at the base of atherosclerosis. *Atherosclerosis* **2008**, *196*, 542–550. [CrossRef] [PubMed]
34. Geerts, W.J.; Vocking, K.; Schoonen, N.; Haarbosch, L.; van Donselaar, E.G.; Regan-Klapisz, E.; Post, J.A. Cobblestone HUVECs: A human model system for studying primary ciliogenesis. *J. Struct. Biol.* **2011**, *176*, 350–359. [CrossRef]
35. Satir, P. Cilia: Before and after. *Cilia* **2017**, *6*. [CrossRef]
36. Egorova, A.D.; van der Heiden, K.; Poelmann, R.E.; Hierck, B.P. Primary cilia as biomechanical sensors in regulating endothelial function. *Differentiation* **2012**, *83*, S56–S61. [CrossRef]
37. Pala, R.; Jamal, M.; Alshammari, Q.; Nauli, S.M. The roles of primary cilia in cardiovascular diseases. *Cells* **2018**, *7*, 233. [CrossRef] [PubMed]
38. Nauli, S.M.; Kawanabe, Y.; Kaminski, J.J.; Pearce, W.J.; Ingber, D.E.; Zhou, J. Endothelial cilia are fluid shear sensors that regulate calcium signaling and nitric oxide production through polycystin-1. *Circulation* **2008**, *117*, 1161–1171. [CrossRef] [PubMed]
39. AbouAlaiwi, W.A.; Ratnam, S.; Booth, R.L.; Shah, J.V.; Nauli, S.M. Endothelial cells from humans and mice with polycystic kidney disease are characterized by polyploidy and chromosome segregation defects through survivin down-regulation. *Hum. Mol. Genet.* **2011**, *20*, 354–367. [CrossRef]
40. Abdul-Majeed, S.; Moloney, B.C.; Nauli, S.M. Mechanisms regulating cilia growth and cilia function in endothelial cells. *Cell. Mol. Life Sci.* **2012**, *69*, 165–173. [CrossRef]
41. Price, R.J.; Owens, G.K.; Skalak, T.C. Immunohistochemical identification of arteriolar development using markers of smooth muscle differentiation. Evidence that capillary arterialization proceeds from terminal arterioles. *Circ. Res.* **1994**, *75*, 520–527. [CrossRef] [PubMed]
42. Murfee, W.L.; Skalak, T.C.; Peirce, S.M. Differential arterial/venous expression of NG2 proteoglycan in perivascular cells along microvessels: Identifying a venule-specific phenotype. *Microcirculation* **2005**, *12*, 151–160. [CrossRef] [PubMed]
43. Reagan, A.M.; Gu, X.; Paudel, S.; Ashpole, N.M.; Zalles, M.; Sonntag, W.E.; Ungvari, Z.; Csiszar, A.; Otalora, L.; Freeman, W.M.; et al. Age-related focal loss of contractile vascular smooth muscle cells in retinal arterioles is accelerated by caveolin-1 deficiency. *Neurobiol. Aging.* **2018**, *71*. [CrossRef] [PubMed]
44. Niu, N.; Xu, S.; Xu, Y.; Little, P.J.; Jin, Z.G. Targeting mechanosensitive transcription factors in atherosclerosis. *Trends Pharmacol. Sci.* **2019**, *40*, 253–266. [CrossRef] [PubMed]
45. Baeyens, N.; Bandyopadhyay, C.; Coon, B.G.; Yun, S.; Schwartz, M.A. Endothelial fluid shear stress sensing in vascular health and disease. *J Clin. Invest.* **2016**, *126*, 821–828. [CrossRef] [PubMed]

46. Wang, S.; Zhang, H.; Wiltshire, T.; Sealock, R.; Faber, J.E. Genetic dissection of the *Canq1* locus governing variation in extent of the collateral circulation. *PLOS One* **2012**, *7*, e31910. [CrossRef] [PubMed]
47. Flurkey, K.; Currer, J.M.; Harrison, D.E. *The Mouse in Biomedical Research*, 2nd ed.; Elsevier: Amsterdam, The Netherlands, 2007; pp. 637–672.
48. Haust, M.D. Endothelial cilia in human aortic atherosclerotic lesions. *Virchows Arch. A* **1987**, *410*, 317–326. [CrossRef]
49. Yamamoto, K.; Fujimoto, S. Endothelial cilium in the capillaries of the human fetal pineal gland. *Microscopy* **1980**, *29*, 256–258.
50. Toomer, K.A.; Fulmer, D.; Guo, L.; Drohan, A.; Peterson, N.; Swanson, P.; Brooks, B.; Mukherjee, R.; Body, S.; Lipschutz, J.H.; et al. A role for primary cilia in aortic valve development and disease. *Dev. Dyn.* **2017**, *246*, 625–634. [CrossRef]
51. Blom, J.N.; Feng, Q. Cardiac repair by epicardial EMT: Current targets and a potential role for the primary cilium. *Pharmacol. Ther.* **2018**, *186*, 114–129. [CrossRef]
52. Bystrevskaya, V.B.; Lichkun, V.V.; Antonov, A.S.; Perov, N.A. An ultrastructural study of centriolar complexes in adult and embryonic human aortic endothelial cells. *Tissue Cell* **1988**, *20*, 493–503. [CrossRef]
53. Lim, Y.C.; McGlashan, S.R.; Cooling, M.T.; Long, D.S. Culture and detection of primary cilia in endothelial cell models. *Cilia* **2015**, *4*, 11. [CrossRef] [PubMed]
54. Pan, J.; Snell, W. The primary cilium: Keeper of the key to cell division. *Cell* **2007**, *129*, 1255–1257. [CrossRef] [PubMed]
55. Boselli, F.; Goetz, J.G.; Charvin, G.; Vermot, J. A quantitative approach to study endothelial cilia bending stiffness during blood flow mechanodetection in vivo. *Methods Cell Biol.* **2015**, *127*, 161–173. [PubMed]
56. Wang, N.; Miao, H.; Li, Y.S.; Zhang, P.; Haga, J.H.; Hu, Y.; Young, A.; Yuan, S.; Nguyen, P.; Wu, C.C.; et al. Shear stress regulation of Krüppellike factor 2 expression is flow pattern-specific. *Biochem. Biophys. Res. Commun.* **2006**, *341*, 1244–1251. [CrossRef] [PubMed]
57. Hierck, B.P.; Van der Heiden, K.; Alkemade, F.E.; Van de Pas, S.; Van Thienen, J.V.; Groenendijk, B.C.; Bax, W.H.; Van der Laarse, A.; Deruiter, M.C.; Horrevoets, A.J.; et al. Primary cilia sensitize endothelial cells for fluid shear stress. *Dev. Dyn.* **2008**, *237*, 725–735. [CrossRef] [PubMed]
58. Hu, X.; De Silva, T.M.; Chen, J.; Faraci, F.M. Cerebral vascular disease and neurovascular injury in ischemic stroke. *Circ. Res.* **2017**, *120*, 449–471. [CrossRef] [PubMed]
59. Dinsmore, C.; Reiter, J.F. Endothelial primary cilia inhibit atherosclerosis. *EMBO Rep.* **2016**, *17*, 156–166. [CrossRef]
60. Sánchez-Duffhues, G.; de Vinuesa, A.G.; Lindeman, J.H.; Mulder-Stapel, A.; DeRuiter, M.C.; Van Munsteren, C.; Goumans, M.J.; Hierck, B.P.; Ten Dijke, P. SLUG is expressed in endothelial cells lacking primary cilia to promote cellular calcification. *Arterioscler. Thromb. Vasc. Biol.* **2015**, *35*, 616–627. [CrossRef]
61. Vion ACAlt, S.; Klaus-Bergmann, A.; Szymborska, A.; Zheng, T.; Perovic, T.; Hammoutene, A.; Oliveira, M.B.; Bartels-Klein, E.; Hollfinger, I.; Rautou, P.E.; et al. Primary cilia sensitize endothelial cells to BMP and prevent excessive vascular regression. *J. Cell. Biol.* **2018**, *217*, 1651–1665. [CrossRef]
62. Chen, X.; Gays, D.; Milia, C.; Santoro, M.M. Cilia control vascular mural cell recruitment in vertebrates. *Cell Rep.* **2017**, *18*, 1033–1047. [CrossRef] [PubMed]
63. Goetz, J.G.; Steed, E.; Ferreira, R.R.; Roth, S.; Ramspacher, C.; Boselli, F.; Charvin, G.; Liebling, M.; Wyart, C.; Schwab, Y.; et al. Endothelial cilia mediate low flow sensing during zebrafish vascular development. *Cell Rep.* **2014**, *6*, 799–808. [CrossRef] [PubMed]
64. Devuyst, O. Variable renal disease progression in autosomal dominant polycystic kidney disease: A role for nitric oxide? *J. Nephrol.* **2003**, *16*, 449–452. [PubMed]
65. Thoma, C.R.; Frew, I.J.; Krek, W. The VHL tumor suppressor: Riding tandem with GSK3beta in primary cilium maintenance. *Cell Cycle* **2007**, *6*, 1809–1813. [CrossRef] [PubMed]
66. Logie, L.; Van Aalten, L.; Knebel, A.; Force, T.; Hastie, C.J.; MacLauchlan, H.; Campbell, D.G.; Gourlay, R.; Prescott, A.; Davidson, J.; et al. Rab-GTPase binding effector protein 2 (RABEP2) is a primed substrate for glycogen synthase kinase-3 (GSK3). *Sci. Rep.* **2017**, *7*, 17682. [CrossRef] [PubMed]

67. Airik, R.; Schueler, M.; Airik, M.; Cho, J.; Ulanowicz, K.A.; Porath, J.D.; Hurd, T.W.; Bekker-Jensen, S.; Schrøder, J.M.; Andersen, J.S.; et al. SDCCAG8 interacts with RAB effector proteins RABEP2 and ERC1 and is required for hedgehog signaling. *PLOS One* **2016**, *11*, e0156081. [CrossRef] [PubMed]
68. Katusic, Z.S.; Austin, S.A. Neurovascular protective function of endothelial nitric oxide—Recent advances. *Circ. J.* **2016**, *80*, 1499–1503. [CrossRef] [PubMed]
69. Zhong, F.; Lee, K.; He, J.C. Role of Krüppel-like factor-2 in kidney disease. *Nephrology* **2018**, *23*, 53–56. [CrossRef] [PubMed]
70. Cheng, Z.; Zou, X.; Jin, Y.; Gao, S.; Lv, J.; Li, B.; Cui, R. The role of KLF4 in Alzheimer's disease. *Front. Cell. Neurosci.* **2018**, *12*, 325. [CrossRef] [PubMed]
71. Sealock, R.; Zhang, H.; Lucitti, J.L.; Moore, S.M.; Faber, J.E. Congenic fine-mapping identifies a major causal locus for variation in the native collateral circulation and ischemic injury in brain and lower extremity. *Circ. Res.* **2014**, *114*, 660–671. [CrossRef]
72. RIGOR. Improving the Quality of NINDS-Supported Preclinical and Clinical Research through Rigorous Study Design and Transparent Reporting. 2012. Available online: http://www.ninds.nih.gov/funding/transparency_in_reporting_guidance.pdf (accessed on 1 May 2019).

7

Isoform-Specific Roles of ERK1 and ERK2 in Arteriogenesis

Nicolas Ricard [1], Jiasheng Zhang [1], Zhen W. Zhuang [1] and Michael Simons [1,2,*]

1 Yale Cardiovascular Research Center, Department of Internal Medicine, Yale University School of Medicine, New Haven, CT 06511, USA; nic.ricard@gmail.com (N.R.); jiasheng.zhang@yale.edu (J.Z.); zhen.zhuang@yale.edu (Z.W.Z.)

2 Department of Cell Biology, Yale University School of Medicine, New Haven, CT 06511, USA

* Correspondence: michael.simons@yale.edu

Abstract: Despite the clinical importance of arteriogenesis, this biological process is poorly understood. ERK1 and ERK2 are key components of a major intracellular signaling pathway activated by vascular endothelial growth (VEGF) and FGF2, growth factors critical to arteriogenesis. To investigate the specific role of each ERK isoform in arteriogenesis, we used mice with a global *Erk1* knockout as well as *Erk1* and *Erk2* floxed mice to delete *Erk1* or *Erk2* in endothelial cells, macrophages, and smooth muscle cells. We found that ERK1 controls macrophage infiltration following an ischemic event. Loss of ERK1 in endothelial cells and macrophages induced an excessive macrophage infiltration leading to an increased but poorly functional arteriogenesis. Loss of ERK2 in endothelial cells leads to a decreased arteriogenesis due to decreased endothelial cell proliferation and a reduced eNOS expression. These findings show for the first time that isoform-specific roles of ERK1 and ERK2 in the control of arteriogenesis.

Keywords: angiogenesis; arteriogenesis; ERK; VEGF; endothelial cells; inflammation; macrophages

---

1. Introduction

Blood vessel development and growth encompasses three distinct biological processes—vasculogenesis, angiogenesis, and arteriogenesis [1]. The term vasculogenesis denotes the formation of the primitive vascular plexus from progenitor cells in embryo and this mode of blood vessel formation is limited to embryonic development. Angiogenesis encompasses the process of new capillary formation from pre-existing capillary beds that involves proliferation, sprouting and, migration of endothelial cells. Finally, arteriogenesis refers to the growth of new arteries and arterioles either de novo or from pre-existing arterial collaterals [2]. Arteriogenesis, the process of new arterial vasculature growth, is critical to the restoration of tissue perfusion following the development of a functionally significant decrease of arterial inflow. It is important to note that compromised arterial inflow results in two distinct events: distal tissue ischemia that leads to local angiogenesis (e.g., angiogenesis along the myocardial infarction border zone) and arteriogenesis that occurs in close proximity to the site of arterial trunk occlusion, a territory that is typically not ischemic [3,4].

While molecular controls of angiogenesis are well understood, events triggering and regulating arteriogenesis are still a matter of intense study and controversy. Vascular endothelial growth factor (VEGF) is the main factor driving angiogenesis in response to tissue hypoxia [5], yet VEGF is equally critical to arteriogenesis [6]. Indeed, disruption of VEGF signaling and, in particular, a reduction in VEGF-induced endothelial ERK1/2 signaling, has been shown to result in decreased arteriogenesis [7].

While angiogenesis involves simple proliferation and sprouting of capillary endothelial cells, arteriogenesis requires a coordinated response that involves multiple cell types that, in addition to endothelial and vascular smooth muscle cells, include a panoply of inflammatory cells including lymphocytes [8,9], natural killer cells [10], macrophages [11], and mast cells [12]. The presence of inflammatory cells (and a local inflammatory response at an arteriogenic site) is critical as these cells serve as the major source of VEGF in the absence of tissue ischemia [13–17].

Endothelial response to VEGF stimulation encompasses a complex series of events that include activation of various intracellular signaling cascades [18]. Of these, activation of ERK1/2 has been directly linked to the extent of arteriogenesis [7]. Remarkably, little is known about the individual contribution of ERK isoforms to this process. Global deletion of *Erk2* is embryonic lethal [19] whereas a global deletion of *Erk1* has no apparent vascular phenotype [20]. Furthermore, endothelial-specific deletion of *Erk2* on the *Erk1* global knockout background is lethal early on in embryonic development due to impaired vascular development [21]. Another key role played by the two ERKs in the adult endothelium is the regulation of vascular normalcy and integrity [22].

In this paper, we focused on the role of ERK1/2 isoforms in adult arteriogenesis. Induction of acute hindlimb ischemia resulted in excessive but poorly functional arteriogenesis in mice with a global deletion of *Erk1* whereas mice with endothelial-specific deletion of *Erk2* exhibited a decreased arteriogenesis. Since arteriogenesis involves a number of cell types, we generated a floxed *Erk1* mouse line and conditionally deleted the gene in macrophages, endothelial, and smooth muscle cells. While endothelial or macrophage deletions of *Erk1* failed to recapitulate the phenotype of the *Erk1*$^{-/-}$ mice, combined deletion of *Erk1* in endothelial cells and macrophages came close to the phenotype in global *Erk1* null mice. Altogether, these results show that endothelial and macrophage *Erk1* is critical to endothelial/macrophage crosstalk and effective adult arteriogenesis.

2. Methods

2.1. Mice

Mapk3$^{-/-}$ mice (denominated *Erk1*$^{-/-}$), *Mapk1*^{tm1Gela}/J mice (denominated *Erk2*$^{Fl/Fl}$), and B6.129P2-Lyz2tm1(cre)Ifo/J mice (denominated LysMCre) were purchased from the Jackson Laboratory. *Cdh5CreER*^{T2} mice were a generous gift from Ralf Adams. Myh11CreER^{T2} mice were a generous gift from Dan Greif. All mice, including the wild type (WT) mice, are *Mus musculus* on a pure C57Bl6 genetic background. *Erk1*$^{Fl/Fl}$ mice were realized by inserting 2 loxP sequences in introns between exons 2 and 3 and exons 8 and 9 of the Erk1 gene. Tamoxifen injections to induce deletion by the Cdh5Cre or Myc11Cre were done with 5 injections of 1.5 mg of tamoxifen on 5 consecutive days. Control mice received the same quantity of tamoxifen. For retinal angiogenesis, 100 µg of tamoxifen were administrated by IP injections starting at P1 to P4. BrdU was injected 2 h prior to euthanasia. Animals were housed and used in accordance with protocols and policies approved by the Yale Institutional Animal Care and Use Committee.

2.2. Endothelial Cells, Macrophages, and Aortic Smooth Muscle Cell Isolations and Quantitative PCR

Endothelial cells were isolated from mouse livers and lungs. Briefly, livers and lungs were collected and digested in a solution of collagenase and dispase (Roche/Sigma Aldrich, St Louis, MO, USA). The suspensions were then washed and filtered. Endothelial cells were isolated using magnetic beads anti-Rat IgG (Invitrogen, Camarillo, CA, USA) previously coated with rat anti-mouse CD31 antibody (BD). After extensive washing, cells were lysed and RNA was isolated using PicoPure RNa isolation kit (ThermoFisher, Waltham, MA, USA) or cultured.

Macrophages were isolated from the peritoneal cavity as previously described [23]. Macrophages were selected using magnetic beads anti-Rat IgG (Invitrogen) previously coated with rat anti-mouse F4/80 antibody (Invitrogen). After extensive washing, cells were lysed, and RNA was isolated using PicoPure RNa isolation kit (ThermoFisher).

Smooth muscle cells were isolated from the aorta. Aortas were collected and digested in 175 U/mL collagenase (Worthington), 1.25 U/mL elastase (Worthington, Lakewood, NJ, USA), and HBSS for 25 to 30 min at 37 °C. Adventitia layer was then pulled out. Media and endothelium were cut and digested in 175 U/mL collagenase and 2.5 U/mL elastase in HBSS for 1 h at 37 °C. Endothelial cells were bound toon beads previously coated with rat anti-mouse CD31 antibody were used and discarded. The remaining smooth muscle cells were lysed and RNA was isolated using PicoPure RNa isolation kit (ThermoFisher).

cDNAs were synthetized with iScript Reverse Transcription Supermix (Bio-Rad, Hercules, CA, USA) and qPCRs were performed using SsoAdvanced Universal SYBR Green Supermix (Bio-Rad).

2.3. *shRNA Infection*

shRNA targeting ERK1 and ERK2 (Sigma-Aldrich, St Louis, MO, USA) were encapsulated into lentivirus that were then. Lentivirus were produced in 293T cells using second generation lentiviral system (Invitrogen).

2.4. *Hindlimb Ischemia Model*

This was done as previously described by our lab [6]. Laser Doppler flow-imaging was carried out using a Moor Infrared Laser Doppler Imager (LDI; Moor Instruments Ltd., Wilmington, DE, USA) under ketamine and xylazine anesthesia.

2.5. *Micro-CT Imaging*

Microcomputed tomography (micro-CT) of the hindlimb vasculature was done by injecting 0.7 mL bismuth contrast solution in the descending aorta and the vasculature was imaged and quantified as previously described [6].

2.6. *Western Blot*

Cells were lysed in RIPA buffer (Boston BioProducts, Ashland, MA, USA). Proteins were titrated using Bio-Rad Protein Assay Dye Reagent (Bio-Rad). A total of 20 ng of proteins were loaded on a 4–12% acrylamide gel (Bio-Rad) and then transferred on a PVDF membrane (Millipore). Primary antibodies used were: F4/80 (Invitrogen), ERK (Cell Signaling, Danvers, MA, USA), and β-actin (Sigma-Aldrich).

2.7. *Immunofluorescent Staining*

Frozen sections were treated with ice cold acetone. Permeabilization was done in triton 0.1%. Primary antibodies were: F4/80 (Invitrogen) and IsolectinB4 (Invitrogen). Pictures were taken using an SP5 confocal microscope (Leica, Allendale, NJ, USA).

2.8. *xCELLigence Real-Time Cell Analysis (RTCA)*

Endothelial cell proliferation was measured by using an xCELLigence RTCA instrument (Roche Diagnostics) and E-plate 16 (a modified 16-well plate, Roche Diagnostics). The E-plate 16 was coated with 0.1% gelatin, loaded with 100 µL cell-free medium, and left in a tissue culture hood for 30 min to reach equilibrium. The E-plate 16 was placed into the RTCA instrument to measure the background impedance. Thereafter, 100 µL cell suspensions with fewer than 3500 cells were added into each well of the E-plate 16, which was then placed in a tissue culture incubator for 30 min to allow cells to settle down before being measured by the RTCA device. The impedance value of E-plate 16 was automatically monitored every 15 min. FGF2 was added at 100 ng/mL.

2.9. *Endothelial Migration*

HUVEC migration was measured in a wound-healing assay, which used ibidi Culture-Inserts (ibidi) to generate the wound. An ibidi Culture-Insert has dimensions of 9 mm × 9 mm× 5 mm (width × length × height) and is composed of two wells. One or two inserts were placed into one well of a six-well plate. After being coated with 0.1% gelatin, both wells of inserts were loaded with 100 μL cell suspension. FGF2 and VEGF were used at 100 ng/mL.

2.10. Statistical Analyses

Statistical tests were performed using the software GraphPad Prism 8.

3. Results

3.1. Erk1 KO Mice Exhibit Excessive but Poorly Functional Arteriogenesis

To assess the role of ERK1 in arteriogenesis, we ligated the common femoral artery (CFA) of *Erk1*$^{-/-}$ mice and assessed blood flow recovery over time using laser Doppler imaging while the anatomical extent of arteriogenesis was studied using micro-CT. While blood flow recovery was reduced in *Erk1*$^{-/-}$ mice compared to wild type (WT) controls (Figure 1A,B), the micro-CT-determined extent of arteriogenesis was dramatically increased (Figure 1C,D). Since macrophages are the critical source of VEGF in this model and since the extent of arteriogenesis generally correlates with the amount of VEGF-A present [24], we used immunocytochemistry to assess the extent of macrophage accumulation in the arteriogenic zone. Staining with an F4/80 antibody of the thigh muscles around the area of CFA, ligation was carried out three and seven days following hindlimb ischemia. There was a marked increase in macrophage tissue infiltration in *Erk1*$^{-/-}$ mice compared to WT mice (Figure 1E). To confirm these findings, we carried out Western blotting using total thigh muscle lysates. In agreement with immunocytochemical findings, we observed a massive increase in F4/80 signal (Figure 1F).

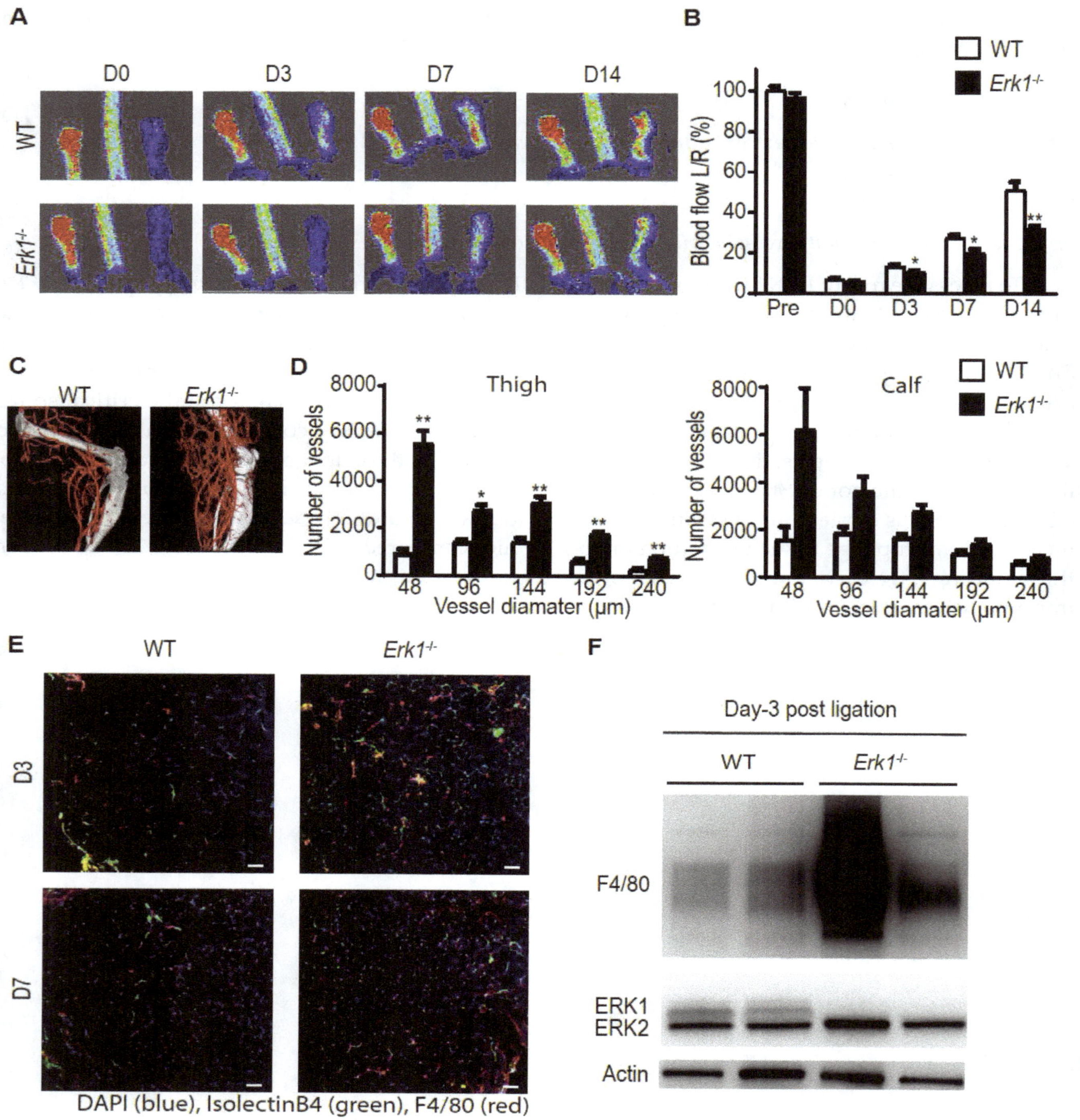

Figure 1. *Erk1*$^{-/-}$ mice exhibit excessive but dysfunctional arteriogenesis. (**A**,**B**) Blood flow recovery after ligation of the CFA in *Erk1*$^{-/-}$ mice assessed by laser-Doppler right after the surgery and 3, 7, and 14 days thereafter. Bar graph represents mean with SEM ($n = 10$ mice) * $p < 0.05$, ** $p < 0.005$ using two-way ANOVA followed by Sidak's multiple comparison test. (**C**,**D**) Quantification of the hindlimb vasculature by micro-CT three weeks after femoral artery ligation. Bar graph represents mean with SEM ($n = 4$ mice) * $p < 0.05$, ** $p < 0.005$ using two-way ANOVA followed by Sidak's multiple comparison test. (**E**,**F**) Macrophage infiltration in the thigh from *Erk1*$^{-/-}$ mice assessed by staining or Western blotting. Scale bar, 50 µm. Bar graph represents mean with SEM ($n = 3$ mice) * $p < 0.05$ using *t*-test.

3.2. *Erk1 Deletions in Endothelial Cells, Macrophages, or Smooth Muscle Cells Do Not Affect Arteriogenesis*

To identify the cell type(s) involved in the defective arteriogenic phenotype seen in *Erk1*$^{-/-}$ mice, we created mice with two intronic loxP sites in the *Erk1* (*Mapk3*) gene (hereafter denominated as *Erk1*$^{Fl/Fl}$ (Figure 2A)). Since endothelial cells are critical to arteriogenesis [6], these mice were crossed with a strain carrying an inducible Cre recombinase under the control of the VE-cadherin promotor (Cdh5CreER^{T2}) [25] generating a Cdh5CreER^{T2};Erk1$^{f/f}$ line (*Erk1*$^{iEC-/-}$). Administration of tamoxifen to eight-week-old *Erk1*$^{Fl/Fl}$ mice resulted in a high efficiency deletion of endothelial *ERK1* (Figure 2B). One week after tamoxifen treatment, common femoral arteries (CFA) of *Erk1*$^{iEC-/-}$ and control mice were ligated. Surprisingly, laser-Doppler assessment of blood flow recovery in *Erk1*$^{iEC-/-}$ mice showed that it was similar to that of WT control mice (Figure 2C,D). We next turned our attention to macrophages. Similarly to Cdh5 CreER^{T2}, LysM Cre [26] was very effective in deleting *Erk1* (Figure 2E). Blood flow recovery after CFA ligation was not impaired compared to WT mice after either *Erk1* gene deletion (Figure 2F,G). We next deleted the *Erk1* gene in smooth muscle cells (SMC) using the Myh11CreER^{T2} driver line [27]. *Erk1* gene was efficiently deleted in SMC (Figure 2H) and this deletion had no effect on the blood flow recovery after CFA (Figure 2I,J).

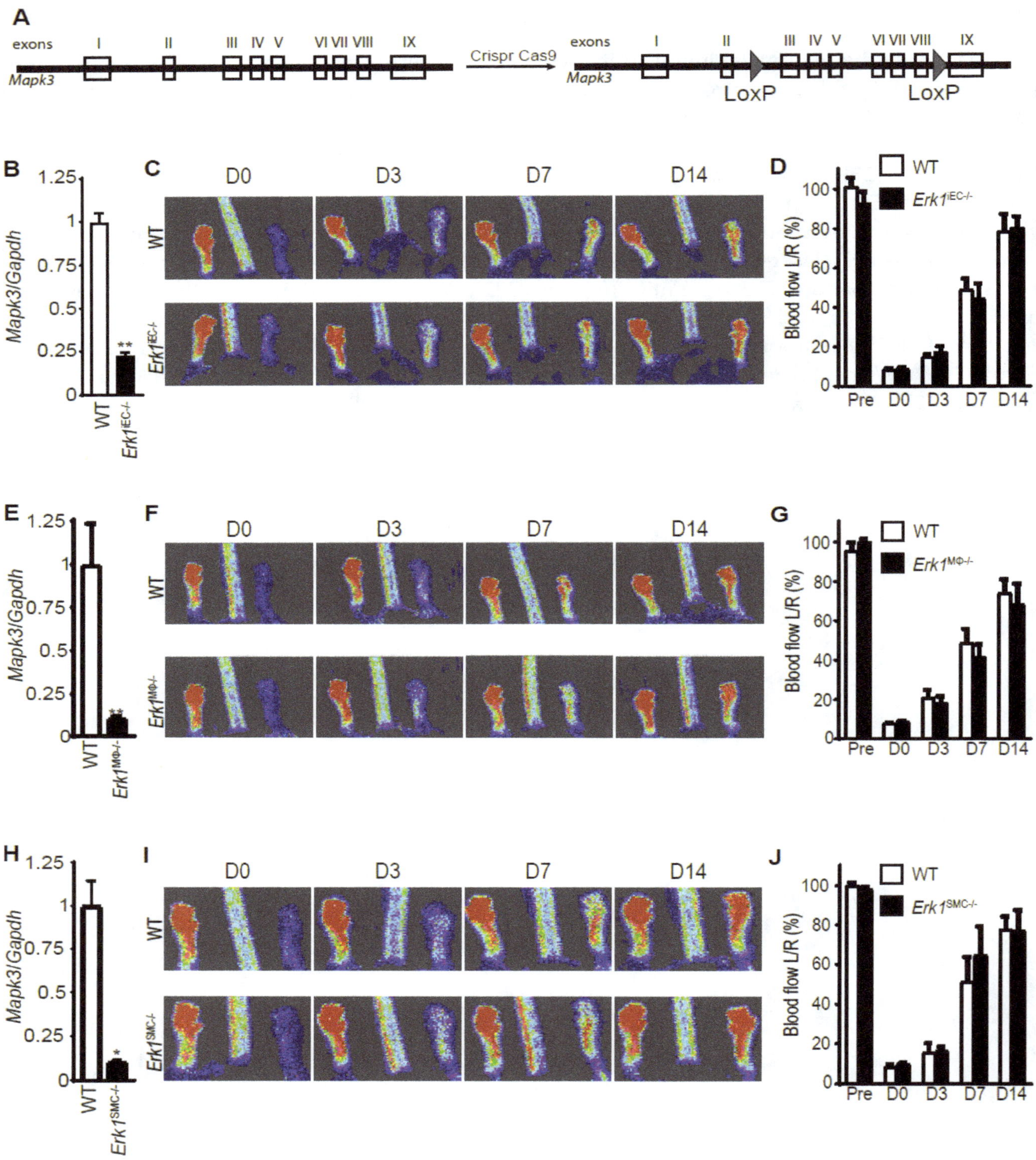

Figure 2. *Erk1* deletions in endothelial cells, macrophages, or smooth muscle cells do not affect arteriogenesis. (**A**) Generation of *Erk1* floxed mice by insertion of LoxP sites between exons 2 and 3 and exons 8 and 9. (**B**) Efficiency of *Erk1* deletion in endothelial cells was assessed by Q-PCR of endothelial cells isolated from mouse livers. Bar graph represents mean with SEM (n = 4 mice) ** $p <$ 0.005 using Mann–Whitney test. (**C**,**D**) Blood flow recovery after ligation of the CFA in $Erk1^{iEC-/-}$ mice assessed by laser Doppler right after the surgery and 3, 7, and 14 days after the surgery. Bar graph represents mean with SEM (n = 8 mice). (**E**) Efficiency of *Erk1* deletion in macrophages was assessed by Q-PCR of peritoneal macrophages. Bar graph represents mean with SEM (n = 4 mice) ** $p < 0.005$ using Mann–Whitney test. (**F**,**G**) Blood flow recovery after ligation of the CFA in $Erk1^{M\Phi-/-}$ mice assessed by laser-Doppler right after the surgery and 3, 7, and 14 days thereafter. Bar graph represents mean with

SEM ($n = 6$ mice). (**H**) Efficiency of *Erk1* deletion in smooth muscle cells was assessed by Q-PCR of smooth muscle cells isolated from the mouse aortas. Bar graph represents mean with SEM ($n = 4$ mice) * $p < 0.05$ using Mann–Whitney test. (**I**,**J**) Blood flow recovery after ligation of the CFA in $Erk1^{SMC-/-}$ mice assessed by laser-Doppler right after the surgery and 3, 7, and 14 days after the surgery. Bar graph represents mean with SEM ($n = 5$ mice).

3.3. *Erk1 Deletions in Endothelial Cells and Macrophages Leads to an Excessive but Poorly Functional Arteriogenesis*

Finally, we bred mice with macrophage- ($Erk1^{M\phi KO}$) and endothelial ($Erk1^{iECKO}$)-specific deletions to generate double knockout mice with ERK1 expression disrupted in both cell types ($Erk1^{iECKO/M\phi KO}$). Induction of hindlimb ischemia in these mice led to impaired blood flow recovery that was similar to that observed in the *Erk1* global null mice (Figure 3A,B) and the anatomical extent of arteriogenesis was increased (Figure 3C,D). We carried out Western blotting using total thigh muscle lysates and we observed a massive increase in F4/80 signal (Figure 3E).

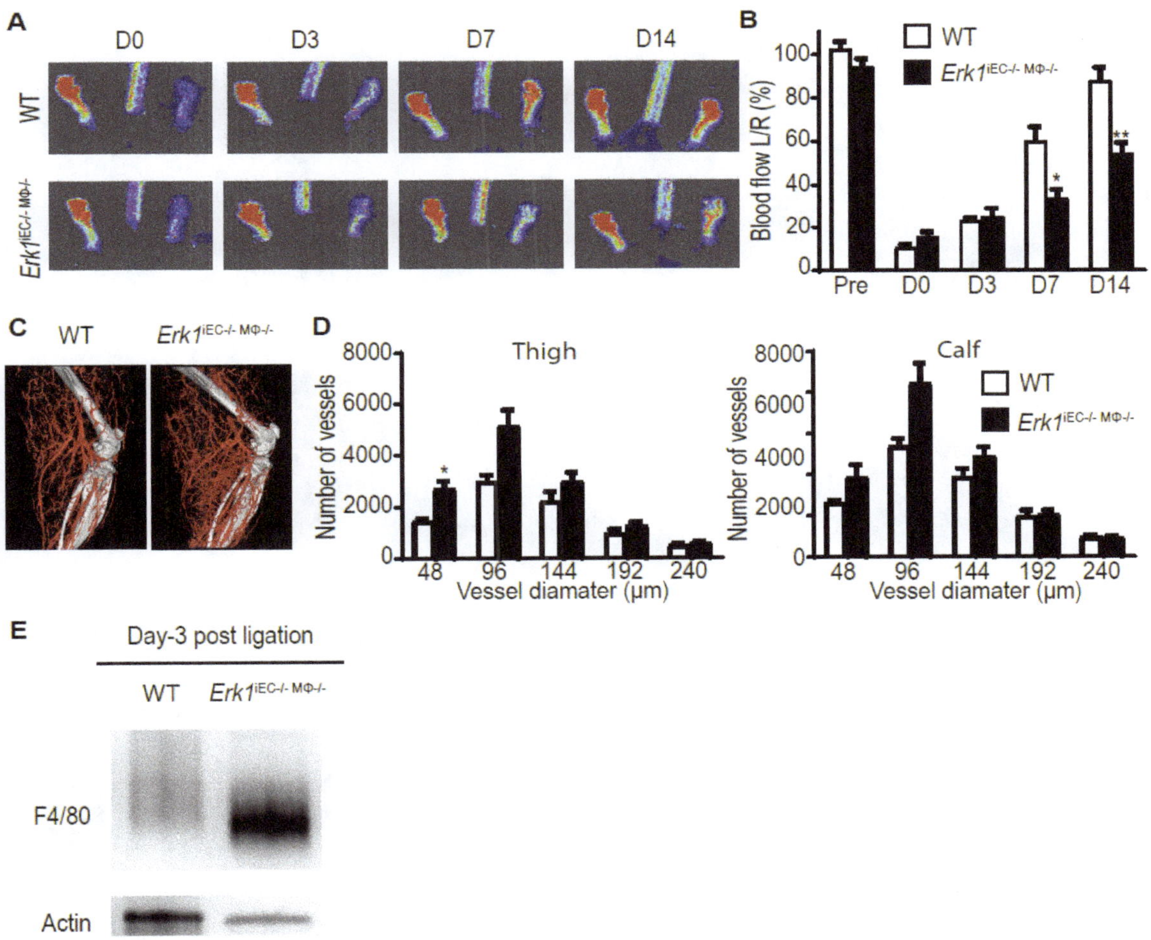

Figure 3. *Erk1* deletion in macrophages and endothelial cells leads to an excessive but poorly functional arteriogenesis. (**A**,**B**) Blood flow recovery after ligation of the femoral artery in $Erk1^{iEC-/-M\phi-/-}$ mice assessed by laser-Doppler right after the surgery and 3, 7, and 14 days thereafter. Bar graph represents mean with SEM ($n = 6$ mice) * $p < 0.05$, ** $p < 0.005$ using two-way ANOVA followed by Sidak's multiple comparison test. (**C**,**D**) Quantification of the hindlimb vasculature by micro-CT three weeks after femoral artery ligation. Bar graph represents mean with SEM ($n = 6$ mice) * $p < 0.05$ using two-way ANOVA followed by Sidak's multiple comparison test. (**E**) Macrophage infiltration in the thigh from $Erk1^{iEC-/-M\phi-/-}$ KO mice assessed by Western blotting. Bar graph represents mean with SEM ($n = 3$ mice) * $p < 0.05$ using *t*-test.

3.4. Erk2 Deletions in Endothelial, but Not Other Cell Types, Decreases Arteriogenesis

We next deleted endothelial *Erk2* (*Mapk1*) using the same Cdh5CreER^{T2} line. As in the case of *Erk1*, the administration of tamoxifen to eight-week-old *Erk2*$^{Fl/Fl}$ mice resulted in high efficiency deletion of the endothelial *Erk2* (Figure 4A). However, unlike the *Erk1*$^{iEC-/-}$ mice, the deletion of endothelial *Erk2* resulted in reduced flow recovery in *Erk2*$^{iEC-/-}$ compared to WT mice (Figure 4B,C). Surprisingly, there was no difference in the anatomical extent of arteriogenesis as determined by micro-CT imaging (Figure 4D,E). Endothelial nitric oxide synthase (eNOS) is a key enzyme producing the vasodilator NO and its activity is critical to arteriogenesis [28]. We found a decreased eNOS expression in *Erk2* KO endothelial cells compared to endothelial cells from WT mice (Figure 4F). We next focused on macrophages. LysM Cre was very effective in deleting *Erk2* in mice (Figure 4G). However, blood flow recovery after CFA ligation was not impaired compared to WT mice after *Erk2* gene deletion (Figure 4H,I). We next deleted the *Erk2* gene in smooth muscle cells using Myh11CreER^{T2} driver line (Figure 4J). *Erk2* deletion had no effect on the blood flow recovery (Figure 4K,L).

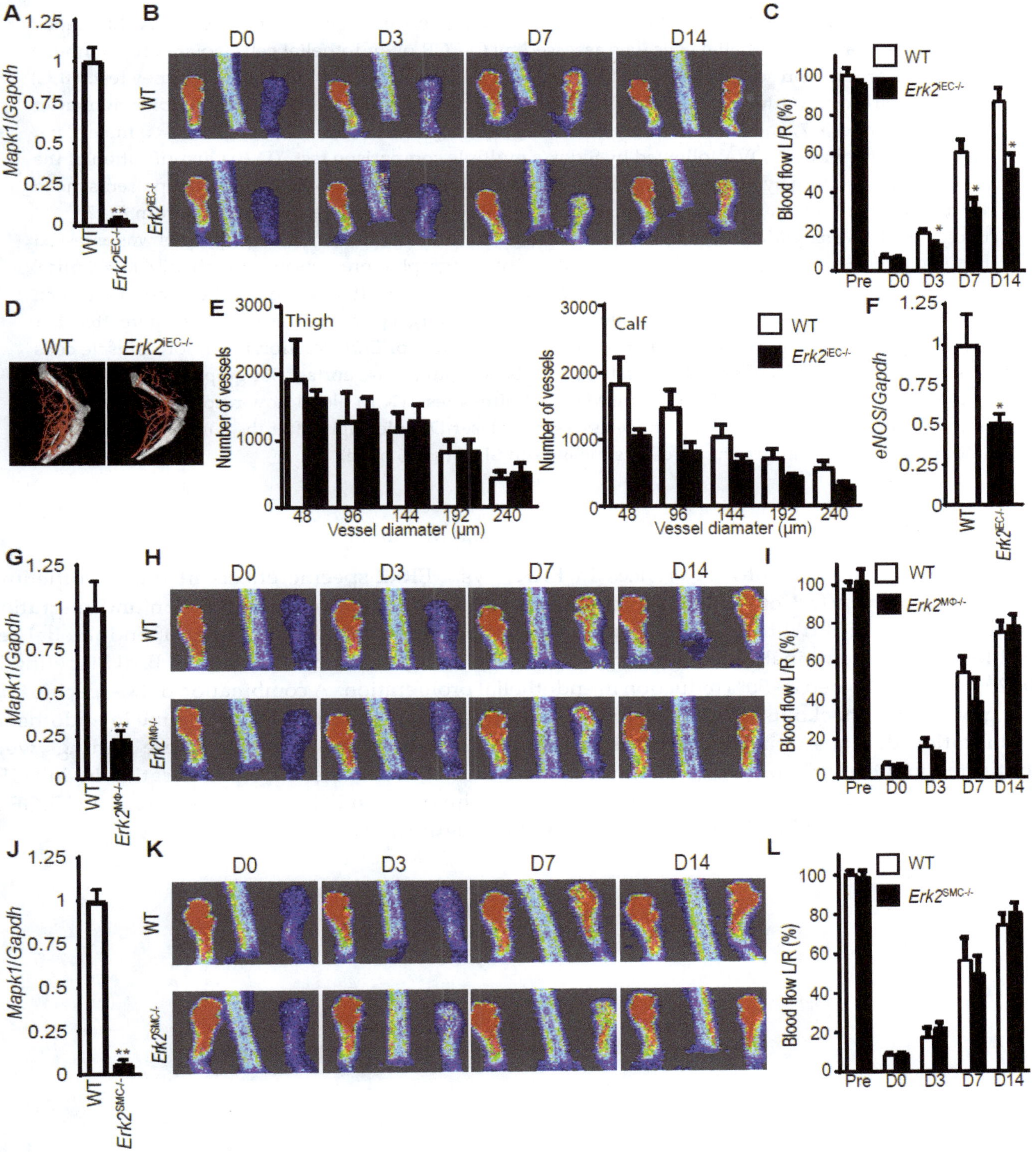

Figure 4. *Erk2* deletion in endothelial cells, but not in other cell types, decreases arteriogenesis. (**A**) Efficiency of *Erk2* deletion in endothelial cells was assessed by Q-PCR of endothelial cells isolated from mouse livers. Bar graph represents mean with SEM ($n = 4$ mice) ** $p < 0.005$ using Mann–Whitney test. (**B**,**C**) Blood flow recovery after ligation of the CFA in *Erk2*$^{iEC-/-}$ mice assessed by laser-Doppler right after the surgery and 3, 7, and 14 days thereafter. Bar graph represents mean with SEM ($n = 5$ mice) * $p < 0.05$ using two-way ANOVA followed by Sidak's multiple comparison test. (**D**,**E**) Quantification of the hindlimb vasculature by micro-CT three weeks after femoral artery ligation. Bar graph represents mean with SEM ($n = 3$ mice). (**F**) eNOS expression in endothelial cells isolated from livers from *Erk2*$^{iEC-/-}$ mice. * $p < 0.05$ using Mann–Whitney test. (**G**) Efficiency of *Erk2* deletion in macrophages was assessed by Q-PCR on macrophages from the peritoneal cavity. Bar graph represents mean with

Erk2 deletion in endothelial cells, but not in other cell types, decreases arteriogenesis. (**A**) Efficiency of *Erk2* deletion in endothelial cells was assessed by Q-PCR of endothelial cells isolated from mouse livers. Bar graph represents mean with SEM ($n = 4$ mice) ** $p < 0.005$ using Mann–Whitney test. (**B**,**C**) Blood flow recovery after ligation of the CFA in $Erk2^{iEC-/-}$ mice assessed by laser-Doppler right after the surgery and 3, 7, and 14 days thereafter. Bar graph represents mean with SEM ($n = 5$ mice) * $p < 0.05$ using two-way ANOVA followed by Sidak's multiple comparison test. (**D**,**E**) Quantification of the hindlimb vasculature by micro-CT three weeks after femoral artery ligation. Bar graph represents mean with SEM ($n = 3$ mice). (**F**) eNOS expression in endothelial cells isolated from livers from $Erk2^{iEC-/-}$ mice. * $p < 0.05$ using Mann–Whitney test. (**G**) Efficiency of *Erk2* deletion in macrophages was assessed by Q-PCR on macrophages from the peritoneal cavity. Bar graph represents mean with SEM ($n = 4$ mice) ** $p < 0.005$ using Mann–Whitney test. (**H**,**I**) Blood flow recovery after ligation of the femoral artery in $Erk2^{M\Phi-/-}$ mice assessed by laser-Doppler right after the surgery and 3, 7, and 14 days thereafter. Bar graph represents mean with SEM ($n = 4$ mice). (**J**) Efficiency of *Erk2* deletion in smooth muscle cells was assessed by Q-PCR of smooth muscle cells isolated from mouse aortas. Bar graph represents mean with SEM ($n = 4$ mice) ** $p < 0.005$ using Mann–Whitney test. (**K**,**L**) Blood flow recovery after ligation of the femoral artery in $Erk2^{SMC-/-}$ mice assessed by laser-Doppler right after the surgery and 3, 7, and 14 days thereafter. Bar graph represents mean with SEM ($n = 6$ mice).

3.5. ERK Isoform Effect on Endothelial Cell Proliferation and Migration

To gain an insight into differences in ERK1- vs. ERk2-specific effects in the endothelium, we examined the effect of either isoform deletion on endothelial cell proliferation and migration. Administration of BrdU to P6 $Erk1^{-/-}$ mice showed no differences in the extent of endothelial cell proliferation in the retinal vasculature vs. WT controls (Figure 5A,B). In contrast, BrdU labeling in $Erk2^{iECKO}$ mice showed a ~50% reduction in endothelial proliferation. A combination of EC-specific *Erk2* and global *Erk1* knockouts ($Erk2^{iECKO}$; $Erk1^{-/-}$ mice) did not result in a further decline in endothelial proliferation demonstrating that *Erk2* is the primary driver of this process. These findings were confirmed in vitro: *Erk2* but not *Erk1* knockdown resulted in decreased EC proliferation in an FGF2 growth assay (Figure 5C). In contrast, both ERKs were involved in EC migration response to VEGF-A or FGF2 stimulation in in vitro cell wounding assays (Figure 5D).

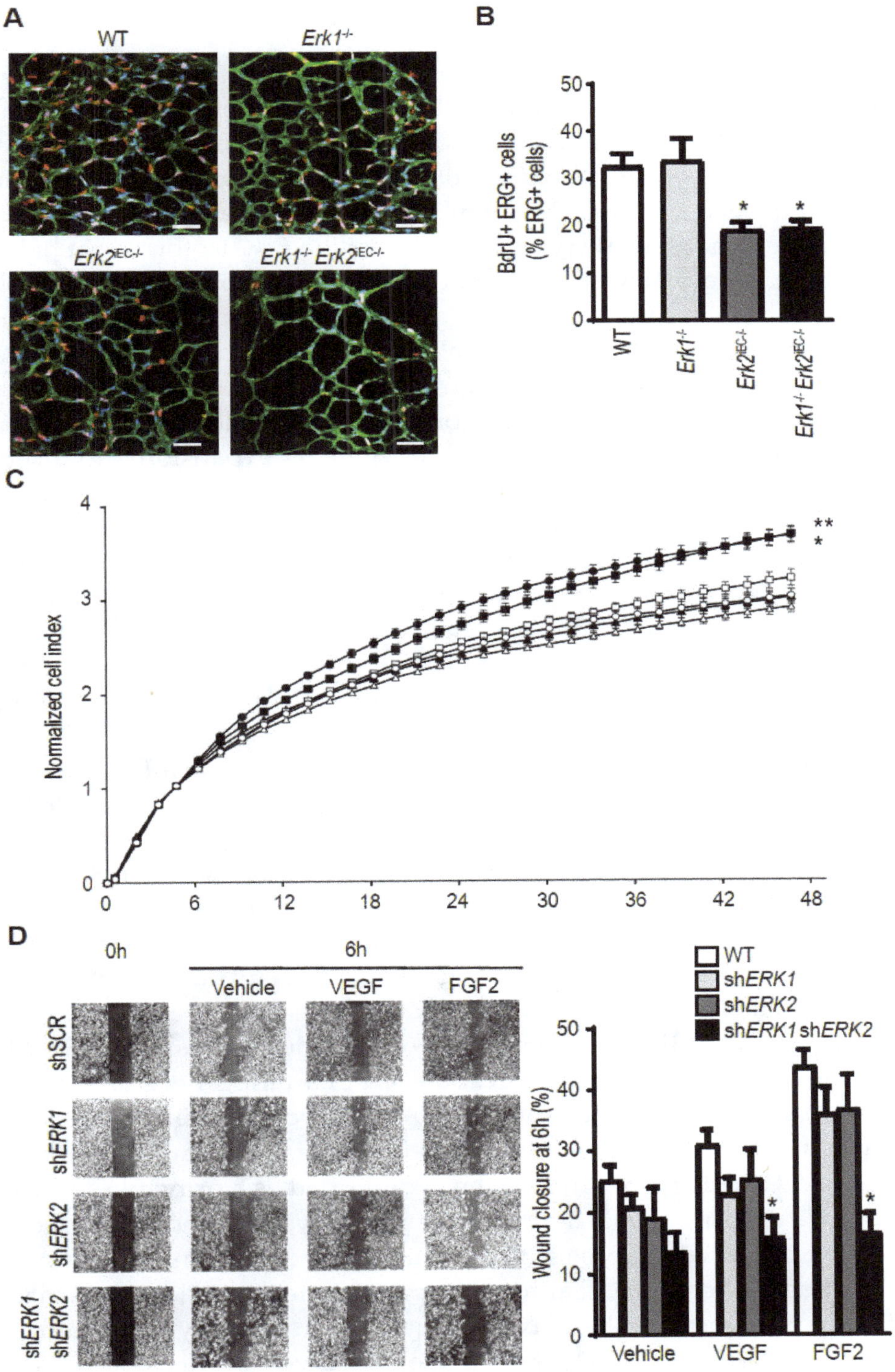

Figure 5. ERK isoform effect on endothelial cell proliferation and migration. (**A**,**B**) Assessment of endothelial cells proliferation in the retina of six-day-old pups by BrdU quantification. * $p < 0.05$ compared to WT using Kruskel–Wallis test with Dunn's multiple comparison test. Scale bar, 50 μm. Bar graph represents mean with SEM ($n = 5$ mice). (**C**) Assessment of proliferation of pulmonary endothelial cells from WT mice (circle), *Erk1*$^{-/-}$ mice (square), or *Erk2*^{iECKO} mice (triangle). White symbols are cells treated with vehicle, and black symbols cells treated with FGF2. Bar graph represents mean with SEM ($n = 6$ wells) * $p < 0.05$, ** $p < 0.005$ compared to WT treated with vehicle using Kruskel–Wallis test with Dunn's multiple comparison test. (**D**) Assessment of migration of HUVEC treated with shRNA scrambled, or against *ERK1*, or against *ERK2* and stimulated with (VEGFA$_{165}$ or FGF2. Bar graph represents mean with SEM ($n = 4$ wells) * $p < 0.05$ compared to siSCR of each condition using Kruskel–Wallis test with Dunn's multiple comparison test.

4. Discussion

The results of this study show that ERK isoforms have a differential effect on arteriogenesis. While a global *Erk1* knockout impaired blood flow recovery due to inefficient arteriogenesis, it took a combination of endothelial- and macrophage-specific knockout of this isoform to match the global deletion phenotype. The principal driver of response appeared to be a large increase in tissue macrophage levels that likely resulted in abnormally high VEGF levels and exuberant, albeit inefficient, arteriogenesis. In contrast, endothelial-specific deletion of the *Erk2* isoform resulted in reduced blood flow recovery even though the anatomical extent of arteriogenesis appeared normal. The culprit in this case was a dramatic reduction in endothelial eNOS expression that led to vasoconstriction. Neither ERK isoform deletion by itself in smooth muscle cells affected either blood flow recovery or arteriogenesis per se, while deletion of both genes resulted in a transient decrease of blood flow recovery.

Arteriogenesis is a process leading to the formation of arteries and arterioles. It can proceed either by remodeling of pre-existing collateral arteries or by expansion and arterialization of the capillary bed [2,5,29]. Arteriogenesis is distinct from angiogenesis, a process defined as sprouting and proliferation of the existing capillary bed [2]. Importantly, the two processes are regulated by distinctly different sets of factors. While hypoxia is the primary driver of angiogenesis, arteriogenesis is induced by a combination of shear stress and other mechanical factors [2,5,30]. At the same time, VEGF, and its subsequent induction of endothelial ERK activation, are crucial to both angiogenesis and arteriogenesis [31–35]. One important distinction, however, is the source of VEGF: while, in angiogenesis, VEGF is produced locally due to tissue ischemia, in arteriogenic settings macrophages are the key source of the growth factor [24].

While the importance of the VEGF/VEGFR2/ERK signaling cascade in both angiogenesis and arteriogenesis has been clearly recognized, how this signaling cascade promotes the two distinct means of vascular growth has been unclear. ERK activation is thought to be involved in the proliferation and migration of endothelial cells. Interestingly, our data indicate that endothelial proliferation is largely controlled by ERK2 while migration is the additive function of both isoforms. These results are in agreement with the study of Lefloch et al. who found that ERK2 controls cell proliferation in NIH 3T3 cells [36]. Other isoforms-specific effects of ERK signaling are regulation of macrophage accumulation by ERK1 and regulation of eNOS expression by ERK2.

Both global and a combination of macrophage- and/endothelial-specific *Erk1* knockouts led to markedly increased macrophage accumulation at the site of arteriogenesis after the common femoral artery ligation that was coupled with exuberant but ineffective arteriogenesis. The critical role macrophages play in arteriogenesis is well established. While the M2 subset (macrophages involved in wounds healing and vascular growth) have been described as a principle source of VEGF [37,38], other cell population, including blood-derived inflammatory cells, and mechanical factors can also contribute [13,39]. The observed increase in tissue macrophage levels in these mutant strains is likely derived from circulating monocytes [11] although a proliferation of resident M2 macrophages cannot be ruled out [39,40]. Endothelial cells play a crucial role in monocyte recruitment by increasing expression of the Notch ligand Dll1 [11], as has been observed in this study. Activation of Notch signaling in recruited monocytes polarizes them to an arteriogenic M2 phenotype [11]. Similarly, haploinsufficiency of *Phd2*, encoding the PHD2 oxygen sensor, leads to an expansion of tissue-resident M2-like macrophages, an increased release in arteriogenic factors, and an improved vascular reperfusion in the hindlimb ischemia model [37]. Here, we found that ERK1 controls endothelial-macrophage crosstalk, and that exacerbated macrophage infiltration increases arteriogenesis extent but decreases arteriogenesis functionality. However, a combination of the macrophage- and endothelial-specific *Erk1* knockout phenotype is not as severe as in the *Erk1* global knockout mice, suggesting that other cell types are also may be involved in the phenotype found in the *Erk1* global knockout mice.

In addition to the Dll1 signaling, endothelial cells also regulate macrophage infiltration via MAPK pathways. There are four distinct MAPK pathways: ERK1/2, ERK5, p38, and JNK. While we show that ERK1 controls macrophage recruitment, p38 MAPK pathway has also been shown to be involved in this process [41]. Indeed, a p38 downstream effector MAP-kinase-activated protein kinase 2 (MK2) induces MCP-1 expression in endothelial cells, which promotes monocyte chemoattraction. Thus, at least two different MAPK pathways are involved in the promotion of macrophage infiltration.

Effective blood flow recovery requires not only expansion of the arterial bed thereby ensuring adequate blood supply, but also effective organization and function of this newly formed vasculature. Interestingly, these processes appear to be differentially regulated. We and others have previously reported a dissociation between the extent of anatomical arteriogenesis and effective blood flow. Thus, a mouse strain with an endothelial loss of NF-kB signaling due to deletion of *Rela* showed increased and disorganized arteriogenesis and decreased tissue perfusion after CFA ligation [42]. This was driven by decreased expression of Dll4 that is NF-kB dependent. Delta-like 4 (Dll4) promotes arterial differentiation and restricts vessel branching by direct endothelial cell–cell signaling. Indeed, a similar phenotype was observed in adult *Dll4*$^{+/-}$ mice. These animals also show reduced blood flow recovery after femoral artery occlusion despite exuberant arteriogenesis [43]. Finally, mice with an endothelial-specific deletion of HIF2α also display increased arteriogenesis abut impaired blood flow recovery in the same hindlimb model [44]. Our description of excessive arteriogenesis yet impaired perfusion in ERK1 null mice adds to this growing body of literature.

In contrast to *Erk1*, *Erk2* knockout in endothelial cells resulted in impaired blood flow recovery despite the normal anatomical extent of arteriogenesis. This is likely due to a decrease in endothelial proliferation combined with decreased expression of eNOS and a corresponding fall in NO production that is critical to the maintenance of arterial tone. Indeed, these observations match a similar decrease in blood flow recovery in endothelial eNOS knockout mice.

ERK1 and ERK2 isoforms share 84% of their amino-acid sequences. ERK1 is larger than ERK2 due to an extension of 17 amino-acids at its N-terminal and two amino-acids at its C-terminal. It has been long a matter of debate whether ERK1 and ERK2 have isoform-specific functions or are totally redundant [45]. ERK2 is expressed at higher levels than ERK1 in most mammalian tissues [46,47]. This difference in expression level may account for the difference in phenotype of the global knockout. Indeed, *Erk1*$^{-/-}$ mice are viable and fertile [20], whereas *Erk2*$^{-/-}$ mice die at an early stage in development [19]. Several studies support the functional redundancy of ERK1 and ERK2. Indeed, deletion of *Erk2* but not *Erk1* affected NIH 3T3 cell proliferation in vitro while overexpression of *Erk1* in *Erk2*-deficient NIH 3T3 cells rescued this proliferation defect [36]. ERK1 can also rescue the loss of ERK2 in vivo. Indeed, overexpression of *Erk1* in *Erk2*$^{-/-}$ mice, generating mice expressing only the ERK1 isoform, fully rescue the developmental defects associated with the loss of ERK2 [47]. We recently published that loss of endothelial *Erk2* in a global *Erk1*$^{-/-}$ background in adult mice is lethal, whereas loss of one of the two isoforms in the endothelium of adult mice has no vascular phenotype [22]. Interestingly, deletion of *Erk2* by a ubiquitously expressed Cre in adult *Erk1*$^{-/-}$ mice is lethal in less than three weeks due to multiple organ failure [48]. However, adult mice with only one allele of ERK regardless of the isoform survive [48]. These results suggest redundant roles between ERK1 and ERK2. On the other hand, other studies suggest isoform-specific functions (review in [45]). Notably, in a model of myocardial ischemia/reperfusion injury, myocardial infarction extent was found to be similar in *Erk1*$^{-/-}$ mice and WT mice [49]. However, mice lacking one *Erk2* allele (*Erk2*$^{+/-}$), developed increased infarct areas compared with WT mice.

In summary, our data demonstrate specific roles of ERK isoforms in endothelial cells. While ERK1 controls macrophage infiltration following an ischemic event, ERK2 primarily controls endothelial cell proliferation and eNOS expression. Both isoforms are involved in regulation of migration.

Author Contributions: N.R. and M.S. designed experiments. J.Z. and Z.W.Z. carried out animal studies. N.R. and M.S. wrote the manuscript. M.S. supervised the study. All authors have read and agreed to the published version of the manuscript.

References

1. Rizzi, A.; Benagiano, V.; Ribatti, D. Angiogenesis versus arteriogenesis. *Rom. J. Morphol. Embryol.* **2017**, *58*, 15–19. [PubMed]

2. Faber, J.E.; Chilian, W.M.; Deindl, E.; Van Royen, N.; Simons, M. A brief etymology of the collateral circulation. *Arterioscler. Thromb. Vasc. Biol.* **2014**, *34*, 1854–1859. [CrossRef] [PubMed]
3. Lee, C.W.; Stabile, E.; Kinnaird, T.; Shou, M.; Devaney, J.M.; Epstein, S.E.; Burnett, M.S. Temporal patterns of gene expression after acute hindlimb ischemia in mice: Insights into the genomic program for collateral vessel development. *J. Am. Coll. Cardiol.* **2004**, *43*, 474–482. [CrossRef] [PubMed]
4. Scholz, D.; Ziegelhoeffer, T.; Helisch, A.; Wagner, S.; Friedrich, C.; Podzuweit, T.; Schaper, W. Contribution of arteriogenesis and angiogenesis to postocclusive hindlimb perfusion in mice. *J. Mol. Cell. Cardiol.* **2002**, *34*, 775–787. [CrossRef] [PubMed]
5. Simons, M.; Eichmann, A. Molecular controls of arterial morphogenesis. *Circ. Res.* **2015**, *116*, 1712–1724. [CrossRef] [PubMed]
6. Moraes, F.; Paye, J.; Mac Gabhann, F.; Zhuang, Z.W.; Zhang, J.; Lanahan, A.A.; Simons, M. Endothelial cell-dependent regulation of arteriogenesis. *Circ. Res.* **2013**, *113*, 1076–1086. [CrossRef]
7. Lanahan, A.A.; Lech, D.; Dubrac, A.; Zhang, J.; Zhuang, Z.W.; Eichmann, A.; Simons, M. Ptp1b is a physiologic regulator of vascular endothelial growth factor signaling in endothelial cells. *Circulation* **2014**, *130*, 902–909. [CrossRef]
8. Stabile, E.; Burnett, M.S.; Watkins, C.; Kinnaird, T.; Bachis, A.; La Sala, A.; Miller, J.M.; Shou, M.; Epstein, S.E.; Fuchs, S. Impaired arteriogenic response to acute hindlimb ischemia in cd4-knockout mice. *Circulation* **2003**, *108*, 205–210. [CrossRef]
9. Stabile, E.; Kinnaird, T.; La Sala, A.; Hanson, S.K.; Watkins, C.; Campia, U.; Shou, M.; Zbinden, S.; Fuchs, S.; Kornfeld, H.; et al. Cd8+ t lymphocytes regulate the arteriogenic response to ischemia by infiltrating the site of collateral vessel development and recruiting cd4+ mononuclear cells through the expression of interleukin-16. *Circulation* **2006**, *113*, 118–124. [CrossRef]
10. Van Weel, V.; Toes, R.E.; Seghers, L.; Deckers, M.M.; De Vries, M.R.; Eilers, P.H.; Sipkens, J.; Schepers, A.; Eefting, D.; Van Hinsbergh, V.W.; et al. Natural killer cells and cd4+ t-cells modulate collateral artery development. *Arterioscler. Thromb. Vasc. Biol.* **2007**, *27*, 2310–2318. [CrossRef]
11. Krishnasamy, K.; Limbourg, A.; Kapanadze, T.; Gamrekelashvili, J.; Beger, C.; Hager, C.; Lozanovski, V.J.; Falk, C.S.; Napp, L.C.; Bauersachs, J.; et al. Blood vessel control of macrophage maturation promotes arteriogenesis in ischemia. *Nat. Commun.* **2017**, *8*, 952. [CrossRef] [PubMed]
12. Ribatti, D. A new role of mast cells in arteriogenesis. *Microvasc. Res.* **2018**, *118*, 57–60. [CrossRef] [PubMed]
13. Li, J.; Hampton, T.; Morgan, J.P.; Simons, M. Stretch-induced vegf expression in the heart. *J. Clin. Investig.* **1997**, *100*, 18–24. [CrossRef] [PubMed]
14. Pipp, F.; Heil, M.; Issbrucker, K.; Ziegelhoeffer, T.; Martin, S.; Van Den Heuvel, J.; Weich, H.; Fernandez, B.; Golomb, G.; Carmeliet, P.; et al. Vegfr-1-selective vegf homologue plgf is arteriogenic: Evidence for a monocyte-mediated mechanism. *Circ. Res.* **2003**, *92*, 378–385. [CrossRef] [PubMed]
15. Morrison, A.R.; Yarovinsky, T.O.; Young, B.D.; Moraes, F.; Ross, T.D.; Ceneri, N.; Zhang, J.; Zhuang, Z.W.; Sinusas, A.J.; Pardi, R.; et al. Chemokine-coupled beta2 integrin-induced macrophage rac2-myosin iia interaction regulates vegf-a mrna stability and arteriogenesis. *J. Exp. Med.* **2014**, *211*, 1957–1968. [CrossRef] [PubMed]
16. Ahn, G.O.; Seita, J.; Hong, B.J.; Kim, Y.E.; Bok, S.; Lee, C.J.; Kim, K.S.; Lee, J.C.; Leeper, N.J.; Cooke, J.P.; et al. Transcriptional activation of hypoxia-inducible factor-1 (hif-1) in myeloid cells promotes angiogenesis through vegf and s100a8. *Proc. Natl. Acad. Sci. USA* **2014**, *111*, 2698–2703. [CrossRef] [PubMed]
17. Heil, M.; Ziegelhoeffer, T.; Pipp, F.; Kostin, S.; Martin, S.; Clauss, M.; Schaper, W. Blood monocyte concentration is critical for enhancement of collateral artery growth. *Am. J. Physiol. Heart Circ. Physiol.* **2002**, *283*, H2411–H2419. [CrossRef]
18. Simons, M.; Gordon, E.; Claesson-Welsh, L. Mechanisms and regulation of endothelial vegf receptor signalling. *Nat. Rev. Mol. Cell. Biol.* **2016**, *17*, 611–625. [CrossRef]
19. Hatano, N.; Mori, Y.; Oh-hora, M.; Kosugi, A.; Fujikawa, T.; Nakai, N.; Niwa, H.; Miyazaki, J.; Hamaoka, T.; Ogata, M. Essential role for erk2 mitogen-activated protein kinase in placental development. *Genes. Cells* **2003**, *8*, 847–856. [CrossRef]

20. Pages, G.; Guerin, S.; Grall, D.; Bonino, F.; Smith, A.; Anjuere, F.; Auberger, P.; Pouyssegur, J. Defective thymocyte maturation in p44 map kinase (erk 1) knockout mice. *Science* **1999**, *286*, 1374–1377.
21. Srinivasan, R.; Zabuawala, T.; Huang, H.; Zhang, J.; Gulati, P.; Fernandez, S.; Karlo, J.C.; Landreth, G.E.; Leone, G.; Ostrowski, M.C. Erk1 and erk2 regulate endothelial cell proliferation and migration during mouse embryonic angiogenesis. *PLoS ONE* **2009**, *4*, e8283. [CrossRef] [PubMed]
22. Ricard, N.; Scott, R.P.; Booth, C.J.; Velazquez, H.; Cilfone, N.A.; Baylon, J.L.; Gulcher, J.R.; Quaggin, S.E.; Chittenden, T.W.; Simons, M. Endothelial erk1/2 signaling maintains integrity of the quiescent endothelium. *J. Exp. Med.* **2019**, *216*, 1874–1890. [CrossRef] [PubMed]
23. Ray, A.; Dittel, B.N. Isolation of mouse peritoneal cavity cells. *J. Vis. Exp.* **2010**. [CrossRef] [PubMed]
24. Ziegelhoeffer, T.; Fernandez, B.; Kostin, S.; Heil, M.; Voswinckel, R.; Helisch, A.; Schaper, W. Bone marrow-derived cells do not incorporate into the adult growing vasculature. *Circ. Res.* **2004**, *94*, 230–238. [CrossRef]
25. Sorensen, I.; Adams, R.H.; Gossler, A. Dll1-mediated notch activation regulates endothelial identity in mouse fetal arteries. *Blood* **2009**, *113*, 5680–5688. [CrossRef]
26. Clausen, B.E.; Burkhardt, C.; Reith, W.; Renkawitz, R.; Forster, I. Conditional gene targeting in macrophages and granulocytes using lysmcre mice. *Transgenic Res.* **1999**, *8*, 265–277. [CrossRef]
27. Wirth, A.; Benyo, Z.; Lukasova, M.; Leutgeb, B.; Wettschureck, N.; Gorbey, S.; Orsy, P.; Horvath, B.; Maser-Gluth, C.; Greiner, E.; et al. G12-g13-larg-mediated signaling in vascular smooth muscle is required for salt-induced hypertension. *Nat. Med.* **2008**, *14*, 64–68. [CrossRef]
28. Lee, M.Y.; Gamez-Mendez, A.; Zhang, J.; Zhuang, Z.; Vinyard, D.J.; Kraehling, J.; Velazquez, H.; Brudvig, G.W.; Kyriakides, T.R.; Simons, M.; et al. Endothelial cell autonomous role of akt1: Regulation of vascular tone and ischemia-induced arteriogenesis. *Arterioscler. Thromb. Vasc. Biol.* **2018**, *38*, 870–879. [CrossRef]
29. Mac Gabhann, F.; Peirce, S.M. Collateral capillary arterialization following arteriolar ligation in murine skeletal muscle. *Microcirculation* **2010**, *17*, 333–347. [CrossRef]
30. Heil, M.; Schaper, W. Influence of mechanical, cellular, and molecular factors on collateral artery growth (arteriogenesis). *Circ. Res.* **2004**, *95*, 449–458. [CrossRef]
31. Shin, M.; Beane, T.J.; Quillien, A.; Male, I.; Zhu, L.J.; Lawson, N.D. Vegfa signals through erk to promote angiogenesis, but not artery differentiation. *Development* **2016**, *143*, 3796–3805. [CrossRef] [PubMed]
32. Kofler, N.M.; Simons, M. Angiogenesis versus arteriogenesis: Neuropilin 1 modulation of vegf signaling. *F1000Prime Rep.* **2015**, *7*, 26. [CrossRef] [PubMed]
33. Lucitti, J.L.; Mackey, J.K.; Morrison, J.C.; Haigh, J.J.; Adams, R.H.; Faber, J.E. Formation of the collateral circulation is regulated by vascular endothelial growth factor-a and a disintegrin and metalloprotease family members 10 and 17. *Circ. Res.* **2012**, *111*, 1539–1550. [CrossRef] [PubMed]
34. Hong, C.C.; Peterson, Q.P.; Hong, J.Y.; Peterson, R.T. Artery/vein specification is governed by opposing phosphatidylinositol-3 kinase and map kinase/erk signaling. *Curr. Biol.* **2006**, *16*, 1366–1372. [CrossRef] [PubMed]
35. Ren, B.; Deng, Y.; Mukhopadhyay, A.; Lanahan, A.A.; Zhuang, Z.W.; Moodie, K.L.; Mulligan-Kehoe, M.J.; Byzova, T.V.; Peterson, R.T.; Simons, M. Erk1/2-akt1 crosstalk regulates arteriogenesis in mice and zebrafish. *J. Clin. Investig.* **2010**, *120*, 1217–1228. [CrossRef]
36. Lefloch, R.; Pouyssegur, J.; Lenormand, P. Single and combined silencing of erk1 and erk2 reveals their positive contribution to growth signaling depending on their expression levels. *Mol. Cell. Biol.* **2008**, *28*, 511–527. [CrossRef]
37. Takeda, Y.; Costa, S.; Delamarre, E.; Roncal, C.; De Oliveira, R.L.; Squadrito, M.L.; Finisguerra, V.; Deschoemaeker, S.; Bruyere, F.; Wenes, M.; et al. Macrophage skewing by phd2 haplodeficiency prevents ischaemia by inducing arteriogenesis. *Nature* **2011**, *479*, 122–126. [CrossRef]
38. Troidl, C.; Jung, G.; Troidl, K.; Hoffmann, J.; Mollmann, H.; Nef, H.; Schaper, W.; Hamm, C.W.; Schmitz-Rixen, T. The temporal and spatial distribution of macrophage subpopulations during arteriogenesis. *Curr. Vasc. Pharmacol.* **2013**, *11*, 5–12. [CrossRef]
39. Li, J.; Brown, L.F.; Hibberd, M.G.; Grossman, J.D.; Morgan, J.P.; Simons, M. VEGF, flk-1, and flt-1 expression in a rat myocardial infarction model of angiogenesis. *Am. J. Physiol.* **1996**, *270*, H1803–H1811. [CrossRef]
40. Jenkins, S.J.; Ruckerl, D.; Cook, P.C.; Jones, L.H.; Finkelman, F.D.; Van Rooijen, N.; MacDonald, A.S.; Allen, J.E. Local macrophage proliferation, rather than recruitment from the blood, is a signature of th2 inflammation. *Science* **2011**, *332*, 1284–1288. [CrossRef]

41. Limbourg, A.; Von Felden, J.; Jagavelu, K.; Krishnasamy, K.; Napp, L.C.; Kapopara, P.R.; Gaestel, M.; Schieffer, B.; Bauersachs, J.; Limbourg, F.P.; et al. Map-kinase activated protein kinase 2 links endothelial activation and monocyte/macrophage recruitment in arteriogenesis. *PLoS ONE* **2015**, *10*, e0138542. [CrossRef] [PubMed]
42. Tirziu, D.; Jaba, I.M.; Yu, P.; Larrivee, B.; Coon, B.G.; Cristofaro, B.; Zhuang, Z.W.; Lanahan, A.A.; Schwartz, M.A.; Eichmann, A.; et al. Endothelial nuclear factor-kappab-dependent regulation of arteriogenesis and branching. *Circulation* **2012**, *126*, 2589–2600. [CrossRef] [PubMed]
43. Cristofaro, B.; Shi, Y.; Faria, M.; Suchting, S.; Leroyer, A.S.; Trindade, A.; Duarte, A.; Zovein, A.C.; Iruela-Arispe, M.L.; Nih, L.R.; et al. Dll4-notch signaling determines the formation of native arterial collateral networks and arterial function in mouse ischemia models. *Development* **2013**, *140*, 1720–1729. [CrossRef] [PubMed]
44. Skuli, N.; Majmundar, A.J.; Krock, B.L.; Mesquita, R.C.; Mathew, L.K.; Quinn, Z.L.; Runge, A.; Liu, L.; Kim, M.N.; Liang, J.; et al. Endothelial hif-2alpha regulates murine pathological angiogenesis and revascularization processes. *J. Clin. Investig.* **2012**, *122*, 1427–1443. [CrossRef]
45. Busca, R.; Pouyssegur, J.; Lenormand, P. Erk1 and erk2 map kinases: Specific roles or functional redundancy? *Front. Cell Dev. Biol.* **2016**, *4*, 53. [CrossRef]
46. Busca, R.; Christen, R.; Lovern, M.; Clifford, A.M.; Yue, J.X.; Goss, G.G.; Pouyssegur, J.; Lenormand, P. Erk1 and erk2 present functional redundancy in tetrapods despite higher evolution rate of erk1. *BMC Evol. Biol.* **2015**, *15*, 179. [CrossRef]
47. Fremin, C.; Saba-El-Leil, M.K.; Levesque, K.; Ang, S.L.; Meloche, S. Functional redundancy of erk1 and erk2 map kinases during development. *Cell. Rep.* **2015**, *12*, 913–921. [CrossRef]
48. Blasco, R.B.; Francoz, S.; Santamaria, D.; Canamero, M.; Dubus, P.; Charron, J.; Baccarini, M.; Barbacid, M. C-Raf, but not B-Raf, is essential for development of K-Ras oncogene-driven non-small cell lung carcinoma. *Cancer Cell* **2011**, *19*, 652–663. [CrossRef]
49. Lips, D.J.; Bueno, O.F.; Wilkins, B.J.; Purcell, N.H.; Kaiser, R.A.; Lorenz, J.N.; Voisin, L.; Saba-El-Leil, M.K.; Meloche, S.; Pouysségur, J.; et al. MEK1-ERK2 signaling pathway protects myocardium from ischemic injury in vivo. *Circulation* **2004**, *109*, 1938–1941. [CrossRef]

8

IL10 Alters Peri-Collateral Macrophage Polarization and Hind-Limb Reperfusion in Mice after Femoral Artery Ligation

Alexander M. Götze [1,*], Christian Schubert [2], Georg Jung [3], Oliver Dörr [4], Christoph Liebetrau [5], Christian W. Hamm [5], Thomas Schmitz-Rixen [3], Christian Troidl [4,†] and Kerstin Troidl [2,3,†]

1 Department of Trauma-, Hand- and Reconstructive Surgery, Johann-Wolfgang-Goethe-University, 60590 Frankfurt am Main, Germany

2 Max-Planck Institute for Heart- and Lung-Research, 61231 Bad Nauheim, Germany; christian.schubert@mpi-bn.mpg.de (C.S.); kerstin.troidl@mpi-bn.mpg.de (K.T.)

3 Department of Vascular and Endovascular Surgery, Johann-Wolfgang-Goethe-University, 60590 Frankfurt am Main, Germany; Georg.Jung@kgu.de (G.J.); schmitz-rixen@em.uni-frankfurt.de (T.S.-R.)

4 Department of Cardiology, Justus-Liebig-University, 35392 Gießen, Germany; oliver.doerr@innere.med.uni-giessen.de (O.D.); c.troidl@kerckhoff-fgi.de (C.T.)

5 Department of Cardiology, Kerckhoff Heart and Thorax Center, 61231 Bad Nauheim, Germany; c.liebetrau@kerckhoff-klinik.de (C.L.); c.hamm@kerckhoff-klinik.de (C.W.H.)

* Correspondence: a.goetze@icloud.com

† These authors contributed equally to this work.

Abstract: Arteriogenesis is a process by which a pre-existing arterioarterial anastomosis develops into a functional collateral network following an arterial occlusion. Alternatively activated macrophages polarized by IL10 have been described to promote collateral growth. This study investigates the effect of different levels of IL10 on hind-limb reperfusion and the distribution of perivascular macrophage activation types in mice after femoral artery ligation (FAL). IL10 and anti-IL10 were administered before FAL and the arteriogenic response was measured by Laser-Doppler-Imaging perioperatively, after 3, 7, and 14 d. Reperfusion recovery was accelerated when treated with IL10 and impaired with anti-IL10. Furthermore, symptoms of ischemia on ligated hind-limbs had the highest incidence after application of anti-IL10. Perivascular macrophages were immunohistologically phenotyped using CD163 and CD68 in adductor muscle segments. The proportion of alternatively activated macrophages ($CD163^+/CD68^+$) in relation to classically activated macrophages ($CD163^-/CD68^+$) observed was the highest when treated with IL10 and suppressed with anti-IL10. This study underlines the proarteriogenic response with increased levels of IL10 and demonstrates an in-vivo alteration of macrophage activation types in the perivascular bed of growing collaterals.

Keywords: arteriogenesis; collateral artery; macrophages; macrophage polarization; M2 macrophages; IL10

---

1. Introduction

Arteriogenesis is the process by which a pre-existing arterioarterial anastomosis develops into a functional collateral network following an arterial occlusion. The remodeling processes involved in collateral vessel growth are complex and are dependent on mechanical, cellular and molecular factors [1]. Several authors have demonstrated the pertinence of monocytes and macrophages in enhancing collateral vessel growth [1–3]. While there is still debate over whether perivascular macrophages are recruited from circulating monocytes or tissue resident precursors, their proarteriogenic effects, however, are still evident [4–6]. Macrophage activation types have become a growing focus in arteriogenesis research, in particular alternatively activated macrophages [7]. Macrophage heterogeneity and plasticity are reflected by their ability to respond to environmental cues giving rise to a spectrum of distinct functional phenotypes or activation states, fulfilling a variety of functions. The extremes of these functional states are commonly defined as M1, M2, or M2-like polarized macrophages [8]. M1 or classically activated macrophages induced by LPS, IFN-γ, and TNF are associated with inflammation and tumor resistance. They differ from M2 macrophages with regard to their arginine metabolism by exhibiting high levels of iNOS and subsequent NO-synthesis, as well as the production of proinflammatory cytokines and chemoattractant proteins. M2/M2-like or alternatively activated macrophages induced by IL4/IL13, immune complexes, agonists of TLR or IL1R, glucocorticoids and IL10, on the other hand, regulate inflammatory responses and promote tissue remodeling, angiogenesis and tumor progression [9]. They are characterized by their arginase/ornithine production, a precursor of cell proliferation, collagen production and ECM remodeling, and the production of anti-inflammatory cytokines [9,10]. While both M1 and M2 macrophages have been shown to contribute to collateral vessel growth, a systemic modulation of known activators of macrophage differentiation demonstrated a determinate proarteriogenic role of M2 macrophages induced by IL10 [11]. This M2 activation phenotype, also referred to as M2c, not only acts as a regulator of immune responses but also as an effector cell of tissue remodeling and repair [9]. It is important to note that the M1/M2 taxonomy of macrophages only represents a limited attempt to categorize the vast variety of functional states observed in vitro. In vivo, this M1/M2 paradigm undermines the complexity of macrophage plasticity and diversity. Functional and phenotypical characteristics of M1 and M2 activation states are not limited to but may instead be shared by more than one macrophage population, allowing them to cater to situational and tissue specific needs. This dogma change has created the need to explore other classifications that more appropriately reflect macrophage behavior in vivo and are subject of current research [12]. Jetten et al. [6] showed that collateral growth was unaffected in mice with a deletion of the IL10 receptor on myeloid cells (IL10R$^{fl/fl}$/LysMCre^{+}), arguing that the M2c activation phenotype is not required in arteriogenesis. When treated with exogenously polarized M2c macrophages, however, an improved reperfusion of collateral vessels compared to untreated IL10R$^{fl/fl}$/LysMCre^{+} mice was still observed. As such, this study investigates the in vivo effect of varying levels of IL10 on arteriogenesis as well as the distribution of macrophage activation types around growing collateral vessels.

2. Results

2.1. Modulation of Blood Concentration Levels of IL10 after Pharmacological Stimulation with IL10 and Anti-IL10

To investigate whether blood concentration levels of endogenous IL10 were affected by an intravenous administration of IL10 or anti-IL10 via tail vein injection, a Mouse Magnetic Luminex Assay was used to determine the blood concentration levels of IL10 prior to (baseline, BL) and 24 h (24 h) after the respective treatments. A control group received NaCl 0.9%. At BL, blood concentration levels of IL10 were below the detection limit of 1.59 pg/mL in all groups. At 24 h, elevated blood concentration levels of IL10 were found only in the IL10 treatment group with 6.35 ± 2.20 pg/mL ($p < 0.05$), indicating that an external administration of IL10 leads to a sustainable change in endogenous blood concentration levels of IL10 for at least 24 h when applied via tail vein injection. Blood concentration levels of IL10 in mice treated with anti-IL10 or NaCl 0.9% remained below the detection limit (Figure 1).

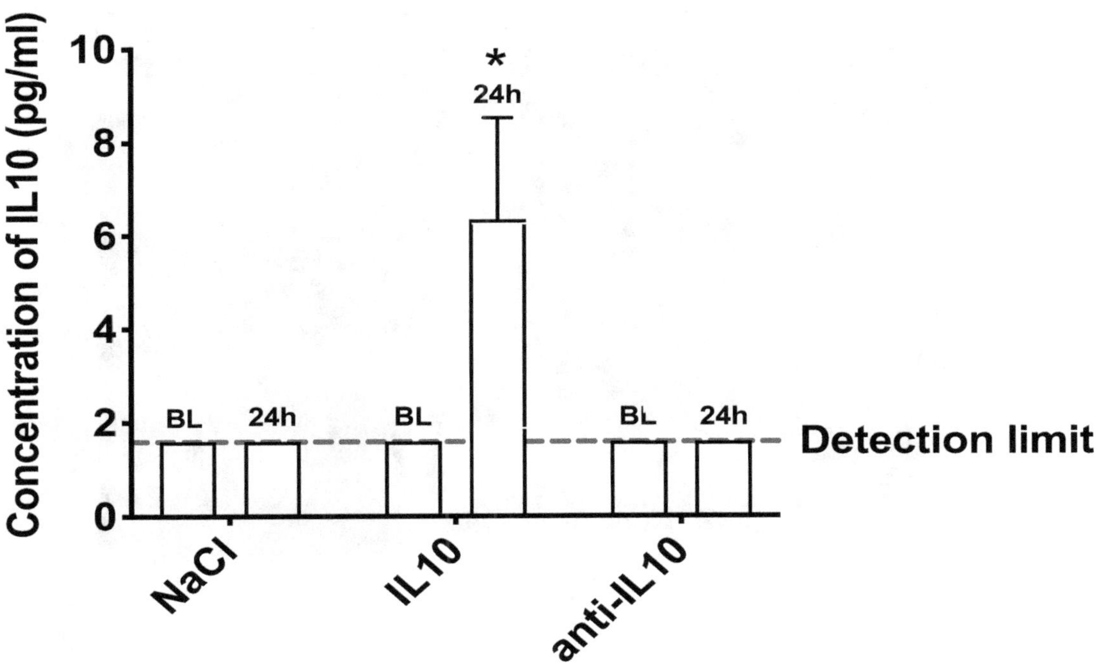

Figure 1. Modulation of blood concentration levels of IL10 after pharmacological stimulation with IL10 and anti-IL10. IL10, anti-IL10, and NaCl were administered via tail vein injection. Blood concentration levels of IL10 were measured before (baseline, BL) and 24 h after pharmacological stimulation. At BL endogenous IL10 levels were below the detection limit of 1.59 pg/mL in all subjects. After an external administration of IL10, blood concentration levels remained significantly increased after 24 h. An effect of anti-IL10 could not be detected, as baseline levels of IL10 remained below the detection limit. * indicates $p < 0.05$; $n = 3$ in each group.

2.2. *Alteration of Macrophage Polarization in the Perivascular Bed of Growing Collateral Vessels after Pharmacological Stimulation with IL10 and Anti-IL10*

Adductor muscle samples were harvested 3 days (3 d) and 7 d after FAL to analyze the effect of a treatment with IL10 and anti-IL10 on the polarization of macrophages in the perivascular bed of growing collateral vessels. The samples were sectioned and stained using antibodies targeting known macrophage markers CD68 and CD163 [11,13] (Figure 2a). The two largest collateral vessels of each section were selected and the ratio of macrophages of the alternatively activated phenotype $CD163^+/CD68^+$ to the classically activated phenotype $CD163^-/CD68^+$ per visual field was calculated. Mice treated with NaCl had a median ratio of $CD163^+/CD68^+$ to $CD163^-/CD68^+$ macrophages of 0.46 (IQR: 0.37–1.20) on day 3 (3 d) and 0.40 (IQR: 0.37–0.55) 7 d after FAL. When treated with IL10 the ratio is skewed towards the alternatively activated phenotype on both 3 d and 7 d after FAL with a ratio of 1.00 (IQR: 0.45–1.44) and 1.19 (IQR: 0.52–1.69). Contrariwise, the ratio is skewed towards the classically activated phenotype after application of anti-IL10 on both 3 d and 7 d after FAL with a ratio of 0.25 (IQR: 0.18–0.35) and 0.27 (IQR: 0.00–0.53), differing significantly from that of the IL10 treatment group ($p < 0.05$) (Figure 2b).

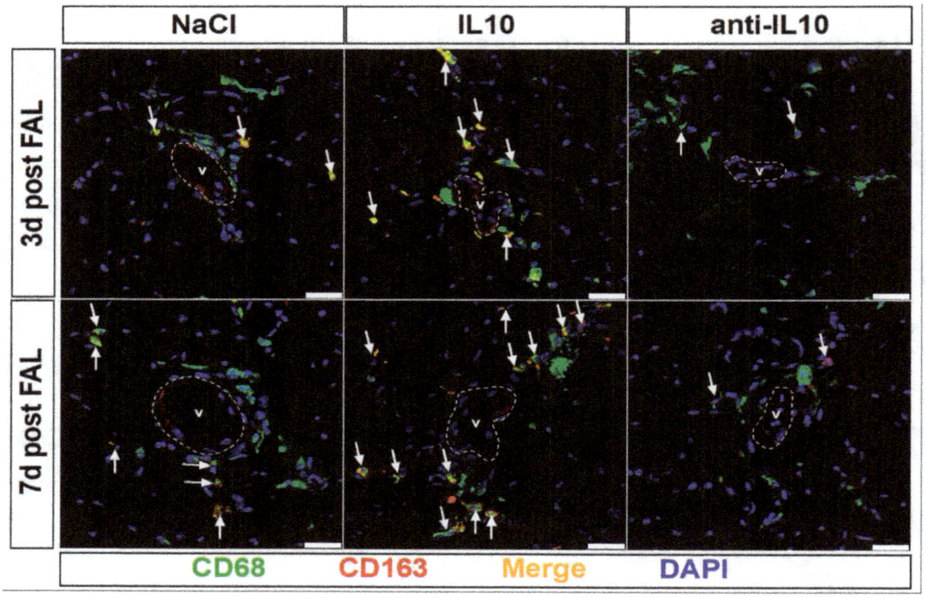

(a)

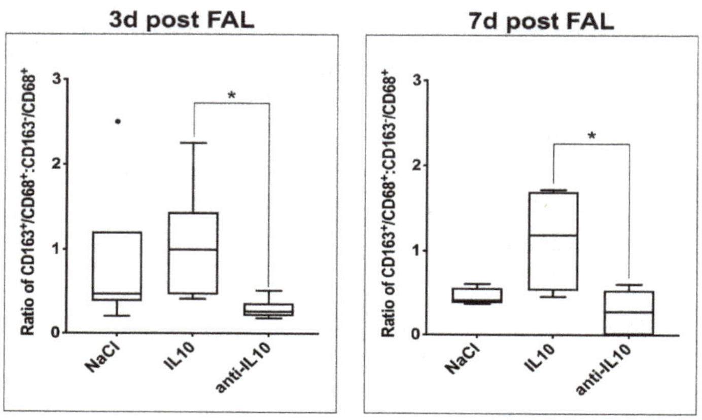

(b)

Figure 2. Alteration of macrophage polarization in the perivascular bed of growing collateral vessels after pharmacological stimulation with IL10 and anti-IL10. (**a**) Confocal micrographs of macrophage differentiation subtypes 3 d and 7 d after FAL. Sections of adductor muscles segments containing growing collateral vessels (V) were stained using DAPI and macrophage differentiation markers CD68 and CD163. The ratio of the alternatively ($CD163^+/CD68^+$) activated phenotype, indicated by white arrows, and classically ($CD163^-/CD68^+$) activated phenotype varies with indicated application. Scale bar: 25μm. (**b**) Quantification of macrophage polarization in the perivascular bed of growing collateral vessels after pharmacological stimulation with IL10 and anti-IL10 3 d and 7 d after FAL. The distribution of macrophage subtypes was skewed towards the alternatively activated phenotype after IL10 application. When anti-IL10 was injected, the opposite effect was observed, and the distribution was skewed towards the classically activated phenotype. * indicates $p < 0.05$; 3 d: $n = 6$ in each group; d7: NaCl and IL10 $n = 4$, anti-IL10: $n = 6$.

2.3. Evaluation of Hind-Limb Perfusion Recovery after FAL and Pharmacological Stimulation with IL10 and Anti-IL10

To assess the effect of varying blood concentration levels of IL10 on growing collateral vessels IL10 and anti-IL10 were externally applied in mice after FAL. Hind-limb perfusion was assessed using Laser-Doppler-Imaging before and shortly after FAL, on 3 d, 7 d, and 14 d and compared to a control group receiving NaCl. Immediately after FAL an acute reduction of hind-limb perfusion was observed in all groups (NaCl: 0.13 ± 0.01, IL10: 0.16 ± 0.03, anti-IL10: 0.13 ± 0.01). Hind-limb reperfusion in the NaCl ($n = 6$) group showed an adequate increase to 0.34 ± 0.04, 0.62 ± 0.07, and 0.62 ± 0.07 on 3 d, 7 d, and 14 d respectively. Elevated blood concentration levels of IL10 led to a significantly higher hind-limb perfusion on 3 d and 14 d ($n = 5$, 3 d: 0.54 ± 0.09, $p < 0.05$, 14 d: 0.83 ± 0.7, $p < 0.05$). Although hind-limb perfusion on 7 d was elevated compared to the control group, the difference was not significant (0.77 ± 0.09, $p = 0.07$) (Figure 3a). Contrariwise, application of anti-IL10 showed a significant impairment of hind-limb perfusion on 7 d ($n = 5$, 0.42 ± 0.4, $p < 0.05$). On 3 d and 14 d, however, no significant difference was observed (3 d: 0.35 ± 0.05, $p = 0.86$, 14d: 0.61 ± 0.07, $p = 0.89$) (Figure 3b).

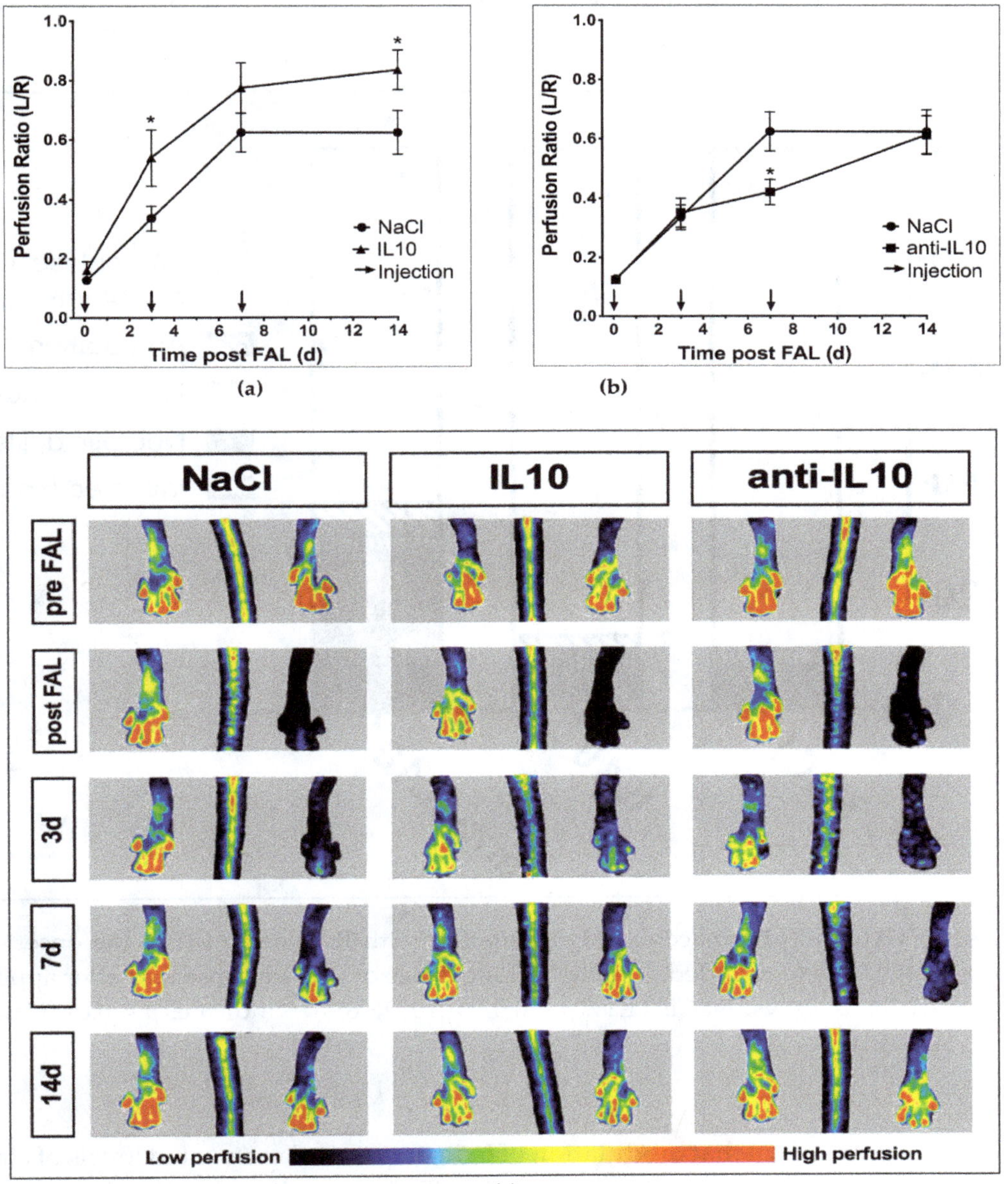

Figure 3. Evaluation of hind-limb perfusion recovery after femoral artery ligation (FAL) and application of IL10 and anti-IL10 (L/R ratio). Hind-limb perfusion was measured prior to and immediately after FAL, on 3 d, 7 d and 14 d. (**a**) IL10 led to a significant acceleration of hind-limb perfusion recovery on 3 d (IL10: 0.54 ± 0.09 vs. NaCl: 0.34 ± 0.04, $p < 0.05$) and 14 d (IL10: 0.83 ± 0.07 vs. NaCl: 0.62 ± 0.07, $p < 0.05$) while (**b**) anti-IL10 led to a brief but significant impairment of hind-limb perfusion recovery on 7 d (anti-IL10: 0.42 ± 0.04 vs. NaCl: 0.62 ± 0.07, $p < 0.05$). (**c**) Representative Laser-Doppler-Images of ligated and non-ligated hind-limbs. *indicates $p < 0.05$; NaCl: $n = 6$, IL10 and anti-IL10: $n = 5$.

2.4. Macroscopic Observations on Ligated Hind-Limbs after FAL and Application of IL10 and Anti-IL10

Ligated hind-limbs were inspected prior to FAL, 3 d and 7 d after FAL. Macroscopic observations associated with an acute ischemia of the affected hind-limb, termed critical ischemic events (CIE), were recorded after FAL and treatment with IL10 and anti-IL10. CIE were categorized as follows: inflamed hind-limb, necrotic digits, necrotic hind-limb and amputation. In total ($n = 115$) CIE occurred in 20%. Necrotic digits were observed most frequently in 65%, followed by a necrotic hind-limb in 17%, an amputation in 13% and an inflamed hind-limb in 4% of CIE. The highest incidence of CIE was observed after application of anti-IL10 (anti-IL10: 37.1% vs. NaCl: 11.1% $p < 0.01$). The incidence of CIE when treated with IL10 was similar to the control group (IL10: 13.6% vs. NaCl: 11.1% $p = 0.73$) (Figure 4).

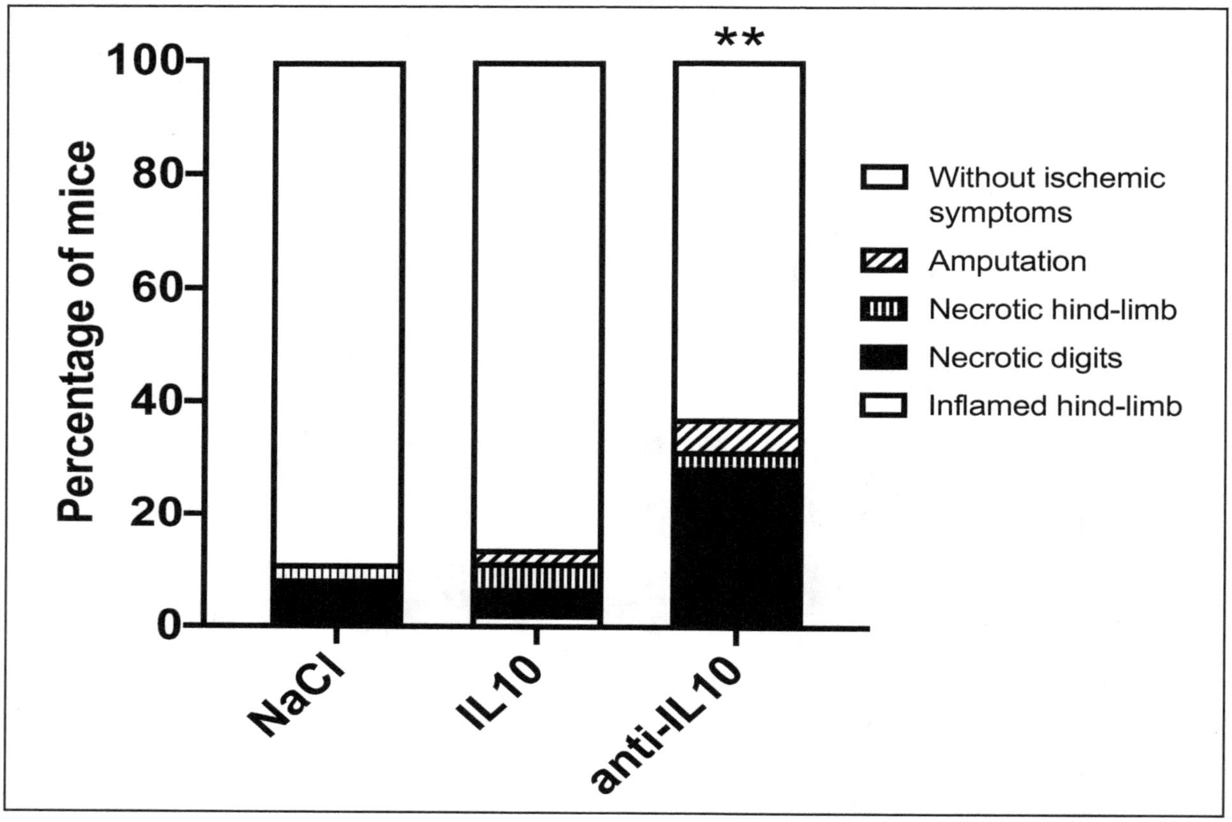

Figure 4. After FAL and pharmacological stimulation with IL10 or anti-IL10 the onset of critical ischemic events (CIE) were recorded. The highest incidence of CIE was observed after application of anti-IL10 (anti-IL10: 37.1% vs. NaCl: 11.1% $p < 0.01$, IL10: 13.6%). **indicates $p < 0.01$; NaCl: $n = 36$, IL10: $n = 44$, anti-IL10: $n = 35$

3. Discussion

In this study we have shown that modulation of IL10, in particular elevated levels of circulating IL10, alters collateral reperfusion after femoral artery ligation (FAL) as well as the distribution of macrophage activation types in the perivascular bed of growing collaterals. Although, the inhibitory effect of an IL10 antibody on circulating IL10 blood levels could not be directly detected due to technical limitations, contrary to elevated levels of circulating IL10, the opposite pertaining to both collateral reperfusion and the distribution of macrophage activation types was observed. The remodeling processes in arteriogenesis involve a controlled destruction of vessel components, activation of endothelial and smooth muscle cell de-differentiation, proliferation and migration, and adventitial restructuring in which monocytes/macrophages were shown to be key orchestrators [1,14]. These seemingly disparate tasks mediated largely by a singular cell type are explained by their heterogeneity and plasticity in response to environmental and situational needs. Previous findings have demonstrated that M1 and M2 macrophages form around growing collateral vessels in a distinct temporal and spatial pattern suggesting a collaborative mechanism of action in collateral artery growth [11]. The M1 phenotype, found proximate to the vessel lumen, is associated with the production of the pro-inflammatory cytokines IL1 and IL6, both described to have autocrine growth effects on vascular smooth muscle cells (VSMC) [15]. Other arteriogenic stimulants expressed by the M1 phenotype include NOS, TNF and MCP-1 [1,2,15,16]. M2 macrophages, on the other hand, are found distal to the vessel lumen [11] and have been ascribed a more prominent role in mediating the growth processes. Takeda et al. [7] showed that improved collateral perfusion after FAL was due to an expansion of the M2 phenotype among tissue-resident macrophages in Phd2 haplodeficient ($Phd2^{+/-}$) mice and that soluble factors secreted by $Phd2^{+/-}$ macrophages in vitro led to increased smooth muscle cell (SMC) proliferation and migration. IL10 is a known activator of the M2c phenotype and we have shown that increased levels of IL10 also led to an improved collateral reperfusion after FAL. Furthermore, an immunohistochemical analysis using the established macrophage polarization marker CD163 [17,18], revealed that perivascular macrophages were proportionally skewed towards the M2 phenotype. The supposed proarteriogenic effects of M2 macrophages induced by IL10 are further supported by the observation that the application of an IL10 antibody led to a transient impairment of collateral reperfusion and was accompanied by an increased onset of ischemic symptoms on ligated hind limbs. Also, the distribution of perivascular macrophages was conversely skewed towards the M1 phenotype. These findings do not undermine the role of M1 macrophages in arteriogenesis. The delayed and transient dip in reperfusion recovery we observed after the application of an IL10 antibody may support the hypothesis, that adluminally located M1 macrophages contribute to collateral vessel growth particularly in early phases through the recruitment of circulating monocytes and expression of arteriogenic relevant cytokines and proteins (IL1, IL6, TNF, NOS, MCP-1). They do, however, highlight the potential role played by M2 macrophages with regard to VSMC differentiation and adventitial restructuring to accommodate the growing collateral vessel. M2 macrophages induced by IL10 secrete high levels of TGFb1, known to stimulate VSMC differentiation and extracellular matrix (ECM) deposition [15,19,20]. They also produce high levels of MMP9 [21], which along with MMP2 was significantly increased in the adventitia of growing coronary collateral vessels [22]. This supports the hypothesis that IL10 induced M2 macrophages may play an active role in the augmentation of adventitial ECM proteolysis and remodeling, thus, facilitating arteriogenic growth. Our findings suggest that varying levels of IL10 in vivo influence collateral reperfusion, which may be explained by a shift in the distribution of macrophages towards the M2 phenotype at the site of collateral growth. From a clinical standpoint, this presents itself as a new therapeutic approach to promote collateral vessel growth in patients suffering from peripheral artery disease. The expression of CD163 on M2 macrophages, however, also poses concerns regarding their use in revascularization therapy. $CD163^{+}$ macrophages in human atherosclerotic lesions were found to increase plaque instability by promoting angiogenesis within areas of intraplaque hemorrhage, in itself thought to be a result of plaque neovascularization and increased microvessel permeability, resulting in a vicious cycle [23]. Seen as a whole, these observations underline the diversity of macrophage functions and activation states with regard to tissue specific cues and needs. A mere distinction between classically activated M1 and alternatively activated M2 macrophages limited by CD163 as an M2 marker alone will not suffice to fully describe the roles played by the macrophage activation states we observed around growing collateral vessels. Further studies utilizing other macrophage markers will be required to elucidate the underlying mechanism involved in our findings. While these remain hypothetical, the results presented in our study shed light on new therapeutic strategies in promoting collateral vessels growth.

4. Materials and Methods

4.1. Animal Models

Animal handling and all experimental procedures carried out were in full compliance with the Directive 2010/63/EU of the European Parliament on protection of animals used for scientific purposes. Approval was given by the responsible local authority, the hessian governmental council for animal protection and handling (permit reference numbers V54-19c20/15-B2/1152, permit date: 23.05.2017). Throughout this study all mice had access to water and food ad libitum.

4.2. Mouse Model of Hind-Limb Ischemia

To evaluate collateral vessel growth perfusion recovery was measured after femoral artery ligation (FAL) using the model described in [24]. For all experiments 10-14 weeks old male C57BL/6 mice from our own breeding program were used with an approximate bodyweight of 30 g. Prior to each experiment all mice were inspected to ensure a healthy state. Anesthesia was performed by intraperitoneal injection using ketamin hydrochloride (120mg/kg bodyweight) and xylazine hydrochloride (16 mg/kg bodyweight). Pre- and post-operative analgesia was performed by subcutaneous injection with buprenorphine (0.1 mg/kg bodyweight). FAL was carried out on the left hind-limb by ligating the femoral artery immediately distal to the origin of the deep femoral branch to redirect blood flow to the collateral arteries. After termination of experiments the mice were euthanized by an anesthetic overdose using ketamin hydrochloride (180mg/kg bodyweight) and xylazine hydrochloride (16 mg/kg bodyweight) followed by exsanguination.

4.3. Pharmacological Stimulation

FAL was performed on C57BL/6 mice. Mice were randomly allocated to each group receiving either recombinant murine interleukin 10 (IL10) (20 μg/kg bodyweight) or purified anti-mouse IL10 antibody (anti-IL10) (0.5 μg/kg bodyweight) diluted in sodium chloride solution (NaCl 0.9%) immediately after FAL, on day 3 and 7 after FAL. The control group received NaCl 0.9%. The application was carried out via intravenous injection into the tail vein. IL10 was purchased from PeproTech (Hamburg, Germany). Anti-IL10 was purchased from BioLegend (Koblenz, Germany).

4.4. Measurement of Blood Concentration Levels of IL10

Retro orbital blood samples were obtained from mice before and 24 h after pharmacological stimulation with IL10 and anti-IL10 as described above. The control group received NaCl 0.9%. Anesthesia war provided as described above. A Mouse Magnetic Luminex Assay (Thermo Fisher Scientific, Waltham, MA, USA) was used to measure the concentration of endogenous IL10 in the blood samples at baseline and 24 h after pharmacological stimulation.

4.5. Hind-limb Perfusion Measurement after Pharmacological Stimulation and FAL

Hind-limb perfusion was assessed and quantified via erythrocyte motion detection through Laser-Doppler-Imaging using a PeriScan PIM3 System (Perimed Instruments, Järfällä, Sweden, Software: LDPIwin for PIM3 3.1.3) before and immediately after FAL, on day 3, 7 and 14 after FAL. For each measurement mice were positioned on a heating plate at 37 °C for 3min prior to and during each measurement to ensure standardized conditions at a distance of 10 cm and a pixel resolution of 256 × 256. A 2 cm × 3 cm area including both feet was scanned and a region of interest (ROI) of approximately 80 mm^2 containing each foot was defined. Mean perfusion (arbitrary units) was used to calculate hind-limb perfusion and expressed as the ligated limb to non-ligated limb ratio as described in [25]. Follow-up measurements were performed under anesthesia as described above.

4.6. *Immunohistochemistry*

Mice were perfused with 10 mL vasodilation buffer (100 μg adenosine, 1 μg sodium nitroprusside, 0.05% BSA in PBS, pH 7.4) followed by 10 mL 4% PFA post mortem. Mm. adductores of ligated hind-limbs were harvested on day 3 after FAL and cryosectioned with a thickness of 10 μm. Immunostaining was performed using the following antibodies: RAT ANTI MOUSE CD68: Alexa Fluor 488 Antibody (AbD Serotec, Düsseldorf, Germany), CD163 (M-96) Antibody (Santa Cruz Biotechnology Inc., Dallas, TX, USA), Donkey anti-Rabbit IgG: Alexa Fluor 546 (Thermo Fisher Scientific, Waltham, MA, USA), DAPI. The two largest collateral vessels were selected. Immunopositive cells were classified as classically activated macrophages ($CD68^+/CD163^-$) or alternatively activated macrophages ($CD68^+/CD163^+$). Confocal imaging was carried out using a Leica SP5 (Wetzlar, Germany). Acquired images were processed with ImageJ Software (National Institutes of Health, Maryland, MD, USA) for further analysis.

4.7. *Data Analysis*

Statistical analysis was performed using Prism (GraphPad Software, San Diego, USA). Data was tested for normality using a D'Agostino-Pearson omnibus normality test. Parametric data is reported as mean ± standard error of mean. Non-parametric data is reported as median (IQR). Unpaired and parametric samples were analyzed using a Student's t-test. Unpaired and non-parametric samples were analyzed using a Mann–Whitney-U test. When more than two groups were compared at different time points, a two-way ANOVA was used for parametric samples followed by a Holm–Sidak's multiple comparison test. For comparison of more than 2 groups with non-parametric samples a Kruskal–Wallis test was used followed by a Dunn's multiple comparison test. Proportions were compared using a Chi-square test. Values of $p < 0.05$ were considered statistically significant.

Author Contributions: Conceptualization, A.M.G., K.T. and C.T.; Data curation, A.M.G.; Formal analysis, A.M.G.; Funding acquisition, C.T.; Investigation, A.M.G., C.S. and K.T.; Methodology, A.M.G., K.T. and C.T.; Project administration, A.M.G.; Resources, K.T. and C.T.; Supervision, K.T. and C.T.; Visualization, A.M.G.; Writing—original draft, A.G.; Writing—review and editing, G.J., O.D., C.L., C.W.H., T.S.-R., K.T., and C.T. All authors have read and agreed to the published version of the manuscript.

Abbreviations

FAL	Femoral artery ligation
CIE	Critical ischemic events
VSMC	Vascular smooth muscle cells
SMC	Smooth muscle cells
ECM	Extracellular matrix

References

1. Heil, M.; Schaper, W. Influence of mechanical, cellular, and molecular factors on collateral artery growth (arteriogenesis). *Circ. Res.* **2004**, *95*, 449–458. [CrossRef] [PubMed]
2. Ito, W.D.; Arras, M.; Winkler, B.; Scholz, D.; Schaper, J.; Schaper, W. Monocyte chemotactic protein-1 increases collateral and peripheral conductance after femoral artery occlusion. *Circ. Res.* **1997**, *80*, 829–837. [CrossRef] [PubMed]
3. Buschmann, I.R.; Hoefer, I.E.; Van Royen, N.; Katzer, E.; Braun-Dulleaus, R.; Heil, M.; Kostin, S.; Bode, C.; Schaper, W. GM-CSF: A strong arteriogenic factor acting by amplification of monocyte function. *Atherosclerosis* **2001**, *159*, 343–356. [CrossRef]
4. Ziegelhoeffer, T.; Fernandez, B.; Kostin, S.; Heil, M.; Voswinckel, R.; Helisch, A.; Schaper, W. Bone marrow-derived cells do not incorporate into the adult growing vasculature. *Circ. Res.* **2004**, *94*, 230–238. [CrossRef] [PubMed]

5. Khmelewski, E.; Becker, A.; Meinertz, T.; Ito, W.D. Tissue resident cells play a dominant role in arteriogenesis and concomitant macrophage accumulation. *Circ. Res.* **2004**, *95*, e56–e64. [CrossRef] [PubMed]
6. Jetten, N.; Donners, M.M.P.C.; Wagenaar, A.; Cleutjens, J.P.M.; Van Rooijen, N.; De Winther, M.P.J.; Post, M.J. Local delivery of polarized macrophages improves reperfusion recovery in a mouse hind limb ischemia model. *PLoS ONE* **2013**, *8*, e68811. [CrossRef]
7. Takeda, Y.; Costa, S.; Delamarre, E.; Roncal, C.; Leite De Oliveira, R.; Squadrito, M.L.; Finisguerra, V.; Deschoemaeker, S.; Bruyere, F.; Wenes, M.; et al. Macrophage skewing by Phd2 haplodeficiency prevents ischaemia by inducing arteriogenesis. *Nature* **2011**, *479*, 122–126. [CrossRef]
8. Mantovani, A.; Biswas, S.K.; Galdiero, M.R.; Sica, A.; Locati, M. Macrophage plasticity and polarization in tissue repair and remodelling. *J. Pathol.* **2013**, *229*, 176–185. [CrossRef]
9. Mantovani, A.; Sica, A.; Sozzani, S.; Allavena, P.; Vecchi, A.; Locati, M. The chemokine system in diverse forms of macrophage activation and polarization. *Trends Immunol.* **2004**, *25*, 677–686. [CrossRef]
10. Mills, C.D.; Ley, K. M1 and M2 macrophages: The chicken and the egg of immunity. *J. Innate Immun.* **2014**, *6*, 716–726. [CrossRef]
11. Troidl, C.; Jung, G.; Troidl, K.; Hoffmann, J.; Mollmann, H.; Nef, H.; Schaper, W.; Hamm, C.W.; Schmitz-Rixen, T. The temporal and spatial distribution of macrophage subpopulations during arteriogenesis. *Curr. Vasc. Pharmacol.* **2013**, *11*, 5–12. [CrossRef] [PubMed]
12. Italiani, P.; Boraschi, D. From monocytes to M1/M2 macrophages: Phenotypical vs. functional differentiation. *Front. Immunol.* **2014**, *5*, 514. [CrossRef] [PubMed]
13. Komohara, Y.; Jinushi, M.; Takeya, M. Clinical significance of macrophage heterogeneity in human malignant tumors. *Cancer Sci.* **2014**, *105*, 1–8. [CrossRef] [PubMed]
14. Schaper, W.; Ito Wulf, D. Molecular mechanisms of coronary collateral vessel growth. *Circ. Res.* **1996**, *79*, 911–919. [CrossRef]
15. Berk, B.C. Vascular smooth muscle growth: Autocrine growth mechanisms. *Physiol. Rev.* **2001**, *81*, 999–1030. [CrossRef] [PubMed]
16. Schaper, W. Collateral circulation: Past and present. *Basic Res. Cardiol.* **2009**, *104*, 5–21. [CrossRef]
17. Micklem, K.; Rigney, E.; Cordell, J.; Simmons, D.; Stross, P.; Turley, H.; Seed, B.; Mason, D. A human macrophage-associated antigen (CD68) detected by six different monoclonal antibodies. *Br. J. Haematol.* **1989**, *73*, 6–11. [CrossRef]
18. Buechler, C.; Ritter, M.; Orsó, E.; Langmann, T.; Klucken, J.; Schmitz, G. Regulation of scavenger receptor CD163 expression in human monocytes and macrophages by pro-and antiinflammatory stimuli. *J. Leukoc. Biol.* **2000**, *67*, 97–103. [CrossRef]
19. O'rourke, S.A.; Dunne, A.; Monaghan, M.G. The Role of macrophages in the infarcted myocardium: Orchestrators of ECM remodeling. *Front. Cardiovasc. Med.* **2019**, *6*, 101. [CrossRef]
20. Royen, N.V.; Hoefer, I.; Buschmann, I.; Heil, M.; Kostin, S.; Deindl, E.; Vogel, S.; Korff, T.; Augustin, H.; Bode, C.; et al. Exogenous application of transforming growth factor beta 1 stimulates arteriogenesis in the peripheral circulation. *FASEB J.* **2002**, *16*, 432–434. [CrossRef]
21. Krzyszczyk, P.; Schloss, R.; Palmer, A.; Berthiaume, F. The role of macrophages in acute and chronic wound healing and interventions to promote pro-wound healing phenotypes. *Front. Physiol.* **2018**, *9*, 419. [CrossRef] [PubMed]
22. Cai, W.-J.; Koltai, S.; Kocsis, E.; Scholz, D.; Kostin, S.; Luo, X.; Schaper, W.; Schaper, J. Remodeling of the adventitia during coronary arteriogenesis. *Am. J. Physiol. Heart Circ. Physiol.* **2003**, *284*, H31–H40. [CrossRef]
23. Guo, L.; Akahori, H.; Harari, E.; Smith, S.L.; Polavarapu, R.; Karmali, V.; Otsuka, F.; Gannon, R.L.; Braumann, R.E.; Dickinson, M.H.; et al. CD163+ macrophages promote angiogenesis and vascular permeability accompanied by inflammation in atherosclerosis. *J. Clin. Investig.* **2018**, *128*, 1106–1124. [CrossRef] [PubMed]
24. Limbourg, A.; Korff, T.; Napp, L.C.; Schaper, W.; Drexler, H.; Limbourg, F.P. Evaluation of postnatal arteriogenesis and angiogenesis in a mouse model of hind-limb ischemia. *Nat. Protoc.* **2009**, *4*, 1737–1748. [CrossRef] [PubMed]
25. Heil, M.; Ziegelhoeffer, T.; Pipp, F.; Kostin, S.; Martin, S.; Clauss, M.; Schaper, W. Blood monocyte concentration is critical for enhancement of collateral artery growth. *Am. J. Physiol. Heart Circ. Physiol.* **2002**, *283*, H2411–H2419. [CrossRef]

9

Assessment of Microvessel Permeability in Murine Atherosclerotic Vein Grafts Using Two-Photon Intravital Microscopy

Fabiana Baganha [1,2], Laila Ritsma [3], Paul H. A. Quax [1,2] and Margreet R. de Vries [1,2,*]

1 Department of Surgery, Leiden University Medical Center, 2333 ZA Leiden, The Netherlands; F.Baganha_Carreiras@lumc.nl (F.B.); P.H.A.Quax@lumc.nl (P.H.A.Q.)

2 Einthoven Laboratory for Experimental Vascular Medicine, Leiden University Medical Center, 2333 ZA Leiden, The Netherlands

3 Department of Cell and Chemical Biology, Leiden University Medical Center, 2333 ZC Leiden, The Netherlands; L.M.A.Ritsma@lumc.nl

* Correspondence: M.R.de_Vries@lumc.nl

Abstract: Plaque angiogenesis and plaque hemorrhage are major players in the destabilization and rupture of atherosclerotic lesions. As these are dynamic processes, imaging of plaque angiogenesis, especially the integrity or leakiness of angiogenic vessels, can be an extremely useful tool in the studies on atherosclerosis pathophysiology. Visualizing plaque microvessels in 3D would enable us to study the architecture and permeability of adventitial and intimal plaque microvessels in advanced atherosclerotic lesions. We hypothesized that a comparison of the vascular permeability between healthy continuous and fenestrated as well as diseased leaky microvessels, would allow us to evaluate plaque microvessel leakiness. We developed and validated a two photon intravital microscopy (2P-IVM) method to assess the leakiness of plaque microvessels in murine atherosclerosis-prone ApoE3*Leiden vein grafts based on the quantification of fluorescent-dextrans extravasation in real-time. We describe a novel 2P-IVM set up to study vessels in the neck region of living mice. We show that microvessels in vein graft lesions are in their pathological state more permeable in comparison with healthy continuous and fenestrated microvessels. This 2P-IVM method is a promising approach to assess plaque angiogenesis and leakiness. Moreover, this method is an important advancement to validate therapeutic angiogenic interventions in preclinical atherosclerosis models.

Keywords: angiogenesis; vessel maturity; vessel permeability; hemorrhage; atherosclerosis; two-photon intravital microscopy

---

1. Introduction

Plaque angiogenesis and plaque hemorrhage are major players in the destabilization and rupture of atherosclerotic lesions [1]. Plaque microvessels increase in numbers via angiogenesis during vulnerable stages of the disease, and microvessels density has been associated with the onset of rupture and clinical manifestations [2,3]. Plaque angiogenesis arises from reduced oxygen availability in the plaque, caused by lesion growth and presence of metabolic active inflammatory cells. Triggered by hypoxia, endothelial cells proliferate and migrate from the vasa vasorum to form microvessels to overcome the oxygen demand in the lesion [1]. However, these plaque microvessels are characterized by poor pericyte coverage, lack of cell junctions, and are highly susceptible to leakage of erythrocytes, leucocytes, and plasma lipids, together described as intraplaque hemorrhage [4,5].

Healthy microvessels are present in most organs and tissues, have a well-organized architecture, act as a protection barrier, and provide nutrients and oxygen by passive diffusion to their surroundings. The type of endothelial lining determines the permeability of the vessel. While in continuous microvessels (abundantly found in the ear skin) the endothelial cell lining is uninterrupted, fenestrated microvessels (found in secreting glands) have more pores to increase molecular diffusion of molecules (up to 66 kDa) without compromising their barrier function [6,7]. Contrarily, microvessels in atherosclerotic lesions in their pathological and immature state are thought to have a compromised barrier function and are as such more permeable [4,8–11].

To date, clinical available imaging techniques to study plaque angiogenesis and subsequent intraplaque hemorrhage, such as PET [12], CT [13], and MRI [14], do not have sufficient spatial resolution to visualize cellular events or image the detailed microvessels network in small size animal models. Two-photon intravital microscopy (2P-IVM), due to its high resolution, can overcome these limitations, allowing detailed 3D reconstructions of plaque angiogenesis and real-time evaluation of target dynamic processes, such as in vivo hemorrhage [7,15,16].

We hypothesized that permeability of healthy continuous and fenestrated microvessels in living mice can be compared to plaque microvessel permeability to assess pathological leakiness. Permeability can be evaluated by quantification of extravasation of 40 kDa-size dextrans [7,17]. It should leak from all vessels [7,17], but is expected to leak more from fenestrated vessels than continuous, and more from pathological vessels than healthy vessels. Moreover, it, is known that capillaries with poor pericytes coverage in context of inflammation can be permeable to large dextrans up to 2000 kDa [17]. Therefore, we also hypothesized that evaluation of 2000 kDa dextran extravasation in the same experimental setting, might be relevant to further assess the pathological permeability.

In this study, we set up an advanced 2P-IVM method to visualize atherosclerotic vein graft (VG) lesions in the neck region of living anesthetized mice. (Figure 1B). With this technique the architecture of adventitial and intimal plaque microvessels in advanced atherosclerotic VG lesions can be visualized (Figure 1C). This model was chosen since in mice, vasa vasorum angiogenesis only occurs at a very old age and most spontaneous atherosclerotic lesions in mice do not show intraplaque angiogenesis [11]. We previously showed that hypercholesterolemic ApoE3*Leiden VG lesions, due to their lesion size and state of hypoxia, present with vasa vasorum derived neovascularization, [8] with the unique characteristic of leaky intimal microvessels and intraplaque hemorrhage [9]. Furthermore, we report a 2P-IVM method to assess vessel permeability by quantification of 40 kDa and 2000 kDa-labeled dextrans extravasation in healthy microvessels and plaque microvessels in real-time (Figure 1D,E). We show that plaque microvessels are pathological more permeable in comparison with healthy continuous and fenestrated microvessels, which advocates for their destabilizing role in plaque rupture.

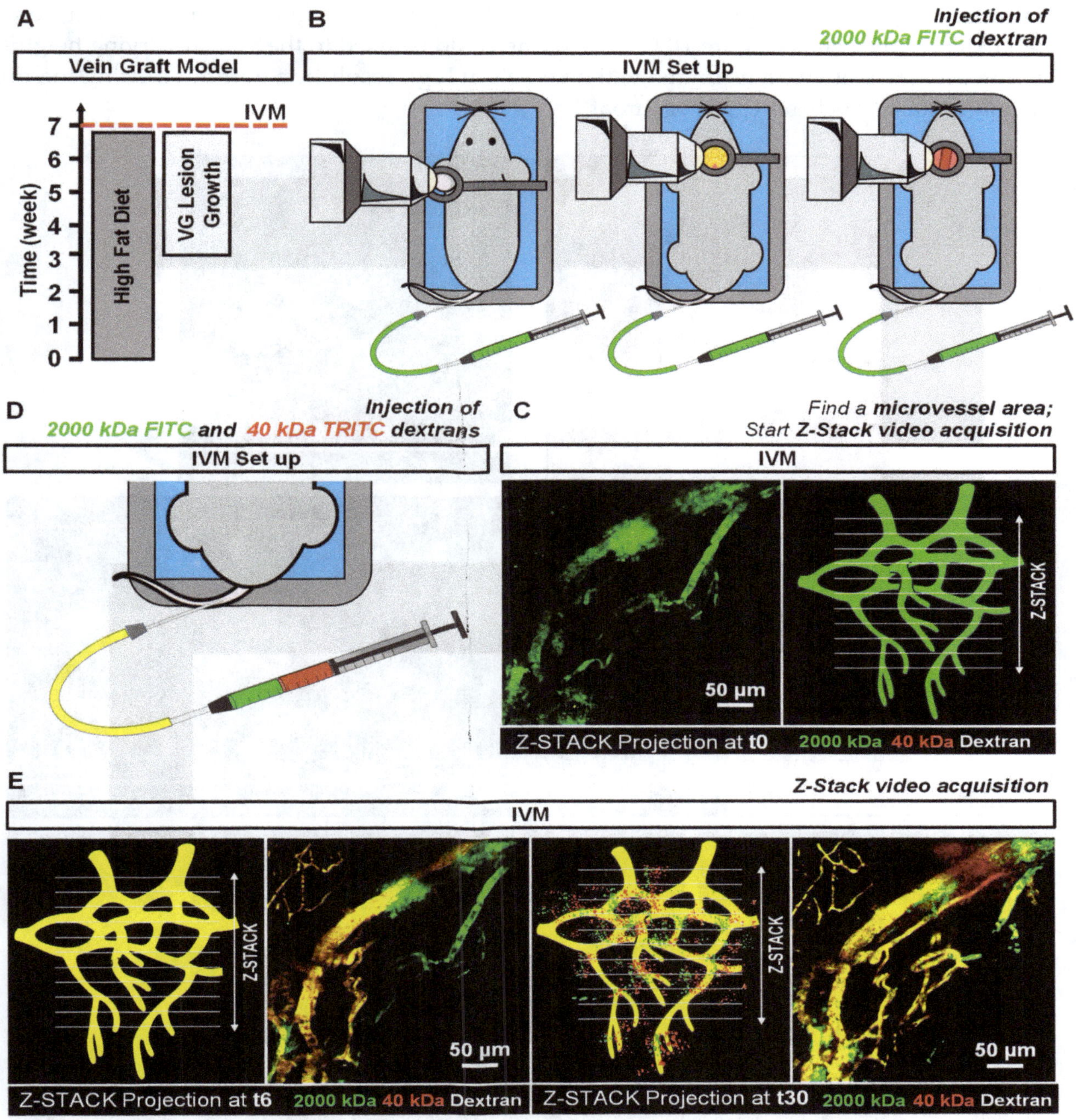

Figure 1. 2P-IVM pipeline to image plaque angiogenesis in advance atherosclerotic lesions and to assess dextrans extravasation in continuous, fenestrated and plaque microvessels. (**A**) After 3 weeks of hypercholesteremic diet, ApoE3*Leiden mice (n = 12) undergo VG surgery. Four weeks later, (**B**) mice are prepared for IVM and plaque microvessels in the VG lesions, continuous microvessels in ear skin, fenestrated microvessels in parotid glands are imaged by injection of 2000 kDa-FITC dextran intravenously. (**C**) Areas of interest are evaluated by time-lapse Z-stack acquisition over 20 min. (**D**,**E**) Injection of 40 kDa-TRITC 2000 kDa-FITC dextran solution is used to assess vessel permeability by quantification of FICT and TRITC fluorescence extravascular intensities in Z-stack projections.

2. Results

2.1. Detection of Plaque Angiogenesis in ApoE3*Leiden Mice Vein Graft Lesions

Plaque angiogenesis was detected by 2P-IVM in advanced atherosclerotic lesions of the ApoE3*Leiden mice VG model by injection of the plasma tracer 2000 kDa-FITC dextran as depicted in Figure 1B,C. Here, we imaged for the first time the VG in the neck using high resolution intravital microscopy. We designed a circular metal frame was designed with a coverslip on top connected to a pole by a stalk (Figure 1B,C). The frame could be fixed to the pole at varying heights by a screw. The thin stalk enabled us to image the vessels at high resolution without putting too much pressure on the sternum/chest region or throat.

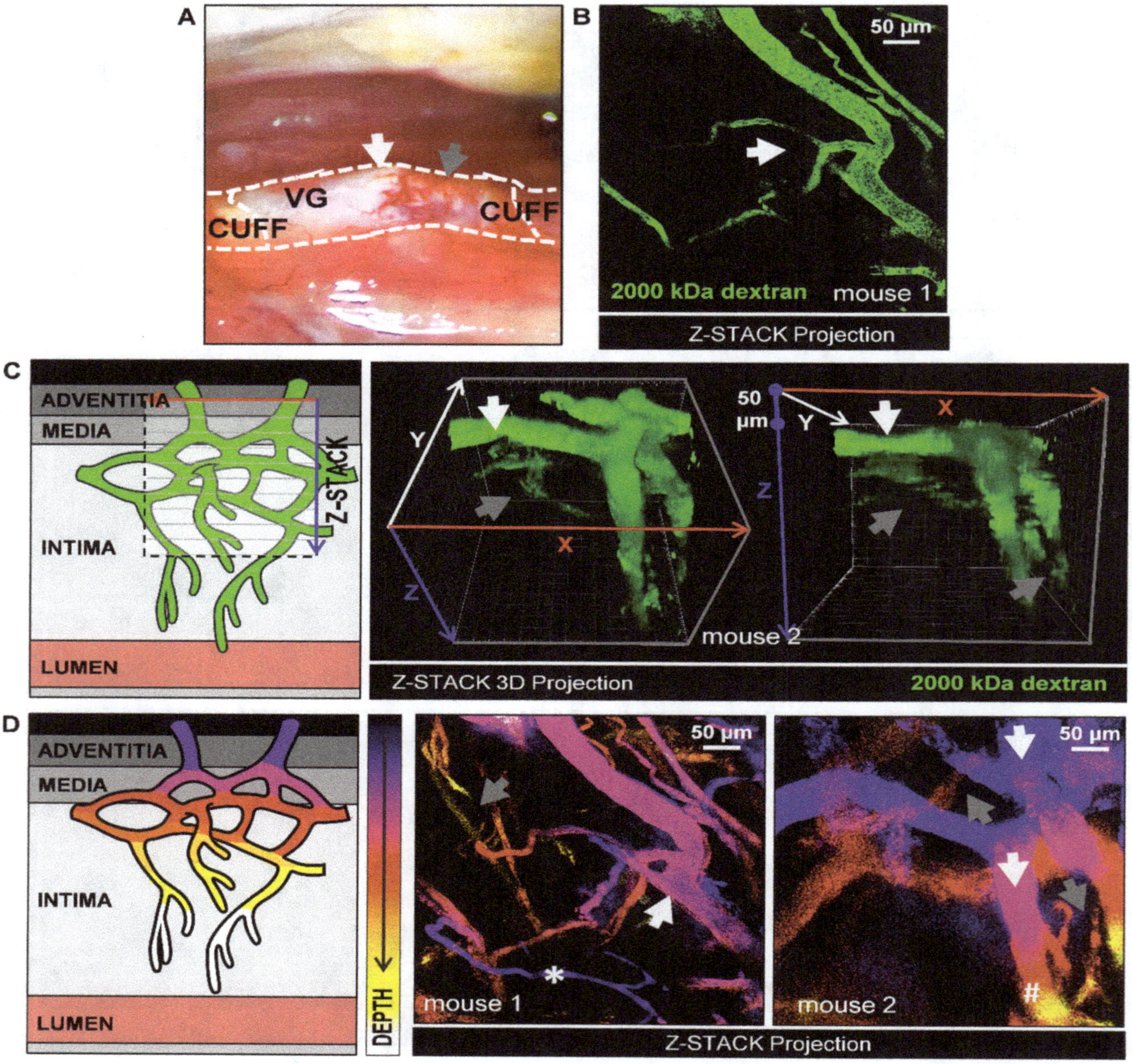

Figure 2. Detection of plaque angiogenesis by 2P-IVM by injection of the plasma tracer 2000 kDa-FITC dextran in atherosclerotic lesions in ApoE3*Leiden mice VGs. (**A**) 28 days after surgery, areas of interest (white arrows: white thick regions, grey arrows: red thin regions) were imaged to study the architecture of plaque microvessels. (**B**) Z-stack projection of plaque microvessels (white arrows: branching). See also Video 1 (total Z-depth of 111 µm, 2 µm step); (**C**) Illustration of Z-stack acquisition in VG lesions and representative Z-stack 3D projections of adventitial (white arrows) and intimal microvessels (grey arrows) from one mouse at two different angles. See also video 2 for 360 view. Note that the large adventitial microvessels are also extending in Z because they are curved around the vein. (**D**) Z-stack projections from two mice with a Z-depth color code filter (white arrows: Adventitial microvessels; grey arrows: Intimal microvessels). Due to the curved nature of the vein: (*) Intimal microvessel is discriminated from adventitial microvessel based on its size, despite being located in a top Z layer; (#) Adventitial microvessel is discriminated from an intimal microvessel based on its size, despite being located in a deeper Z layer.

Thick white fatty atherosclerotic regions were observed along the conduit (Figure 2A). Compared to red thin lesion regions, these white regions show a prominent presence of microvessels. Therefore, white fatty thick spots were chosen to image the architecture of plaque angiogenesis (Figure 2B). FITC signal was homogenously distributed within the intravascular space of the microvessels with no signs of blood flow obstructions. Branching features, characteristic of immature or angiogenic vessels [18] were also observed (Figure 2B and Video 1). In video 1, a 111-μm deep z-stack projection of the image of Figure 2B is shown. This video offers an in depth view of the plaque microvessels throughout the adventitia, media, and intima.

Using 3D stack projections, vasa vasorum angiogenesis is observed throughout the lesion depth (Figure 2C and Video 2). Vasa vasorum angiogenesis expands towards hypoxic plaque areas, (intima) and these intimal microvessels were observed to be narrower than most preexisting adventitial vessels. Bigger adventitial microvessels were usually detected at 50–100 μm depth and narrower intimal microvessel structures, from >100 μm. Accordingly, size and depth were required to discriminate adventitial microvessels from intimal microvessels.

To easily visualize this in a single image, Z depth color coding was used (Figure 2D). As an example of the different variations seen in mice, two examples are given (mouse 1 and mouse 2). Here, vessels which are located deep in Z (in the intimal layer) are differently colored from vessels located high in Z (adventitial layer). Adventitial microvessels are shown in a blue to purple color gradient (Figure 2D, grey arrows) while intimal microvessels are shown in a red to yellow color gradient (Figure 2D, white arrows).

Due to the curved nature of the vein graft, some microvessels not match the color-code (* and #). Indeed, a thin vessel (*) is excluded as an adventitial microvessel based on its caliber, despite being located in a top Z layer. In addition, a thick microvessel (#) is partially located in the deeper Z layers. As can be appreciated in the 3D rendering (Figure 2C), the thick vessel is curved around the vein graft, and therefore extending into the deeper Z layer, and should be excluded as an intimal microvessel. As shown by the represented examples, vessel depth, microvessel caliber, and 3D rendering have to be considered to distinguish adventitial and intimal microvessels.

2.2. *Evaluation of Dextran in Microvessels*

To determine the amplitude and speed at which dextrans become visible in the various microvessels, we first injected mice with 2000 kDa-FITC to detect the microvessels and assess a region of interest, and then injected mice with a mixture of 2000 kDa-FITC and 40 kDa-TRITC dextran during timelapse imaging. We plotted the relative fluorescence intensity (RFI, normalized to t6) of 2000 kDa-FITC and 40 kDa-TRITC dextran over time for continuous (Figure 3A), fenestrated (Figure 3B), and plaque microvessels (Figure 3C).

Residual 2000 kDa-FITC fluorescence from the first injection ($t \leq 5$) was observed in all groups (Figure 3A–C). As shown in Figure 2D, residual FITC RFI at t5 is similar between the groups (Figure 3D).

As expected, after injection of 2000 kDa-FICT and 40 kDa-TRITC dextrans at t5, intravascular FITC RFI increases significantly until t6 in all groups, as demonstrated in Figure 3D (continuous microvessels: $p < 0.0001$, fenestrated microvessels: $p = 0.0007$, plaque microvessels: $p = 0.0106$). TRITC RFI increased even more than FITC RFI, as depicted in Figure 3E, most likely due to the residual FITC from the first injection (continuous microvessels: $p < 0.0001$, fenestrated microvessels: $p < 0.0001$, plaque microvessels: $p < 0.0001$).

During the next 24 image recordings, intravascular FITC and TRITC signal remained stable (~1) in all groups (Figure 3A–C). As shown in Figure 3D,E, FITC and TRITC RFI between t6 and t30 did not differ between continuous, fenestrated and plaque microvessels. Representative sequences of FITC and TRITC fluorescence intensities in continuous, fenestrated and plaque microvessels, observed in real-time, at t5 and t6, are shown in Figure 3F.

Thus, tail vein-injected dextrans appear quickly and with the same dynamics in the various microvessels, and remain so in similar concentration throughout the course of imaging.

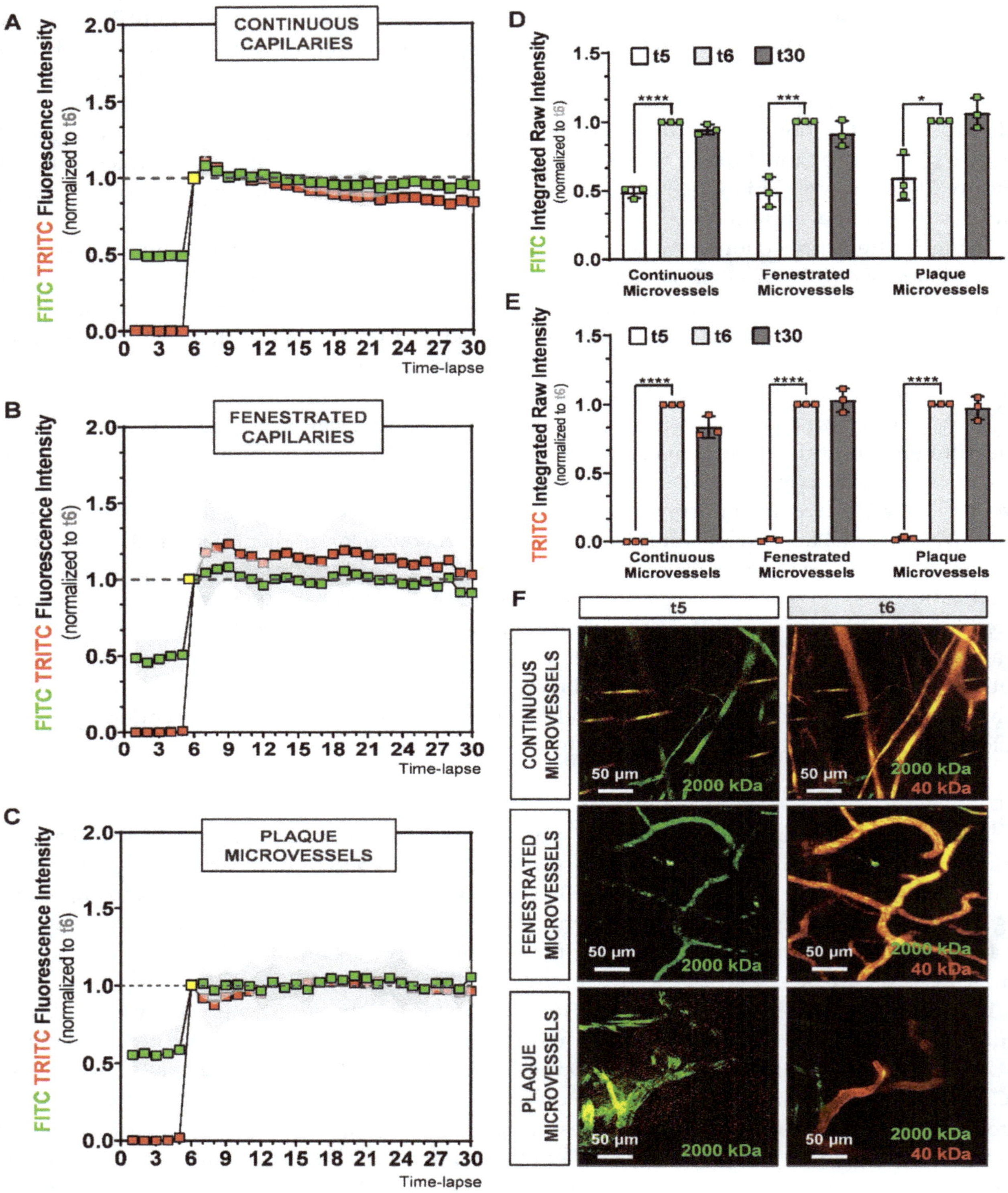

Figure 3. Evaluation of time-lapse imaging of 2000 kDa-FITC and 40 kDa-TRITC RFI inside the microvessel structures of (**A**) continuous, (**B**) fenestrated and (**C**) plaque microvessels. (**D**,**E**) Quantification of FITC and TRITC intravascular RFI at time-lapse 5, 6 and 30. (**F**) Representative max-projection of FITC and TRITC signal in continuous, fenestrated and plaque microvessels at t5 and t6. Data presented as mean ± SD. * $p \leq 0.05$, *** $p \leq 0.001$, **** $p \leq 0.0001$ by 1-way-ANOVA.

2.3. Evaluation of Dextran Extravasation into the Extravascular Space

Next, we determined if it was possible to visualize dextran extravasation from the vasculature. In the same time-lapse movies as used for Figure 3, we measured the extravascular RFI (normalized to t6) for 2000 kDa-FITC and 40 kDa-TRITC dextran for continuous (Figure 4A), fenestrated (Figure 4B), and plaque (Figure 4C) microvessels.

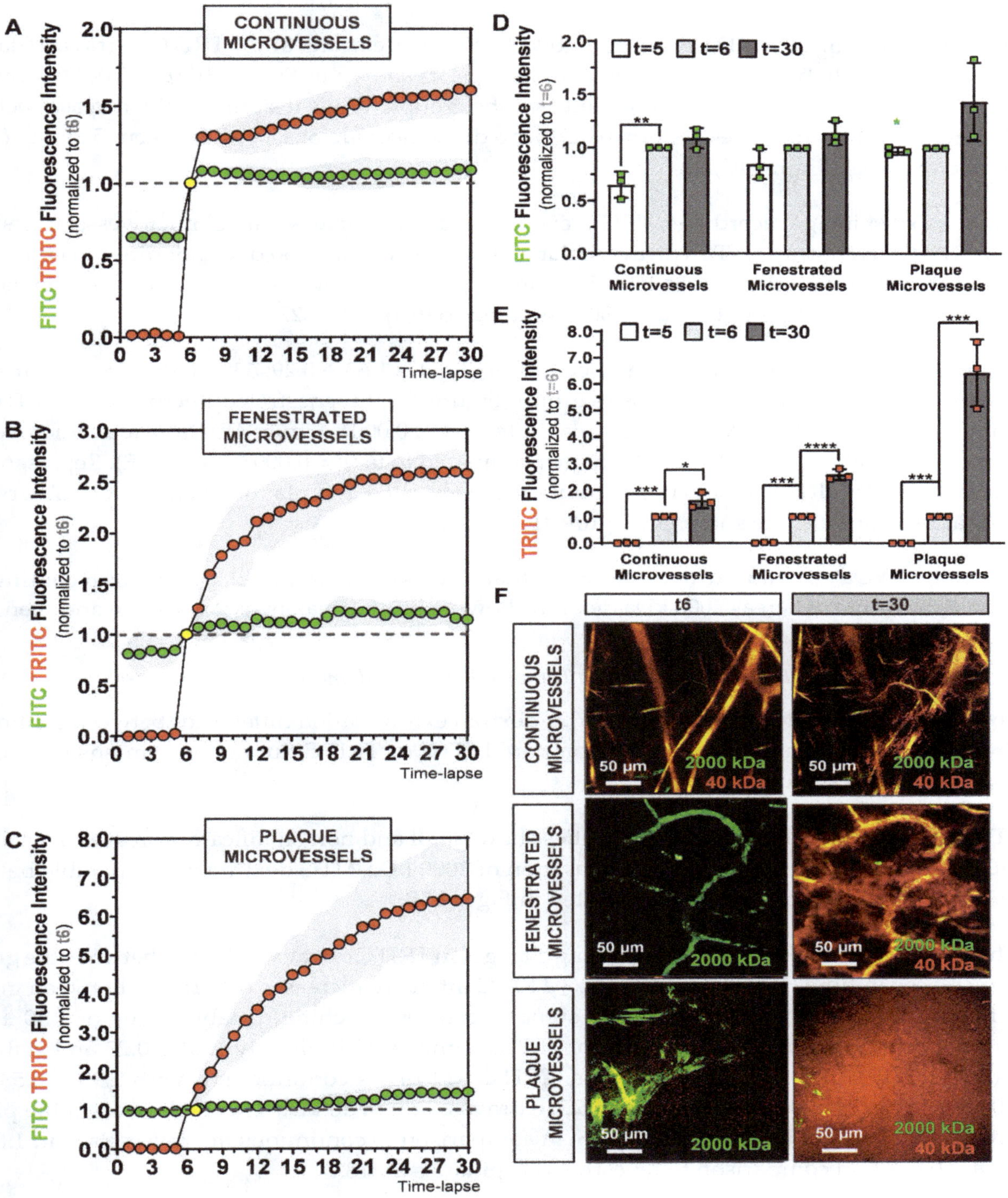

Figure 4. Evaluation of time-lapse imaging of 2000 kDa-FITC and 40 kDa-TRITC RFI outside the microvessel structures of (**A**) continuous, (**B**) fenestrated and (**C**) plaque microvessels. (**D**,**E**) Quantification of FITC and TRITC extravascular RFI at time-lapse 5, 6 and 30. (**F**) Representative max-projection of FITC and TRITC signal in continuous, fenestrated and plaque microvessels at t6 and t30. Data presented as mean ± SD. * $p \leq 0.05$, ** $p \leq 0.001$, *** $p \leq 0.001$, **** $p \leq 0.0001$ by 1-way-ANOVA; Green star (* $p \leq 0.05$): FITC RFI at t5 between continuous and plaque microvessels.

Residual fluorescence from the 2000 kDa-FITC first injection ($t \leq 5$) was detected in all groups in the extravascular space as shown in Figure 4A–C. FITC RFI at t5 is different between continuous and plaque microvessels groups (0.652 ± 0.14 vs. 0.973 ± 0.14, $p = 0.0274$, Figure 4D, green star).

After injection of 2000 kDa-FICT and 40 kDa-TRITC dextrans at t5, TRITC extravascular RFI increases significantly between t5 and t6 in all groups, as shown in Figure 3E ($p < 0.001$). However, FITC extravascular RFI (Figure 3D) varies between the groups. While it significantly increases between t5 and t6 in continuous microvessels ($p = 0.0274$), no differences are observed between t5 and t6 (~1) in plaque microvessels (Figure 4C,D).

In the next 24 image recordings, TRITC extravascular RFI increases in all microvessels, as shown in Figure 4A–C. In contrast, FITC extravascular RFI between t6 and t30 does not differ in continuous and fenestrated microvessels, (Figure 3D). However, in plaque microvessels, a trend towards an increase in FITC extravascular RFI is detected at t30 compared to t6, ($p = 0.0827$, Figure 4D).

Importantly, the mean TRITC extravascular RFI at t30 is 1.63 ± 0.29, 63% higher in comparison to t6 ($p = 0.01$) in the continuous microvessels group (Figure 4E). In fenestrated microvessels, TRITC RFI mean at t30 is 2.58 ± 0.21, 158% higher compared to t6 ($p < 0.0001$, Figure 4E). In plaque microvessels, TRITC mean intensity is 6.64 ± 1.27, 564% higher compared to t6 ($p = 0.0003$, Figure 4E). Representative sequences of FITC and TRITC signal in continuous, fenestrated and plaque microvessels, observed in real-time at t0, t6 and t30 are shown in Figure 4F.

Overall, 40 kDa dextran extravasates more than 2000 kDa dextran. 40 kDa dextran continues to extravasate over time, whereas 2000 kDa dextran shows an initial peak in extravasation and then stops.

2.4. Comparison Dextrans Extravasation in Continuous, Fenestrated and Plaque Microvessels

To better understand 2000 kDa and 40 kDa dextran extravasation differences between continuous, fenestrated and plaque microvessels, we compared FITC or TRITC fluorescence intensities outside the vessel structures (Figure 5).

FITC extravascular fluorescence intensities show small and non-significant increases over time in all groups as depicted in Figure 5A. Extravasation of 2000 kDa-FITC dextran is comparable between the groups at t18, t24, and t30 as demonstrated in Figure 5B.

The 40 kDa dextran profile displays, strong changes in TRITC extravascular RFI between the groups, which increases in time (Figure 5C). After t6, TRITC intensity increases differently between groups. While in continuous microvessels, TRITC signal increases, reaching a stable value of 1.30 ± 0.10, at t8, in the fenestrated microvessels group, TRITC signal at t8 is already 1.60 ± 0.23 and stabilizes at t18 (2.38 ± 0.19). In plaque microvessels, TRITC RFI raises continuously, with 1.98 ± 0.53 at t8 and 5.03 ± 1.13 at t18. As shown in Figure 5D, extravasation of 40 kDa TRITC-dextran in the plaque microvessels was 3.4-fold higher ($p = 0.0016$) in comparison to continuous microvessels, and 1.8-fold higher ($p = 0.0072$) in comparison to fenestrated capillaries at t18.

At the end of the observation period (t30), TRITC RFI was 1.60 ± 0.29 in continuous microvessels, 2.58 ± 0.11 in fenestrated microvessels and 6.42 ± 1.27 in plaque microvessels ($n = 3$). Extravasation of 40 kDa TRITC-dextran in plaque microvessels was four-fold higher ($p = 0.0006$) compared to continuous microvessels and 2.5-fold higher ($p = 0.0020$) compared to fenestrated capillaries. Thus, continuous, fenestrated, and plaque microvessels are all permeable to 40 kDa size-dextrans but follow different and vessel specific extravasation curves. Importantly, plaque microvessels show the largest permeability.

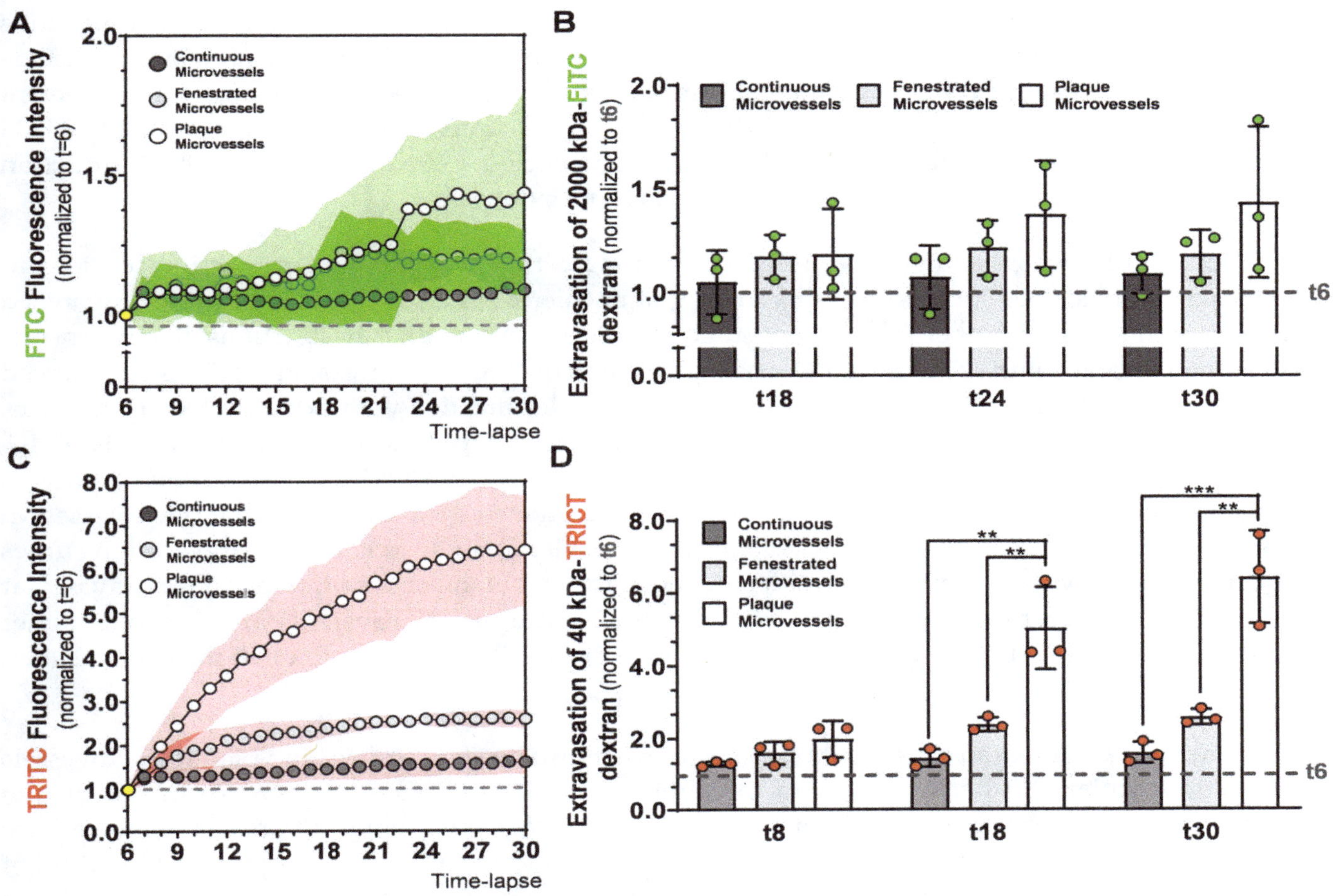

Figure 5. Evaluation of 2000 kDa-FITC and 40 kDa-TRITC dextrans extravasation in continuous, fenestrated and plaque microvessels. Time dependent evolution of (**A**) FITC and (**C**) TRITC extravascular RFI between groups. Comparison of (**B**) 2000 kDa and (**D**) 40 kDa extravasation at different timepoint between groups. Data presented as mean ± SD (SD is expressed as a green (**A**) or red (**C**) cloud). ** $p \leq 0.001$, *** $p \leq 0.001$, by 1-way-ANOVA.

3. Discussion

In this study, we used 2P-IVM to visualize adventitial and intimal plaque microvessels in advanced atherosclerotic lesions in ApoE3*Leiden VGs. In this model, a non-diseased caval vein from a donor mouse is used as an interposition in the carotid artery of a hypercholesterolemic ApoE3*Leiden mouse, within 28 day an atherosclerotic lesion forms with adventitial and intimal plaque microvessels with various forms of maturity [8,9]. We report a 2P-IVM method to evaluate plaque microvessels leakiness in vivo, by comparing the extravasation of 40 kDa dextran in healthy, continuous, and fenestrated, as well as diseased, plaque microvessels. We demonstrated in real-time, that microvessels in advanced atherosclerotic lesions in VGs are pathologically permeable.

By injecting 2000 kDa-FITC dextrans, we were able to observe in vivo microvessels networks throughout the adventitia, media and extending into the intimal layer of the VG lesion. Larger vessels were detected in the adventitia layer, while more narrow vessel structures were detected further deep in the plaque. We here confirm in vivo the abundant presence of intimal microvessels in advance atherosclerotic lesions in the ApoE3*Leiden VG model that was previously shown with histology [8,9]. This is a rare feature seldomly seen in other atherosclerotic mouse models [19,20]. These microvessel networks are characterized by typical vessel features of ongoing angiogenesis, as observed by the irregular microvessel architecture with accentuated turns and branching. Moreover, using 3D and color-depth Z-Stack projections, we demonstrate how vasa vasorum angiogenesis evolves throughout the lesion including the intima.

Fenestrated microvessels (observed in salivary glands) are more permeable than continuous microvessels (located in the ears) due to their increased number of pores, which drives faster molecule diffusion [6,7]. Accordingly, we observed that continuous and fenestrated microvessels follow different 40 kDa dextran extravasation signatures. While in continuous microvessels, extravasation of 40 kDa dextran reached a stable value rapidly in the observation period, extravasation of the 40 kDa dextran in fenestrated microvessels took more time and was more extensive.

Healthy microvessels have a well-organized architecture that acts as a protection barrier but which does let molecules such as nutrients cross. Plaque microvessels, in contrast, have a disorganized structure with a lack of proper pericyte coverage, diminished VE-cadherins junctions, heterogeneous basement membrane and show an unbalance in angiopoietin 1 and 2 expression [9]. This unbalanced architecture leads to dysfunctionality as shown by their co-localization with extravasated erythrocytes and inflammatory cells, in part explained by the increased expression of VCAM-1 and ICAM-1, as previously described by histological analysis [8,9]. By comparing 40 kDa extravasation patterns in healthy microvessels with the plaque microvessels, we demonstrate in real-time, that microvessels in advanced atherosclerotic lesions are pathological permeable. Their 40 kDa-FITC extravasation curves of the plaque microvessels were clearly different and at the end of the observation period, extravascular 40 kDa dextran was four-fold higher compared to continuous microvessels and 2.5-fold higher compared to fenestrated microvessels. This increased permeability can contribute to the extravasation of erythrocytes and leukocytes which drive plaque instability [4].

In the 2000 kDa dextran extravasation patterns in continuous, fenestrated, and plaque microvessels FITC extravascular RFI between t6 and t30 showed a trend towards an increase in the plaque microvessels. FITC extravascular RFI at t30 was similar between the groups. The reason why we were not able to detect different FITC extravascular RFI at t30 might be related to the immature nature of the plaque microvessels. Recent studies have shown that microvessels with an immature structure drive macromolecules accumulation by the enhanced permeability and retention (EPR) effect [21,22].

In this study, we used two injections of 2000 kDa dextran with the same fluorescent dye (FITC), with the first to visualize blood flow and the second to quantify vessel permeability. After the second injection, FITC intravascular RFI increased significantly between t5 and t6, in all groups. However, FITC extravascular RFI between t5 and t6, only increased significantly in continuous microvessels and did not differ in plaque microvessels. Moreover, when we compared FITC extravascular residual fluorescence (from the first injection) at t5 between groups, it was significantly higher in plaque microvessels compared to continuous microvessels.

Therefore, it is possible that 2000 kDa dextran (from the first injection) accumulates in the extravascular space of plaque microvessels due to the EPR effect, thereby decreasing signal differences during quantification of 2000 kDa extravasation in the second injection. In future approaches that aim to quantify extravasation patterns of macromolecules (such as 2000 kDa dextrans) other methods (e.g., dextrans with differently colored dyes) to detect blood flow should be considered.

Nevertheless, this 2P-IVM imaging methodology allows direct imaging of adventitial and intimal microvessels but also the quantification of the permeability of the microvessels by 40 kDa extravasation in a more realistic test environment compared to post-mortem tissue. Moreover, this technique could be easily adapted to further investigated the dynamics of intraplaque angiogenesis and intraplaque hemorrhage. By injecting fluorescent-labelled cells (such as erythrocytes or inflammatory cells), their extravasation, transmigration, and interaction with the endothelium could easily be monitored and quantified in vivo. Therefore, this 2P-IVM method is a promising approach to validate therapeutic angiogenic interventions targeting advance atherosclerosis in preclinical models in real-time.

4. Materials and Methods

4.1. Animals

All experiments were carried out with approval of the Animal Welfare Committee of the Leiden Medical University Center (28 March 2018; approval number 116002106645-18-096) and in compliance the Directive 2010/63/EU of the European Parliament. Male ApoE3*Leiden mice (n = 12), 10–16 weeks old, were fed with a high-cholesterol inducing diet (2.5% cholesterol and 0.05% cholate *w/w*, AB diets, Woerden, The Netherlands) during all the experiment. Mice were housed under standard laboratory conditions and received food and water ad libitum.

4.2. Vein Graft Surgery

VG surgery consists of the interposition of the caval vein from a donor mouse in the carotid artery of a recipient mouse, as described before [8]. In brief, the recipient mouse was fixed in a supine position, and an incision was made in the neck. The parotid glands were put aside exposing the right carotid artery. Next, the carotid artery was ligated and cut in middle, a cuff was placed at both ends of the arterial segments. Subsequently, the ends were everted over the cuffs and ligated. The vena cava was harvested from the donor mouse and positioned between the carotid artery by sleeving it over the cuffs and tightened with 8/0 sutures. Pulsatile flow through the venous conduit confirms a successful procedure. Finally, the parotid gland is put back in position and the skin is sutured. Within 28 days after the surgery, the VG lesions develop from a few cell layers at the start of the engraftment, to a massive thickened vessel wall [23].

Mice were anesthetized (intraperitoneally) with 5 mg/kg of midazolam (Roche Diagnostics, Basel, Switzerland), 0.5 mg/kg of dexmedetomidine (Orion Corporation, Espoo, Finland) and 0.05 mg/kg of fentanyl (Janssen Pharmaceutical, Beerse, Belgium). After the surgery, the anesthesia was antagonized with 2.5 mg/kg of atipamezole (Orion Corporation,) and 0.5 mg/kg of flumazenil (0.5 mg/kg, Fresenius Kabi, Bad Homburg vor der Höhe, Germany). Then, 0.1 mg/kg of buprenorphine (MSD Animal Health, Boxmeer, The Netherlands) was given for pain relief.

4.3. Two-Photon Intravital Microscopy

Four weeks after the surgery (Figure 1A), mice (n = 12) were anesthetized and prepared for intravital imaging on a Zeiss LSM 710 NLO upright multiphoton microscope equipped with a Mai Tai Deep See multiphoton laser (690–1040 nm).

Neck and ear regions were shaved, and a catheter was placed in the tail vein for intravenous injections. To image fenestrated microvessels (in the parotid glands) and plaque microvessels (in the VGs), mice were placed in a supine position on an inset located under the microscope (Figure 1B). Parotid glands were extracorporated, and VGs were carefully exposed from the surrounding connective tissue. To image continuous microvessels (in the ear skin), mice were placed in prone position on the inset (Figure 1B). In both positions, temperature was controlled and breathing was monitored. On top of the target tissue, a metal frame was placed. This metal frame was specially designed to allow the use of a water immersion objective (W Plan Apochromat 20×/1.0 DIC M27 75 mm objective) in the different tissues of the mouse body (Figure 1B).

To select areas of interest in the different microvessels types (continuous, fenestrated and plaque), mice were injected with 50 μL of 100 mg/mL FITC-conjugated 2000 kDa dextran (a blood tracer), via the vein catheter (Figure 1B). These areas were imaged by cycles of time-lapse Z-stacks (40 s each) over 20 min by multiphoton excitation at 488 nm (FITC) and 555 nm (TRITC). Emission was collected by two LSM PMTs at 500–558 nm (FITC) and 578–700 nm (TRITC). At the 5th frame of the time-lapse (t5) a mixture of 100 μL of a 100 mg/mL 40 kDa Dextran-TRITC (42874, Sigma-Aldrich, Zwijndrecht, The Netherlands) and 2000 kDa Dextran-FITC (FD2000S, Sigma-Aldrich, Zwijndrecht, The Netherlands) solution was injected to assess vessel permeability in real-time in all the groups (Figure 1C).

To study plaque angiogenesis in particular, a separate group of three mice was used to study the architecture of intimal and adventitial microvessels. Then, 50–150 μm depth Z-stacks were acquired by multiphoton excitation at 488 nm, after injection of 50 μL 100 mg/mL FITC-conjugated 2000 kDa dextran, via the tail vein catheter. Directly after imaging, all mice were euthanized by exsanguination.

4.4. Data Analysis

4.4.1. Quantification of FITC and TRITC Fluorescence Integrated Density Inside and Outside the Vessel Structures

To quantify FITC and TRITC fluorescence integrated density inside and outside the vessel structures, we converted 2P-IVM time-lapse acquisition files in maximal intensity Z-stack projections (RBG). Based on the literature, 2000 kDa-size dextrans are less prone to extravasate in microvascular structures due to their big size [17]. Therefore, we used the FITC channel to apply a tight automatic threshold and define vessel structures surface, denominated as Vessel Mask. Vessel Mask comprises all pixels inside the vessel value as 1 (defined by the automatic threshold) and all the pixels outside the vessel value as 0, at all the timelapsess. The Outside Mask was created via inversion. Both Vessel Mask and Outside Mask were then multiplied by the FITC and TRITC channel, generating four additional files: FITC pixels inside the vessel, FITC pixels outside the vessel, TRITC pixels inside the vessel, TRITC pixels outside the vessel.

For the all the six files, relative fluorescence intensity (RFI) was calculated by RawIntegrated density function. Since the area between intravascular and extravascular space are different between mice and organs, FITC and TRITC integrated densities were divided by the number of pixels of theVessel Mask or Outside Mask. Subsequently, FITC and TRITC fluorescence integrated densities reflect all the pixel intensities inside or outside the vessel structures. Since 40 kD and 2000 kDa dextran injection was detected intravitally at the 6th frame of the time-lapse (t6), FITC and TRITC fluorescence integrated intensities, intra and extravascular, were normalized to t6 values, and plotted in XY graphs.

4.4.2. Video Processing of FITC and TRITC Fluorescence Time-Lapse Series Acquired by 2P-IVM

To evaluate 40 kDa and 2000 kDa dextran extravasation patterns, we generated video time-lapse series of maximal FITC and TRITC fluorescence Z-stack projections. 2000 kDa dextran is visualized in the green channel and 40 kDa dextran is visualized in the red channel.

Plaque microvessels in advanced atherosclerotic VG lesions were processed by maximal FITC fluorescence Z-stack projections. Moreover, we generated 3D stack projections using Imaris 3D rendering software (Imaris, Zurich, Switzerland). In both renderings 2000 kDa-FITC dextran is visualized in the green channel.

To distinguish between adventitial and intimal microvessels, we used the temporal color-coding plugin in ImageJ FIJI that used a color LUT based on Z-depth and projects this in a maximum projection image.

4.5. Statistical Analysis

Results are shown as mean ± standard deviation error (SD). One-way ANOVA was used to compare differences between groups. Differences were considered significant when $p^{*} \leq 0.05$, $p^{**} \leq 0.01$, $p^{***} \leq 0.001$ or $p^{****} \leq 0.001$.

Author Contributions: Conception and design of the work: F.B. and L.R.; Animal surgeries and data acquisition: F.B., L.R. and M.R.d.V.; Data analysis: F.B. and L.R.; The first draft of the manuscript was written by F.B., and revised by M.R.d.V., P.H.A.Q. and L.R. Supervision: M.R.d.V. and P.H.A.Q. All authors have read and agreed to the published version of the manuscript.

Abbreviations

2P-IVM Two-photon intravital microscopy
RFI Relative fluorescence intensity

References

1. Parma, L.; Baganha, F.; Quax, P.H.A.; De Vries, M.R. Plaque angiogenesis and intraplaque hemorrhage in atherosclerosis. *Eur. J. Pharmacol.* **2017**, *816*, 107–115. [CrossRef]
2. Sluimer, J.C.; Daemen, M.J. Novel concepts in atherogenesis: Angiogenesis and hypoxia in atherosclerosis. *J. Pathol.* **2009**, *218*, 7–29. [CrossRef] [PubMed]
3. Kalucka, J.; Bierhansl, L.; Wielockx, B.; Carmeliet, P.; Eelen, G. Interaction of endothelial cells with macrophages—Linking molecular and metabolic signaling. *Pflügers Arch. Eur. J. Physiol.* **2017**, *469*, 473–483. [CrossRef]
4. De Vries, M.R.; Quax, P.H. Plaque angiogenesis and its relation to inflammation and atherosclerotic plaque destabilization. *Curr. Opin. Lipidol.* **2016**, *27*, 499–506. [CrossRef]
5. Pérez-Medina, C.; Binderup, T.; Lobatto, M.E.; Tang, J.; Calcagno, C.; Giesen, L.; Wessel, C.H.; Witjes, J.; Ishino, S.; Baxter, S.; et al. In Vivo PET Imaging of HDL in Multiple Atherosclerosis Models. *JACC Cardiovasc. Imaging* **2016**, *9*, 950–961. [CrossRef] [PubMed]
6. Stan, R.V.; Tse, D.; Deharvengt, S.J.; Smits, N.C.; Xu, Y.; Luciano, M.R.; McGarry, C.L.; Buitendijk, M.; Nemani, K.V.; Elgueta, R.; et al. The Diaphragms of Fenestrated Endothelia: Gatekeepers of Vascular Permeability and Blood Composition. *Dev. Cell* **2012**, *23*, 1203–1218. [CrossRef]
7. Ono, S.; Egawa, G.; Kabashima, K. Regulation of blood vascular permeability in the skin. *Inflamm. Regen.* **2017**, *37*, 1–8. [CrossRef]
8. De Vries, M.R.; Niessen, H.W.M.; Löwik, C.W.G.M.; Hamming, J.F.; Jukema, J.W.; Quax, P.H.A. Plaque Rupture Complications in Murine Atherosclerotic Vein Grafts Can Be Prevented by TIMP-1 Overexpression. *PLoS ONE* **2012**, *7*, e47134. [CrossRef]
9. De Vries, M.R.; Parma, L.; Peters, H.A.B.; Schepers, A.; Hamming, J.F.; Jukema, J.W.; Goumans, M.-J.; Guo, L.; Finn, A.V.; Virmani, R.; et al. Blockade of vascular endothelial growth factor receptor 2 inhibits intraplaque haemorrhage by normalization of plaque neovessels. *J. Intern. Med.* **2019**, *285*, 59–74. [CrossRef] [PubMed]
10. Marsch, E.; Theelen, T.L.; Demandt, J.A.; Jeurissen, M.; Van Gink, M.; Verjans, R.; Janssen, A.; Cleutjens, J.P.; Meex, S.J.R.; Donners, M.M.; et al. Reversal of Hypoxia in Murine Atherosclerosis Prevents Necrotic Core Expansion by Enhancing Efferocytosis. *Arter. Thromb. Vasc. Biol.* **2014**, *34*, 2545–2553. [CrossRef]
11. Rademakers, T.; Douma, K.; Hackeng, T.M.; Post, M.J.; Sluimer, J.C.; Daemen, M.J.; Biessen, E.A.; Heeneman, S.; Van Zandvoort, M. Plaque-Associated Vasa Vasorum in Aged Apolipoprotein E–Deficient Mice Exhibit Proatherogenic Functional Features In Vivo. *Arter. Thromb. Vasc. Biol.* **2013**, *33*, 249–256. [CrossRef] [PubMed]
12. Alie, N.; Eldib, M.; Fayad, Z.A.; Mani, V. Inflammation, Atherosclerosis, and Coronary Artery Disease: PET/CT for the Evaluation of Atherosclerosis and Inflammation. *Clin. Med. Insights Cardiol.* **2014**, *8*, 13–21. [CrossRef] [PubMed]
13. Tsujita, K.; Kaikita, K.; Araki, S.; Yamada, T.; Nagamatsu, S.; Yamanaga, K.; Sakamoto, K.; Kojima, S.; Hokimoto, S.; Ogawa, H. In Vivo optical coherence tomography visualization of intraplaque neovascularization at the site of coronary vasospasm: A case report. *BMC Cardiovasc. Disord.* **2016**, *16*, 1–4. [CrossRef] [PubMed]
14. Neeman, M. Perspectives: MRI of angiogenesis. *J. Magn. Reson.* **2018**, *292*, 99–105. [CrossRef]
15. Taqueti, V.R.; Jaffer, F.A. High-resolution molecular imaging via intravital microscopy: Illuminating vascular biology in vivo. *Integr. Biol.* **2013**, *5*, 278–290. [CrossRef]
16. Ritsma, L.; Ponsioen, B.; Van Rheenen, J. Intravital imaging of cell signaling in mice. *IntraVital* **2012**, *1*, 2–10. [CrossRef]
17. Egawa, G.; Nakamizo, S.; Natsuaki, Y.; Doi, H.; Miyachi, Y.; Kabashima, K. Intravital analysis of vascular permeability in mice using two-photon microscopy. *Sci. Rep.* **2013**, *3*, srep01932. [CrossRef]

18. Rattigan, S. Faculty Opinions recommendation of In vivo imaging shows abnormal function of vascular endothelial growth factor-induced vasculature. *Hum. Gene Ther.* **2007**, 515–524. [CrossRef]
19. Eriksson, E.E. Intravital Microscopy on Atherosclerosis in Apolipoprotein E–Deficient Mice Establishes Microvessels as Major Entry Pathways for Leukocytes to Advanced Lesions. *Circulation* **2011**, *124*, 2129–2138. [CrossRef]
20. Perrotta, P.; Pintelon, I.; De Vries, M.R.; Quax, P.H.; Timmermans, J.-P.; De Meyer, G.R.; Martinet, W. Three-Dimensional Imaging of Intraplaque Neovascularization in a Mouse Model of Advanced Atherosclerosis. *J. Vasc. Res.* **2020**, *57*, 348–354. [CrossRef]
21. Debefve, E.; Cheng, C.; Schaefer, S.; Yan, H.; Ballini, J.-P.; Bergh, H.V.D.; Lehr, H.-A.; Ruffieux, C.; Ris, H.-B.; Krueger, T. Photodynamic therapy induces selective extravasation of macromolecules: Insights using intravital microscopy. *J. Photochem. Photobiol. B* **2010**, *98*, 69–76. [CrossRef] [PubMed]
22. Maeda, H.; Wu, J.; Sawa, T.; Matsumura, Y.; Hori, K. Tumor vascular permeability and the EPR effect in macromolecular therapeutics: A review. *J. Control. Release* **2000**, *65*, 271–284. [CrossRef]
23. Lardenoye, J.H.; de Vries, M.R.; Lowik, C.W.; Xu, Q.; Dhore, C.R.; Cleutjens, J.P.; van Hinsbergh, V.W.; van Bockel, J.H.; Quax, P.H. Accelerated Atherosclerosis and Calcification in Vein Grafts: A Study in Apoe*3 Leiden Transgenic Mice. *Circ. Res.* **2002**, *7*, 577–584. [CrossRef] [PubMed]

10

The Extraordinary Role of Extracellular RNA in Arteriogenesis, the Growth of Collateral Arteries

Anna-Kristina Kluever [1], Anna Braumandl [1], Silvia Fischer [2], Klaus T. Preissner [2] and Elisabeth Deindl [1,*]

[1] Walter-Brendel-Center of Experimental Medicine, University Hospital, Ludwig-Maximilians-University, 81377 Munich, Germany; A.Kluever@campus.lmu.de (A.-K.K.); Anna.Braumandl@med.uni-muenchen.de (A.B.)

[2] Institute of Biochemistry, Medical School, Justus-Liebig-University, 35392 Giessen, Germany; Silvia.Fischer@biochemie.med.uni-giessen.de (S.F.); klaus.t.preissner@biochemie.med.uni-giessen.de (K.T.P.)

* Correspondence: elisabeth.deindl@med.uni-muenchen.de

Abstract: Arteriogenesis is an intricate process in which increased shear stress in pre-existing arteriolar collaterals induces blood vessel expansion, mediated via endothelial cell activation, leukocyte recruitment and subsequent endothelial and smooth muscle cell proliferation. Extracellular RNA (eRNA), released from stressed cells or damaged tissue under pathological conditions, has recently been discovered to be liberated from endothelial cells in response to increased shear stress and to promote collateral growth. Until now, eRNA has been shown to enhance coagulation and inflammation by inducing cytokine release, leukocyte recruitment, and endothelial permeability, the latter being mediated by vascular endothelial growth factor (VEGF) signaling. In the context of arteriogenesis, however, eRNA has emerged as a transmitter of shear stress into endothelial activation, mediating the sterile inflammatory process essential for collateral remodeling, whereby the stimulatory effects of eRNA on the VEGF signaling axis seem to be pivotal. In addition, eRNA might influence subsequent steps of the arteriogenesis cascade as well. This article provides a comprehensive overview of the beneficial effects of eRNA during arteriogenesis, laying the foundation for further exploration of the connection between the damaging and non-damaging effects of eRNA in the context of cardiovascular occlusive diseases and of sterile inflammation.

Keywords: arteriogenesis; VEGF; extracellular RNA; shear stress; endothelial activation; mast cell degranulation; macrophages; sterile inflammation; collateral artery growth; TACE

---

1. Introduction

Cardiovascular diseases such as ischemic heart disease, stroke or peripheral arterial occlusive disease are a major public health burden, accounting for approximately 30% of deaths worldwide in 2017 [1]. These diseases are commonly treated with percutaneous coronary interventions involving stents or with coronary bypass surgery. Interestingly enough, the body has a natural non-invasive way of forming a bypass around an occluded vessel called arteriogenesis. During arteriogenesis, blood flow is redirected through preexisting collateral arterioles upon occlusion of a supplying artery [2]. The main stimulus to initiate arteriogenesis in the pre-existing arteriolar vessels is increased fluid shear stress, which subsequently leads to endothelial cell activation, leukocyte extravasation and vessel wall (endothelial and smooth muscle cell) proliferation, substantially increasing the luminal diameter and restoring perfusion [2]. Whilst many of the steps leading to leukocyte extravasation and vessel growth have been uncovered, the crucial missing link of how intravascular shear stress is translated into local endothelial activation and vascular cell growth remained unknown.

Extracellular RNA (eRNA) released upon increased fluid shear stress during arteriogenesis in vivo has recently been suggested to be this missing link by initiating the cascade of arteriogenesis through vascular endothelial growth factor (VEGF)/VEGF receptor 2 (VEGFR2) signaling [3]. eRNA is released from cells upon cellular stress or damage and is mainly composed of rRNA [3,4]. Other forms of extracellular RNA such as microRNA have also been suggested to have a regulatory effect on collateral remodeling during arteriogenesis through modulation of intracellular signaling pathways; however, whether this effect is positive or negative seems to depend on the specific microRNA [5–8]. In terms of cardiovascular disease, eRNA released upon cellular damage has proven to have adverse effects in, e.g., ischemia/reperfusion injury, transplantation or atherosclerosis by mediating vascular edema, thrombus formation and inflammation [9–14]. This review aims to further elucidate the beneficial role of eRNA during the various stages of arteriogenesis.

2. The Role of eRNA in Arteriogenesis

2.1. eRNA Acts as a Translator of Shear Stress during Arteriogenesis through an Endothelial Mechanosensory Complex

The initiating stimulus for collateral remodeling in arteriogenesis is increased arteriolar fluid shear stress as a result of the occlusion of the main supplying artery [15]. In sharp contrast to other forms of vessel growth such as vasculogenesis or angiogenesis, vessel remodeling in arteriogenesis is stimulated by mechanical forces rather than by conditional factors such as hypoxia or ischemia [15,16]. Various mechanisms for shear stress sensing in endothelial cells have been described such as mechano-sensitive ion channels or the entire cytoskeleton transmitting changes in membrane tension (tensegrity architecture) [17]. However, it has recently been suggested that shear stress is in fact translated into endothelial cell activation through a mechanosensory complex, which was previously found to be located on endothelial cells in murine aortas predominantly at sites of non-laminar blood flow [18]. This complex comprises platelet endothelial cell adhesion molecule 1 (PECAM-1), vascular endothelial cell cadherin (VE-cadherin) and VEGFR2, whereby PECAM-1 acts as a mechano-sensor and together with VE-cadherin mediates VEGFR2 activation and subsequent intracellular signaling (Figure 1) [18]. VE-cadherin is an essential component of the endothelial adherens junction, mediating interactions with cytoskeletal anchoring molecules, and has been demonstrated to promote endothelial cell survival by enhancing VEGF-A signaling via VEGFR2 and subsequent phosphatidylinositol-3-OH-kinase activation as well as by activating protein kinase B (Akt) [19,20]. PECAM-1, also an adhesion molecule, has been shown to be involved in collateral remodeling in arteriogenesis as deficiency of PECAM-1 led to an attenuated increase in collateral luminal diameter and leukocyte recruitment to the perivascular space in a murine model of peripheral arteriogenesis [21]. Interestingly, in mice deficient in PECAM-1, the diameter of preexisting collaterals was larger than in wildtype mice; however, the number of preexisting collateral arterioles was comparable in both groups [21]. The signaling pathways activated by this mechanosensory complex that could also be highly relevant in arteriogenesis include (1) VEGFR2 activation, crucial for endothelial proliferation and von Willebrand factor (vWF) release, (2) nuclear factor κB (NFκB) activation, important for enhancing cytokine release and adhesion molecule expression, and (3) phosphatidylinositol-3-OH-kinase and protein kinase B (Akt) activation, essential for promoting endothelial cell survival [18].

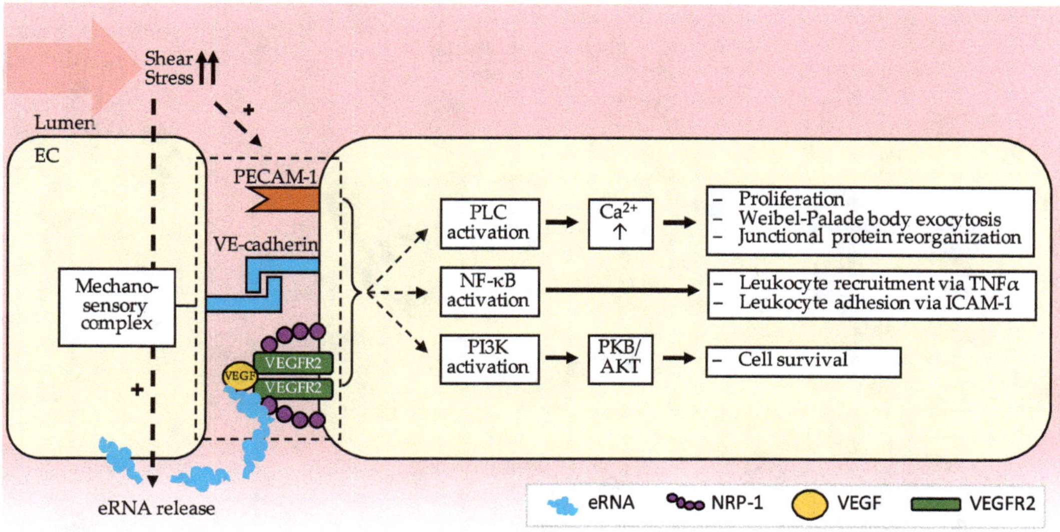

Figure 1. Proposed signaling mechanism downstream of the mechano-sensory complex composed of PECAM-1 (Platelet endothelial cell adhesion molecule (1), VE-cadherin (Vascular endothelial cadherin) and VEGFR2 (Vascular endothelial growth factor receptor (2) which could be relevant in arteriogenesis. eRNA released from EC (endothelial cells) upon shear stress enhances binding of VEGF to VEGFR2 and NRP-1 (Neuropilin-1) thus inducing the signaling mechanisms leading to endothelial cell activation and proliferation as well as leukocyte recruitment and adhesion. The intracellular compartment (EC) is depicted in yellow, the extracellular vessel lumen in red. Arrows indicate the various steps of the signaling pathways. [NF-κB (nuclear factor 'kappa-light-chain-enhancer' of activated B-cells); PI3K (Phosphoinositide 3-kinases); PLC (Phospholipase C); PKB/AKT (Protein kinase B)].

2.1.1. eRNA Initiates Arteriogenesis by Locally Enhancing VEGF/VEGFR2 Signaling

VEGF is a glycoprotein produced by a variety of cell types including leukocytes such as neutrophils or monocytes [22–25] and is critically involved in enhancing endothelial cell proliferation, permeability, and angiogenesis [26–28]. The role of VEGF in arteriogenesis remained uncertain for a long time; however, it has now been established that its downstream signaling events are crucial for this process [3,25]. While it has been demonstrated that the expression of the isoform VEGF-A is not increased in collateral vessels during the process of arteriogenesis and that administration of additional VEGF does not significantly improve collateral vessel development [16,29], antibodies blocking either VEGF or the cognate receptor (VEGFR2) have been shown to interfere greatly with vessel remodeling [25,30,31]. This indicates that VEGFR2 signaling is relevant in arteriogenesis but that endogenous VEGF levels are sufficient for this process [25]. Under physiological conditions, the activation of VEGFR2 induces its dimerization and subsequent tyrosine kinase auto-phosphorylation and endocytosis, thus activating phospholipase C (PLC) and raising intracellular calcium levels [32]. These intracellular signaling events ultimately lead to endothelial activation including the release of Weibel–Palade bodies. Hereby, the co-receptor neuropilin-1 (NRP-1) plays an essential role in linking VEGF and its receptor and in enhancing subsequent intracellular signaling (Figure 2) [32]. In vitro and in vivo studies have demonstrated that NRP-1 is also relevant in arteriogenesis [33,34], whereby its cytoplasmic domain mediates both the co-endocytosis of NRP-1 and VEGFR2 as well as its interaction with synectin [32–34]. These results indicate that the VEGF/VEGFR2 system plays a part in arteriogenesis; nevertheless, they do not explain how VEGFR2 is locally activated in collaterals upon increased shear stress. This is where eRNA comes into play.

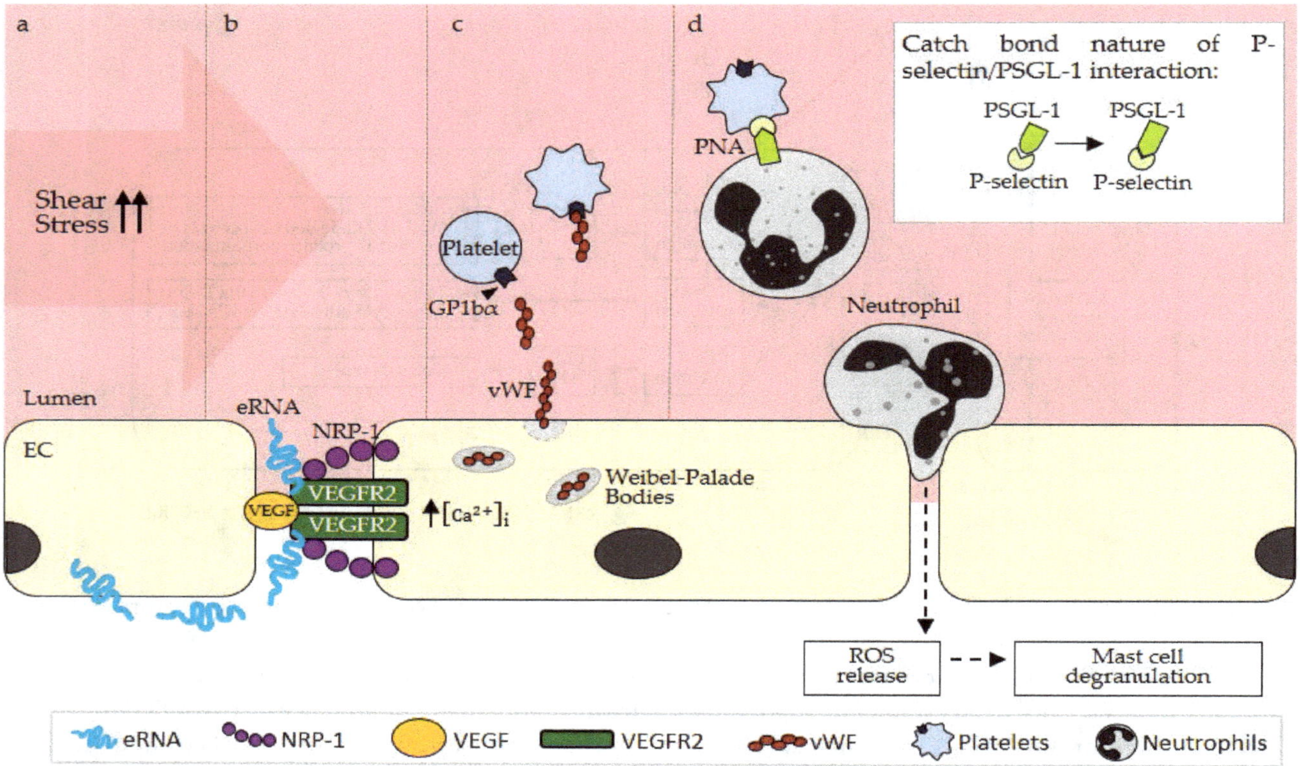

Figure 2. (**a**) Shear stress-induced activation of endothelial cells (EC) leads to the release of eRNA (extracellular RNA) on their abluminal side. (**b**) eRNA enhances the binding of VEGF (vascular endothelial growth factor) to NRP-1 (neuropilin (1) thus promoting VEGFR2 (VEGF Receptor (2) intracellular signaling. (**c**) VEGFR2 mediated raise of intracellular Ca^{2+} leads to the exocytosis of Weibel–Palade bodies and vWF (von Willebrand factor) release, which activates platelets via their GP1bα (Glycoprotein 1bα) receptor. (**d**) Upon activation, platelets express P-selectin, which subsequently binds its ligand PSGL-1 (P-selectin glycoprotein ligand-1) on neutrophils, inducing the formation of PNAs (platelet-neutrophil aggregates). The bond between P-selectin and PSGL-1 induces a deformational change, which promotes binding in these molecules (catch bond nature). PNA formation enhances neutrophil extravasation followed by ROS (reactive oxygen species) release which promotes mast cell degranulation. The intracellular compartment (EC) is depicted in yellow, the extracellular vessel lumen in red. Arrows indicate the subsequent steps during arteriogenesis.

VEGFR2 activation and signaling have been demonstrated to be involved in mediating the pro-inflammatory and permeability-enhancing effects of eRNA on endothelial cells. Binding studies of eRNA to different VEGF isoforms ($VEGF_{165}$ and $VEGF_{121}$) confirmed that eRNA directly interacts with VEGF, most likely via its heparin binding domain [12]. Whilst eRNA does not alter the expression of either VEGF [12] or of VEGFR2 in vitro [35], it has been shown to enhance the binding of VEGF to NRP-1 in vitro [35]. The formation of this complex of eRNA with VEGF, NRP-1 and VEGFR2 thus promotes PLC-dependent intracellular signaling mechanisms. Since eRNA is released from endothelial cells upon shear stress in vitro [3], it was proposed that eRNA could also play a role in the early steps of arteriogenesis by activating the VEGF/VEGFR2 signaling pathway and thereby inducing endothelial activation. Accordingly, in a murine model of peripheral arteriogenesis, eRNA—mostly rRNA—was found to be released from endothelial cells of developing collaterals, which were exposed to increased shear stress, on their abluminal side [3]. The levels of VEGF bound to the glycocalyx of endothelial cells might be sufficient for initial local signaling induced by eRNA; however, as collateral remodeling progresses, leukocytes might take over the role of supplying VEGF [24,25]. Crucially, this shear stress-induced release of eRNA during arteriogenesis is not related to cellular injury, as no lactate dehydrogenase was released into cell supernatants in vitro [3]. In contrast, eRNA, which is involved in other pathological situations such as stroke, was liberated mostly as a result of tissue damage [9,12]. eRNA seems to play a stimulatory part in arteriogenesis as treatment of mice with RNA-degrading RNase1 led to a smaller increase in luminal diameter of the growing collateral vessels compared to saline-treated control mice and also impaired perfusion recovery in vivo [3,36]. In contrast, administration of DNase or inactive RNase1 did not alter perfusion recovery [3], supporting the notion that the observed effects of RNase1 resulted from the hydrolysis of eRNA rather than from other functions of the endonuclease. In accordance with this, the administration of an RNase inhibitor improved perfusion recovery as well [3], which is highly relevant since eRNA is rapidly degraded in the circulation by RNases under physiological conditions [37]. Therefore, eRNA released upon increased fluid shear stress seems to play a pivotal role in the early processes of arteriogenesis by mediating endothelial cell activation through an enhanced VEGF/NRP-1/VEGFR2 interaction and subsequent intracellular signaling.

2.1.2. Contribution of eRNA in the Promotion of Collateral Remodeling through Stimulation of Endothelial NFκB Signaling

The extravasation of leukocytes, particularly of monocytes, is critical in arteriogenesis, since the cytokines and growth factors released by these cells are essential stimulators of endothelial and smooth muscle cell proliferation [38,39]. eRNA has previously been established as a strong promoter of leukocyte adhesion and extravasation, especially of monocytes, as demonstrated in a murine cremaster model and a murine model of atherosclerosis [11,14]. This pro-inflammatory effect was also confirmed in the process of arteriogenesis [3], where RNase1 treatment reduced the extravasation of neutrophils and monocytes in vivo [3]. In this case, no change in blood levels of leukocytes was observed [3], indicating that eRNA affects local cell interactions but not the systemic cell count. Physiologically and in arteriogenesis, leukocyte transmigration is facilitated by the interaction between endothelial adhesion molecules such as intercellular adhesion molecule 1 (ICAM-1) and leukocyte ligands such as macrophage-1 antigen (Mac-1) [40,41]. The expression of ICAM-1 has independently been shown to be upregulated on the one hand by fluid shear stress in vitro and in vivo [42,43] and on the other hand by eRNA in vitro [14,44]. In an in vivo model of peripheral arteriogenesis, the effects of eRNA on endothelial cell signaling were also demonstrated to be relevant for subsequent leukocyte adhesion, as inhibition of eRNA through RNase administration reduced the perivascular macrophage count to a similar degree as seen in ICAM-1 deficient mice [3].

Two possible ways through which eRNA might affect the expression of ICAM-1 are through stimulation of the NFκB or of the VEGFR2 signaling pathways. VEGF has been shown to induce the upregulation of ICAM-1 in a transgenic mouse model of psoriasis [45], whereby its effects on ICAM-1 expression were demonstrated to be the result of an enhanced VEGF/NRP-1 interaction in a retinal mouse model [46]. Since eRNA enhances the formation of an activated VEGF/NRP-1/VEGFR2 complex during arteriogenesis, it might promote the expression of adhesion molecules on endothelial cells through this avenue of signaling. Nevertheless, eRNA has also been shown to promote the activity of NFκB, which also enhances ICAM-1 expression [47], by inducing the phosphorylation of the cytoplasmic inhibitor of κB (IκB) in vitro [14]. The role of NFκB signaling in arteriogenesis has not yet been studied in detail; however, this pathway was found to be continuously activated in situations of disturbed blood flow such as in atherosclerosis [18]. Furthermore, an increase in the nuclear translocation of NFκB and hence an increase in the expression of its target genes was observed in a rat mesenteric model of collateral growth [48]. Moreover, NFκB is also able to induce the expression of VEGF [49], suggesting that there might be an interplay between these two avenues of signaling in mediating the effects of eRNA on endothelial activation during arteriogenesis.

2.2. eRNA Is Relevant for Mast Cell Degranulation during Arteriogenesis by Stimulating vWF Release and PNA Formation

2.2.1. eRNA Mediates vWF Release from Endothelial Weibel–Palade Bodies by Promoting VEGF/ VEGFR2 Signaling

Through its stimulatory effect on VEGF/VEGFR2 signaling, eRNA mediates endothelial activation and the release of vWF from Weibel–Palade bodies, which is essential for subsequent platelet activation and platelet-neutrophil aggregate (PNA) formation in arteriogenesis (Figure 2). Endothelial cell activation as seen in arteriogenesis is characterized to a large extent by a loss of vascular barrier function, luminal expression of adhesion molecules for leukocytes and release of cytokines and pro-coagulatory molecules [50]. eRNA has been associated with all of these events, since it mediates hyper-permeability and vascular edema formation under conditions of ischemia/reperfusion injury or transplantation by disrupting endothelial tight junctions and since it promotes thrombus formation by activating the contact phase system of intrinsic coagulation [4,10,12,13]. In the inflammatory setting of arteriogenesis where eRNA plays such a prominent role, this raises the question of how thrombus formation is inhibited, which will be discussed at a later stage of this review. In addition to these pro-inflammatory and pro-coagulatory effects, eRNA also stimulates the exocytosis of endothelial cell storage granules, designated as Weibel–Palade bodies, which contain vWF, P-Selectin and other cytokines [51–53], as indicated by increased vWF release from endothelial cells upon eRNA exposure in vitro [35]. The exocytosis of Weibel–Palade bodies can also be induced by various other stimuli including thrombin, VEGF and reactive oxygen species (ROS) [54–56]. Weibel–Palade body exocytosis by eRNA was inhibited by an antibody against VEGF [35], suggesting that eRNA stimulates vWF release from endothelial cells via VEGF/VEGFR2 signaling as described above [12]. In the context of arteriogenesis, the ability of eRNA to induce endothelial activation and vWF release via VEGFR2 activation was confirmed, since RNase1 treatment in a murine model of peripheral arteriogenesis decreased luminal vWF levels to a similar extent as seen with vWF deficiency or VEGFR2 inhibition [3].

2.2.2. eRNA-Mediated vWF Release Is Pivotal for PNA Formation

vWF is an adhesive and prothrombotic glycoprotein, constitutively produced by endothelial cells and released from endothelial Weibel–Palade bodies upon cell stimulation. It forms large and ultralarge multimers and plays a key role in the tethering and adhesion of platelets to the injured vessel wall, particularly under fluid shear stress conditions [57,58]. In arteriogenesis, the release of vWF and its interaction with platelets have been demonstrated as pivotal, triggering the activation of platelets and the formation of PNAs (Figure 2) [59,60]. PNAs in turn have been implicated in the recruitment and priming of neutrophils during inflammatory processes and were shown to be relevant for the release of reactive oxygen species (ROS) [61], both of which are relevant in arteriogenesis [60,62]. Following neutrophil extravasation and ROS release, perivascular mast cells are activated and the subsequent extravasation of leukocytes and their release of cytokines and growth factors are increased. In this way, the proliferation of endothelial cells and smooth muscle cells is stimulated, collateral vessels are able to expand, and perfusion can be sufficiently restored. PNAs are also crucial for the formation of neutrophil extracellular traps (NETs), comprising the entire decondensated chromatin of neutrophils, whose formation has also been induced following stimulation of neutrophils with extracellular nucleic acids [63]. In the context of arteriogenesis, though, the formation of NETs has not yet been described. However, since the application of DNase had no effect on perfusion recovery in vivo [3], one can assume that even if NETs are formed during arteriogenesis, they would not have a negative effect on vessel remodeling.

While free platelets do not usually interact with vWF, they are able to transiently bind to vWF via their receptor glycoprotein Ibα (GPIbα) under high fluid shear stress, resulting in platelet activation and adhesion [64]. GPIbα also binds to other pro-coagulatory factors such as thrombin or factors XI and FXII as well as to adhesion molecules such as P-selectin or Mac-1 on immune cells, thereby facilitating cell-cell contacts [65]. Interestingly, the vWF-GPIbα interaction appears to be optimal at high fluid shear stress, a condition which is predominantly found in arterioles [64–66], which is also where vessel remodeling takes places during arteriogenesis. This seems to be due to the fact that shear stress induces conformational changes in the vWF multimers [64], which then facilitate their interactions with platelets. These interactions are also vital in the high shear stress setting of arteriogenesis, where both platelet deficiency and GPIbα deficiency resulted in reduced perfusion recovery in vivo [59]. Once platelets are activated through vWF/GPIbα binding, they express P-selectin on their surface, which is subsequently able to bind to the corresponding P-selectin glycoprotein ligand-1 (PSGL-1) on neutrophils [67,68], enabling the formation of PNAs [60]. The expression of P-selectin has been demonstrated to be increased by shear stress as well [67], and additionally, it was suggested that the resulting adhesive bonds between P-selectin and PSGL-1 are stronger under high fluid shear stress owing to the catch bond nature of selectins [40]. P-selectin and PSGL-1 seem to mediate the interactions of platelets with neutrophils at higher rates of shear stress in vitro, while integrin-mediated interactions seem to be more relevant at lower levels of fluid shear stress [69]. The formation of PNAs was also observed in vivo in the high fluid shear stress setting of arteriogenesis, whereby this binding of platelets to neutrophils was abolished in GPIbα knock-out mice [59], underlining the relevance of vWF release and binding to GPIbα for PNA formation in arteriogenesis.

This important step during collateral remodeling might also be influenced indirectly by eRNA, marking another point where eRNA could play a role during arteriogenesis. In a murine model of arteriogenesis, RNase1 treatment decreased the formation of PNAs to a similar extent as was seen in mice which were either deficient in vWF or treated with a VEGFR2 inhibitor [3], suggesting that VEGF/VEGFR2-dependent eRNA-mediated effects on vWF release also ultimately affect PNA formation. Critically, the administration of RNase1 did not change the blood levels of platelets or neutrophils [3], indicating that eRNA-mediated effects are not systemic but localized to collaterals and do not involve enhanced release of effector cells from the bone marrow. In addition, activated platelets are able to trigger the expression of P-selectin on endothelial cells, thus enabling leukocyte rolling along the activated vessel wall [70]. Such transient interactions of platelets with endothelial cells were also observed in arteriogenesis [59]. In summary, the release of vWF from endothelial Weibel–Palade bodies is a critical step in arteriogenesis as vWF subsequently leads to the activation of platelets and the formation of PNAs, and these processes depend on eRNA, which enhances VEGF/VEGFR2 signaling and endothelial activation.

2.2.3. The Possible Role of ADAMTS13 in the Suppression of Thrombus Formation in Arteriogenesis

The activation of platelets together with the secretion of highly reactive multimeric vWF from endothelial cells under inflammatory conditions during the process of arteriogenesis would provide an ideal setting for thrombus formation. Yet, such an outcome has never been observed, and it remains to be studied in which way local thrombus formation is inhibited during arteriogenesis. Following activation of endothelial cells and the initial release of vWF in a multimeric form to promote platelet adhesion under flow, the readily coagulable nature of these large vWF multimers needs to be weakened at a later phase to prevent the formation of microthrombi [71]. vWF can be cleaved via limited proteolysis by the circulating plasma metalloprotease ADAMTS13 (a disintegrin and metalloprotease with a thrombospondin type 1 motif, member 13) [57]. The deficiency of this protease has been associated with a thrombotic pathology known as thrombotic thrombocytopenic purpura [72]. The interaction between vWF and ADAMTS13 was revealed to be increased under high shear stress in vitro and was maintained even after shear stress was eliminated [58,73]. This effect has been attributed to unfolding of the vWF molecule from a globular to an elongated form upon exposure to shear stress and subsequent exposition of scissile bonds for cleavage by ADAMTS13 [57]. Cleavage of vWF by ADAMTS13 could therefore be a potential mechanism through which thrombus formation could be inhibited in arteriogenesis. In fact, platelet adhesion and aggregation reactions were increased in the arterioles of ADAMTS13-deficient mice compared to wild-type mice; however, this situation could be reversed by the administration of recombinant ADAMTS13 [74]. Furthermore, in a murine model of stroke, ADAMTS13 deficiency was associated with impaired angiogenesis and brain capillary perfusion [75]. The pro-angiogenic properties of ADAMTS13 have been proposed to be due to the phosphorylation of VEGFR2 and upregulation of VEGF, both in vivo and in vitro [75,76], which was also reflected by the fact that an in vitro siRNA-induced knockdown of ADAMTS13 reduced VEGF levels in the cell lysate as well as endothelial proliferation [77]. ADAMTS13 therefore seems to influence VEGF signaling, and since the effect of eRNA on this signaling pathway has proven to be pivotal in arteriogenesis, there might be a link between eRNA and ADAMTS13 in arteriogenesis as well. Yet, the exact role of ADAMTS13 during this process still needs to be assessed.

2.2.4. eRNA is Relevant for Mast Cell Degranulation Following PNA Formation

Following PNA formation, the extravasation of neutrophils is mediated through urokinase-type plasminogen activator (uPA) [60], which, in contrast to tissue plasminogen activator, has been shown to be vital for the transmigration of leukocytes during arteriogenesis in vivo [62]. The subsequent release of NADPH oxidase 2 (Nox2)-derived ROS from neutrophils is crucial for inducing mast cell degranulation [60], whereby neutrophils in PNAs were shown to produce more ROS than non-complexed neutrophils [61]. Both the surface expression of uPA as well as ROS formation via Nox2 were reduced in P-selectin-deficient and PSGL-1-deficient cells in vitro [60], underlining the importance of PNAs in triggering the steps leading to mast cell degranulation in arteriogenesis. Perivascular mast cells in turn have been established as key players during collateral remodeling and have been suggested to act in three ways: (1) by releasing cytokines, which promote the recruitment of growth factor producing leukocytes, (2) by themselves supplying growth factors for the growing collateral, and (3) by activating matrix metalloproteases (MMPs), responsible for extracellular matrix remodeling (Figure 3) [60]. Mast cell degranulation in arteriogenesis has also been shown to be promoted following eRNA stimulation of endothelial VEGF/VEGFR2 signaling, as RNase1 administration impaired mast cell degranulation in an in vivo model of arteriogenesis to a comparable degree as VEGFR2 inhibition and vWF deficiency did without affecting the perivascular mast cell count [3].

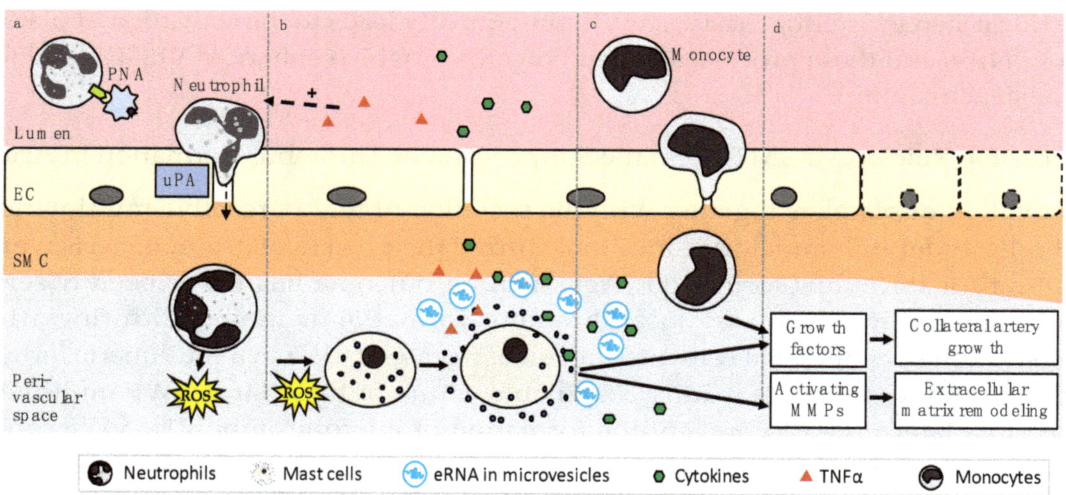

Figure 3. (**a**) PNA (platelet neutrophil aggregate) formation leads to uPA (Urokinase-type plasminogen activator) mediated neutrophil extravasation and subsequent ROS (reactive oxygen species) release. (**b**) ROS, released from neutrophils, initiates mast cell degranulation and consecutive release of cytokines, growth factors and eRNA in microvesicles. (**c**) eRNA and cytokine (especially MCP-1) mediated recruitment and extravasation of monocytes enhances local inflammatory processes leading to (**d**) collateral artery growth (arteriogenesis) and extracellular matrix remodeling. The extracellular vessel lumen is depicted in red, EC in yellow, SMC in orange, and the perivascular space in gray. Arrows indicate the subsequent steps during arteriogenesis. [EC: endothelial cells; SMC: smooth muscle cells].

2.3. eRNA Released from Mast Cells Provides a Second Stimulatory Boost for Collateral Remodeling

As previously described, eRNA released by endothelial cells upon cellular stress such as fluid shear stress has been attributed an essential role as the translator of shear stress into endothelial activation during the initial stages of collateral remodeling. However, eRNA is rapidly degraded by circulating RNases and could thus only unfold its actions over a short period of time [37]. Arteriogenesis, on the contrary, is a chronic process. Mast cells, whose degranulation is stimulated by the downstream effects of endothelial cell-derived eRNA, also release eRNA in the form of microvesicles concomitantly with degranulation [44]. This release of eRNA has been shown to promote local inflammatory processes and leukocyte extravasation [44]. Microvesicles (MV) are a type of extracellular vesicles that have been described to be released from a variety of cell types including endothelial cells, leukocytes, platelets and mast cells [78–81], often upon cell stress [82], to be involved in cell communication and inflammation including during angiogenesis [82,83], and to be selectively enriched with different types of RNA [84]. Microvesicles/microparticles are generated via budding from the cell membrane and can reach a diameter of up to 1000 nm, whereas exosomes, another type of extracellular vesicle, are released via exocytosis and are generally smaller than 100 nm [82]. In the context of arteriogenesis, this additional release of eRNA in microvesicles might act as a booster of the initial effects mediated by endothelial cell-derived eRNA. What remains to be determined is the exact mechanism through which mast cell-derived eRNA unfolds its effects. However, it is plausible that it also stimulates VEGF/VEGFR2 signaling in endothelial cells. This is supported by the fact that various leukocytes including neutrophils and monocytes, whose extravasation is critical in arteriogenesis, secrete VEGF and have been demonstrated to do so in arteriogenesis [22–25]. In addition, treatment of endothelial cells with MVs derived from mast cells potentiated the release of vWF from endothelial cells just as endothelial cell-derived eRNA did [44]. Besides acting as a positive feedback mechanism for endothelial activation, an important effect of mast cell-derived eRNA might also be the stimulation of the expression of adhesion molecules on endothelial cells as was shown for ICAM-1 in vitro [44]—potentially through VEGFR2 or NFκB signaling.

Furthermore, eRNA released by mast cells might also directly influence leukocyte adhesion, transmigration and cytokine/chemokine release such as of TNFα or MCP-1 during arteriogenesis and might thus amplify the budding local inflammatory response. TNFα is a key pro-inflammatory cytokine released by a variety of cell types including granulocytes, macrophages and smooth muscle cells and is able to enhance leukocyte adhesion, coagulation, and endothelial permeability [85–87]. Its ability to promote MCP-1 expression and monocyte extravasation are extremely relevant in arteriogenesis [88], as is its stimulation of neutrophil and T-cell extravasation [60,89–91]. In a murine model of peripheral arteriogenesis, the inhibition of TNFα lead to reduced perfusion recovery and, in a rabbit model, to a decrease in luminal vessel diameter, smooth muscle cell proliferation and leukocyte extravasation [92,93]. MCP-1 has been established as a major trigger of monocyte recruitment and accelerator of collateral growth during arteriogenesis [94–97], and key sources of this chemokine include macrophages, endothelial cells and smooth muscle cells [98–100]. eRNA was found to promote the release of TNFα from monocytes by activating the TNFα converting enzyme (TACE/ADAM17), which releases soluble TNFα from its membrane-bound form [101]. The inhibition of TACE reduced both the eRNA-mediated release of TNFα in vitro and the adhesion of leukocytes following eRNA administration in vivo [14]. This effect of eRNA on TACE activation in macrophages in vitro was found to involve NFκB signaling [102]. The effects of eRNA on TACE activity in arteriogenesis have not yet been explored; however, it would be interesting to see if eRNA released by mast cells could stimulate the release of TNFα via TACE and thus boost the local inflammatory response. Nevertheless, both TNFα and eRNA were demonstrated to have similar effects on cell adhesion to the endothelium in murine cremaster venules in the context of arteriogenesis [3,14]. The stimulatory effect of eRNA on cell adhesion was abolished by pre-treatment with a VEGFR2 inhibitor (Semaxanib), again highlighting that eRNA enhances VEGFR2 activation, whereas the TNFα-mediated effect was not diminished by pre-treatment with Semaxanib [3], since the release of TNFα occurs at a later stage of arteriogenesis following VEGFR2 activation and signaling. The expression of MCP-1, on the other hand, was increased by MV-derived eRNA from mast cells in vitro [44]. eRNA released by mast cells might therefore activate TACE and thus stimulate TNFα and subsequent MCP-1 release in arteriogenesis, thereby enhancing the local inflammatory response and leukocyte transmigration. In addition, NFκB, whose activation can be stimulated by eRNA as previously touched upon, can also induce the expression of pro-inflammatory cytokines such as TNFα [103], suggesting that mast cell-derived eRNA might also promote local inflammation through this avenue of signaling. However, the exact ways through which this second release of eRNA enhances leukocyte extravasation and collateral remodeling during arteriogenesis still have to be confirmed.

At this point, it is interesting to note that eRNA administration in vitro was shown to prompt a shift in macrophage polarization towards the pro-inflammatory M1 phenotype with an upregulation of pro-inflammatory cytokines such as TNFα and a concurrent downregulation of anti-inflammatory cytokines [104]. In the context of arteriogenesis, the pro-inflammatory M1 macrophage phenotype is important during the initial stages of vessel remodeling, which would correlate with the release of eRNA during arteriogenesis and would suggest that the previously described eRNA-induced shift in macrophage polarization could also occur during arteriogenesis, whilst the anti-inflammatory M2 phenotype is more relevant during later stages of vessel remodeling [105].

3. eRNA in Other Forms of Vessel Growth

The role of eRNA in other forms of vessel growth, namely vasculogenesis and angiogenesis, has not been studied in great detail so far. In vasculogenesis, tRNA and rRNA were found to stimulate the formation of new vessels and the leukocyte differentiation of embryonic bodies via increased VEGF signaling and ROS generation [106]. VEGF signaling is crucial in vasculogenesis [107], and upon eRNA exposure, the expression of $VEGF_{165}$, NRP-1 and other hypoxia related factors such as HIF-1α was increased [106]. ROS formation was also enhanced after eRNA administration [106], which is significant, since the interplay between intracellular VEGF signaling and ROS generation is a central issue of embryoid body differentiation [108]. In angiogenesis, the focus has been more on the stimulatory role of endogenous RNases namely of angiogenin, also known as hRNase5, as a strong promoter of endothelial cell proliferation through its effects on rRNA and ribosome synthesis and its regulatory role in translation during cellular stress [109,110].

4. Conclusions

The remodeling of pre-existing arteriolar collaterals during arteriogenesis is a complex process requiring the highly-coordinated interplay of different leukocytes to promote endothelial and smooth muscle cell proliferation and to ultimately establish perfusion. eRNA has been demonstrated to translate fluid shear stress into endothelial activation during arteriogenesis, further stimulating vWF release, PNA formation, mast cell degranulation and leukocyte recruitment, culminating in the beneficial process of arteriogenesis to promote perfusion recovery. In contrast to the beneficial role of eRNA in arteriogenesis, eRNA has been formerly established as a damaging or pathological factor in a variety of cardiovascular diseases based upon its modulation of endothelial cell and leukocyte function, whereby administration of RNase1 was demonstrated to serve as a tissue- and vessel-protective regimen. It remains to be established which particular molecular interactions and binding partners as well as which putative cellular receptors for eRNA appear to be responsible for its either adverse or beneficial functions in the cardiovascular system.

Author Contributions: Writing—Original Draft Preparation, A.-K.K. and A.B.; Writing—Review & Editing, S.F., K.T.P. and E.D.

Abbreviations

ADAMTS13 A disintegrin and metalloprotease with a thrombospondin type 1 motif, member 13
eRNA Extracellular RNA
ICAM-1 Intercellular adhesion molecule 1
Mac-1 Macrophage-1 antigen
MCP-1 Monocyte chemoattractant protein 1
MMP Matrix metalloprotease
MV Microvesicle
NFkB Nuclear factor kB
Nox2 NADPH oxidase 2
NRP-1 Neuropilin-1
PECAM-1 Platelet endothelial cell adhesion molecule 1
PLC Phospholipase C
PNA Platelet-neutrophil aggregate
ROS Reactive oxygen species
TACE TNFa converting enzyme
TNFa Tumor necrosis factor a
uPA Urokinase-type plasminogen activator
VE-cadherin Vascular endothelial cell cadherin
VEGF Vascular endothelial growth factor
VEGFR2 Vascular endothelial growth factor receptor 2
vWF Von Willebrand factor

References

1. GBD 2017 Causes of Death Collaborators. Global, regional, and national age-sex-specific mortality for 282 causes of death in 195 countries and territories, 1980-2017: A systematic analysis for the Global Burden of Disease Study 2017. *Lancet* **2018**, *392*, 1736–1788. [CrossRef]
2. Deindl, E.; Schaper, W. The art of arteriogenesis. *Cell Biochem. Biophys.* **2005**, *43*, 1–15. [CrossRef]
3. Lasch, M.; Kleinert, E.C.; Meister, S.; Kumaraswami, K.; Buchheim, J.I.; Grantzow, T.; Lautz, T.; Salpisti, S.; Fischer, S.; Troidl, K.; et al. Extracellular RNA released due to shear stress controls natural bypass growth by mediating mechanotransduction in mice. *Blood* **2019**, *134*, 1469–1479. [CrossRef] [PubMed]
4. Cabrera-Fuentes, H.A.; Ruiz-Meana, M.; Simsekyilmaz, S.; Kostin, S.; Inserte, J.; Saffarzadeh, M.; Galuska, S.P.; Vijayan, V.; Barba, I.; Barreto, G.; et al. RNase1 prevents the damaging interplay between extracellular RNA and tumour necrosis factor-alpha in cardiac ischaemia/reperfusion injury. *Thromb. Haemost.* **2014**, *112*, 1110–1119. [CrossRef] [PubMed]
5. Zhu, L.P.; Zhou, J.P.; Zhang, J.X.; Wang, J.Y.; Wang, Z.Y.; Pan, M.; Li, L.F.; Li, C.C.; Wang, K.K.; Bai, Y.P.; et al. MiR-15b-5p Regulates Collateral Artery Formation by Targeting AKT3 (Protein Kinase B-3). *Arterioscler. Thromb. Vasc. Biol.* **2017**, *37*, 957–968. [CrossRef] [PubMed]
6. Guan, Y.; Cai, B.; Wu, X.; Peng, S.; Gan, L.; Huang, D.; Liu, G.; Dong, L.; Xiao, L.; Liu, J.; et al. microRNA-352 regulates collateral vessel growth induced by elevated fluid shear stress in the rat hind limb. *Sci. Rep.* **2017**, *7*, 6643. [CrossRef] [PubMed]
7. Heuslein, J.L.; McDonnell, S.P.; Song, J.; Annex, B.H.; Price, R.J. MicroRNA-146a Regulates Perfusion Recovery in Response to Arterial Occlusion via Arteriogenesis. *Front. Bioeng. Biotechnol.* **2018**, *6*, 1. [CrossRef]
8. Lei, Z.; van Mil, A.; Brandt, M.M.; Grundmann, S.; Hoefer, I.; Smits, M.; El Azzouzi, H.; Fukao, T.; Cheng, C.; Doevendans, P.A.; et al. MicroRNA-132/212 family enhances arteriogenesis after hindlimb ischaemia through modulation of the Ras-MAPK pathway. *J. Cell. Mol. Med.* **2015**, *19*, 1994–2005. [CrossRef]
9. Stieger, P.; Daniel, J.M.; Tholen, C.; Dutzmann, J.; Knopp, K.; Gunduz, D.; Aslam, M.; Kampschulte, M.; Langheinrich, A.; Fischer, S.; et al. Targeting of Extracellular RNA Reduces Edema Formation and Infarct Size and Improves Survival After Myocardial Infarction in Mice. *J. Am. Heart Assoc.* **2017**, *6*. [CrossRef]
10. Kleinert, E.; Langenmayer, M.C.; Reichart, B.; Kindermann, J.; Griemert, B.; Blutke, A.; Troidl, K.; Mayr, T.; Grantzow, T.; Noyan, F.; et al. Ribonuclease (RNase) Prolongs Survival of Grafts in Experimental Heart Transplantation. *J. Am. Heart Assoc.* **2016**, *5*. [CrossRef]

11. Simsekyilmaz, S.; Cabrera-Fuentes, H.A.; Meiler, S.; Kostin, S.; Baumer, Y.; Liehn, E.A.; Weber, C.; Boisvert, W.A.; Preissner, K.T.; Zernecke, A. Role of extracellular RNA in atherosclerotic plaque formation in mice. *Circulation* **2014**, *129*, 598–606. [CrossRef] [PubMed]
12. Fischer, S.; Gerriets, T.; Wessels, C.; Walberer, M.; Kostin, S.; Stolz, E.; Zheleva, K.; Hocke, A.; Hippenstiel, S.; Preissner, K.T. Extracellular RNA mediates endothelial-cell permeability via vascular endothelial growth factor. *Blood* **2007**, *110*, 2457–2465. [CrossRef] [PubMed]
13. Kannemeier, C.; Shibamiya, A.; Nakazawa, F.; Trusheim, H.; Ruppert, C.; Markart, P.; Song, Y.; Tzima, E.; Kennerknecht, E.; Niepmann, M.; et al. Extracellular RNA constitutes a natural procoagulant cofactor in blood coagulation. *Proc. Natl. Acad. Sci. USA* **2007**, *104*, 6388–6393. [CrossRef] [PubMed]
14. Fischer, S.; Grantzow, T.; Pagel, J.I.; Tschernatsch, M.; Sperandio, M.; Preissner, K.T.; Deindl, E. Extracellular RNA promotes leukocyte recruitment in the vascular system by mobilising proinflammatory cytokines. *Thromb. Haemost.* **2012**, *108*, 730–741. [CrossRef] [PubMed]
15. Pipp, F.; Boehm, S.; Cai, W.J.; Adili, F.; Ziegler, B.; Karanovic, G.; Ritter, R.; Balzer, J.; Scheler, C.; Schaper, W.; et al. Elevated fluid shear stress enhances postocclusive collateral artery growth and gene expression in the pig hind limb. *Arterioscler. Thromb. Vasc. Biol.* **2004**, *24*, 1664–1668. [CrossRef] [PubMed]
16. Deindl, E.; Buschmann, I.; Hoefer, I.E.; Podzuweit, T.; Boengler, K.; Vogel, S.; van Royen, N.; Fernandez, B.; Schaper, W. Role of ischemia and of hypoxia-inducible genes in arteriogenesis after femoral artery occlusion in the rabbit. *Circ. Res.* **2001**, *89*, 779–786. [CrossRef]
17. Busse, R.; Fleming, I. Regulation of endothelium-derived vasoactive autacoid production by hemodynamic forces. *Trends Pharmacol. Sci.* **2003**, *24*, 24–29. [CrossRef]
18. Tzima, E.; Irani-Tehrani, M.; Kiosses, W.B.; Dejana, E.; Schultz, D.A.; Engelhardt, B.; Cao, G.; DeLisser, H.; Schwartz, M.A. A mechanosensory complex that mediates the endothelial cell response to fluid shear stress. *Nature* **2005**, *437*, 426–431. [CrossRef]
19. Shay-Salit, A.; Shushy, M.; Wolfovitz, E.; Yahav, H.; Breviario, F.; Dejana, E.; Resnick, N. VEGF receptor 2 and the adherens junction as a mechanical transducer in vascular endothelial cells. *Proc. Natl. Acad. Sci. USA* **2002**, *99*, 9462–9467. [CrossRef]
20. Carmeliet, P.; Lampugnani, M.G.; Moons, L.; Breviario, F.; Compernolle, V.; Bono, F.; Balconi, G.; Spagnuolo, R.; Oosthuyse, B.; Dewerchin, M.; et al. Targeted deficiency or cytosolic truncation of the VE-cadherin gene in mice impairs VEGF-mediated endothelial survival and angiogenesis. *Cell* **1999**, *98*, 147–157. [CrossRef]
21. Chen, Z.; Rubin, J.; Tzima, E. Role of PECAM-1 in arteriogenesis and specification of preexisting collaterals. *Circ. Res.* **2010**, *107*, 1355–1363. [CrossRef] [PubMed]
22. Gong, Y.; Koh, D.R. Neutrophils promote inflammatory angiogenesis via release of preformed VEGF in an in vivo corneal model. *Cell Tissue Res.* **2010**, *339*, 437–448. [CrossRef] [PubMed]
23. Ramanathan, M.; Giladi, A.; Leibovich, S.J. Regulation of vascular endothelial growth factor gene expression in murine macrophages by nitric oxide and hypoxia. *Exp. Biol. Med.* **2003**, *228*, 697–705. [CrossRef] [PubMed]
24. Morrison, A.R.; Yarovinsky, T.O.; Young, B.D.; Moraes, F.; Ross, T.D.; Ceneri, N.; Zhang, J.; Zhuang, Z.W.; Sinusas, A.J.; Pardi, R.; et al. Chemokine-coupled beta2 integrin-induced macrophage Rac2-Myosin IIA interaction regulates VEGF-A mRNA stability and arteriogenesis. *J. Exp. Med.* **2014**, *211*, 1957–1968. [CrossRef] [PubMed]
25. Lautz, T.; Lasch, M.; Borgolte, J.; Troidl, K.; Pagel, J.I.; Caballero-Martinez, A.; Kleinert, E.C.; Walzog, B.; Deindl, E. Midkine Controls Arteriogenesis by Regulating the Bioavailability of Vascular Endothelial Growth Factor A and the Expression of Nitric Oxide Synthase 1 and 3. *EBioMedicine* **2018**, *27*, 237–246. [CrossRef] [PubMed]
26. Connolly, D.T.; Heuvelman, D.M.; Nelson, R.; Olander, J.V.; Eppley, B.L.; Delfino, J.J.; Siegel, N.R.; Leimgruber, R.M.; Feder, J. Tumor vascular permeability factor stimulates endothelial cell growth and angiogenesis. *J. Clin. Investig.* **1989**, *84*, 1470–1478. [CrossRef] [PubMed]
27. Yuan, F.; Chen, Y.; Dellian, M.; Safabakhsh, N.; Ferrara, N.; Jain, R.K. Time-dependent vascular regression and permeability changes in established human tumor xenografts induced by an anti-vascular endothelial growth factor/vascular permeability factor antibody. *Proc. Natl. Acad. Sci. USA* **1996**, *93*, 14765–14770. [CrossRef]
28. Leung, D.W.; Cachianes, G.; Kuang, W.J.; Goeddel, D.V.; Ferrara, N. Vascular endothelial growth factor is a secreted angiogenic mitogen. *Science* **1989**, *246*, 1306–1309. [CrossRef]

29. Pipp, F.; Heil, M.; Issbrucker, K.; Ziegelhoeffer, T.; Martin, S.; van den Heuvel, J.; Weich, H.; Fernandez, B.; Golomb, G.; Carmeliet, P.; et al. VEGFR-1-selective VEGF homologue PlGF is arteriogenic: Evidence for a monocyte-mediated mechanism. *Circ. Res.* **2003**, *92*, 378–385. [CrossRef]
30. Lloyd, P.G.; Prior, B.M.; Li, H.; Yang, H.T.; Terjung, R.L. VEGF receptor antagonism blocks arteriogenesis, but only partially inhibits angiogenesis, in skeletal muscle of exercise-trained rats. *Am. J. Physiol. Heart Circ. Physiol.* **2005**, *288*, H759–H768. [CrossRef]
31. Toyota, E.; Warltier, D.C.; Brock, T.; Ritman, E.; Kolz, C.; O'Malley, P.; Rocic, P.; Focardi, M.; Chilian, W.M. Vascular endothelial growth factor is required for coronary collateral growth in the rat. *Circulation* **2005**, *112*, 2108–2113. [CrossRef] [PubMed]
32. Koch, S.; Claesson-Welsh, L. Signal transduction by vascular endothelial growth factor receptors. *Cold Spring Harb. Perspect. Med.* **2012**, *2*, a006502. [CrossRef] [PubMed]
33. Lanahan, A.; Zhang, X.; Fantin, A.; Zhuang, Z.; Rivera-Molina, F.; Speichinger, K.; Prahst, C.; Zhang, J.; Wang, Y.; Davis, G.; et al. The neuropilin 1 cytoplasmic domain is required for VEGF-A-dependent arteriogenesis. *Dev. Cell* **2013**, *25*, 156–168. [CrossRef] [PubMed]
34. Lanahan, A.A.; Hermans, K.; Claes, F.; Kerley-Hamilton, J.S.; Zhuang, Z.W.; Giordano, F.J.; Carmeliet, P.; Simons, M. VEGF receptor 2 endocytic trafficking regulates arterial morphogenesis. *Dev. Cell* **2010**, *18*, 713–724. [CrossRef] [PubMed]
35. Fischer, S.; Nishio, M.; Peters, S.C.; Tschernatsch, M.; Walberer, M.; Weidemann, S.; Heidenreich, R.; Couraud, P.O.; Weksler, B.B.; Romero, I.A.; et al. Signaling mechanism of extracellular RNA in endothelial cells. *FASEB J.* **2009**, *23*, 2100–2109. [CrossRef]
36. Landre, J.B.; Hewett, P.W.; Olivot, J.M.; Friedl, P.; Ko, Y.; Sachinidis, A.; Moenner, M. Human endothelial cells selectively express large amounts of pancreatic-type ribonuclease (RNase 1). *J. Cell. Biochem.* **2002**, *86*, 540–552. [CrossRef]
37. Tsui, N.B.; Ng, E.K.; Lo, Y.M. Stability of endogenous and added RNA in blood specimens, serum, and plasma. *Clin. Chem.* **2002**, *48*, 1647–1653.
38. Arras, M.; Ito, W.D.; Scholz, D.; Winkler, B.; Schaper, J.; Schaper, W. Monocyte activation in angiogenesis and collateral growth in the rabbit hindlimb. *J. Clin. Investig.* **1998**, *101*, 40–50. [CrossRef]
39. Hoefer, I.E.; Grundmann, S.; van Royen, N.; Voskuil, M.; Schirmer, S.H.; Ulusans, S.; Bode, C.; Buschmann, I.R.; Piek, J.J. Leukocyte subpopulations and arteriogenesis: Specific role of monocytes, lymphocytes and granulocytes. *Atherosclerosis* **2005**, *181*, 285–293. [CrossRef]
40. Ley, K.; Laudanna, C.; Cybulsky, M.I.; Nourshargh, S. Getting to the site of inflammation: The leukocyte adhesion cascade updated. *Nat. Rev. Immunol.* **2007**, *7*, 678–689. [CrossRef]
41. Hoefer, I.E.; van Royen, N.; Rectenwald, J.E.; Deindl, E.; Hua, J.; Jost, M.; Grundmann, S.; Voskuil, M.; Ozaki, C.K.; Piek, J.J.; et al. Arteriogenesis proceeds via ICAM-1/Mac-1- mediated mechanisms. *Circ. Res.* **2004**, *94*, 1179–1185. [CrossRef] [PubMed]
42. Scholz, D.; Ito, W.; Fleming, I.; Deindl, E.; Sauer, A.; Wiesnet, M.; Busse, R.; Schaper, J.; Schaper, W. Ultrastructure and molecular histology of rabbit hind-limb collateral artery growth (arteriogenesis). *Virchows Arch.* **2000**, *436*, 257–270. [CrossRef] [PubMed]
43. Morigi, M.; Zoja, C.; Figliuzzi, M.; Foppolo, M.; Micheletti, G.; Bontempelli, M.; Saronni, M.; Remuzzi, G.; Remuzzi, A. Fluid shear stress modulates surface expression of adhesion molecules by endothelial cells. *Blood* **1995**, *85*, 1696–1703. [CrossRef] [PubMed]
44. Elsemuller, A.K.; Tomalla, V.; Gartner, U.; Troidl, K.; Jeratsch, S.; Graumann, J.; Baal, N.; Hackstein, H.; Lasch, M.; Deindl, E.; et al. Characterization of mast cell-derived rRNA-containing microvesicles and their inflammatory impact on endothelial cells. *FASEB J.* **2019**, *33*, 5457–5467. [CrossRef] [PubMed]
45. Xia, Y.P.; Li, B.; Hylton, D.; Detmar, M.; Yancopoulos, G.D.; Rudge, J.S. Transgenic delivery of VEGF to mouse skin leads to an inflammatory condition resembling human psoriasis. *Blood* **2003**, *102*, 161–168. [CrossRef] [PubMed]
46. Wang, J.; Wang, S.; Li, M.; Wu, D.; Liu, F.; Yang, R.; Ji, S.; Ji, A.; Li, Y. The Neuropilin-1 Inhibitor, ATWLPPR Peptide, Prevents Experimental Diabetes-Induced Retinal Injury by Preserving Vascular Integrity and Decreasing Oxidative Stress. *PLoS ONE* **2015**, *10*, e0142571. [CrossRef]
47. Numata, T.; Ito, T.; Maeda, T.; Egusa, C.; Tsuboi, R. IL-33 promotes ICAM-1 expression via NF-kB in murine mast cells. *Allergol. Int.* **2016**, *65*, 158–165. [CrossRef]

48. Unthank, J.L.; McClintick, J.N.; Labarrere, C.A.; Li, L.; Distasi, M.R.; Miller, S.J. Molecular basis for impaired collateral artery growth in the spontaneously hypertensive rat: Insight from microarray analysis. *Physiol. Rep.* **2013**, *1*, e0005. [CrossRef]
49. Huang, S.; Pettaway, C.A.; Uehara, H.; Bucana, C.D.; Fidler, I.J. Blockade of NF-kappaB activity in human prostate cancer cells is associated with suppression of angiogenesis, invasion, and metastasis. *Oncogene* **2001**, *20*, 4188–4197. [CrossRef]
50. Hunt, B.J.; Jurd, K.M. Endothelial cell activation. A central pathophysiological process. *Bmj (Clin. Res. Ed.)* **1998**, *316*, 1328–1329. [CrossRef]
51. Wagner, D.D.; Olmsted, J.B.; Marder, V.J. Immunolocalization of von Willebrand protein in Weibel-Palade bodies of human endothelial cells. *J. Cell Biol* **1982**, *95*, 355–360. [CrossRef] [PubMed]
52. McEver, R.P.; Beckstead, J.H.; Moore, K.L.; Marshall-Carlson, L.; Bainton, D.F. GMP-140, a platelet alpha-granule membrane protein, is also synthesized by vascular endothelial cells and is localized in Weibel-Palade bodies. *J. Clin. Investig.* **1989**, *84*, 92–99. [CrossRef] [PubMed]
53. Utgaard, J.O.; Jahnsen, F.L.; Bakka, A.; Brandtzaeg, P.; Haraldsen, G. Rapid secretion of prestored interleukin 8 from Weibel-Palade bodies of microvascular endothelial cells. *J. Exp. Med.* **1998**, *188*, 1751–1756. [CrossRef] [PubMed]
54. Matsushita, K.; Yamakuchi, M.; Morrell, C.N.; Ozaki, M.; O'Rourke, B.; Irani, K.; Lowenstein, C.J. Vascular endothelial growth factor regulation of Weibel-Palade-body exocytosis. *Blood* **2005**, *105*, 207–214. [CrossRef] [PubMed]
55. Vischer, U.M.; Jornot, L.; Wollheim, C.B.; Theler, J.M. Reactive oxygen intermediates induce regulated secretion of von Willebrand factor from cultured human vascular endothelial cells. *Blood* **1995**, *85*, 3164–3172. [CrossRef]
56. Van den Biggelaar, M.; Hernandez-Fernaud, J.R.; van den Eshof, B.L.; Neilson, L.J.; Meijer, A.B.; Mertens, K.; Zanivan, S. Quantitative phosphoproteomics unveils temporal dynamics of thrombin signaling in human endothelial cells. *Blood* **2014**, *123*, e22–e36. [CrossRef]
57. Crawley, J.T.; de Groot, R.; Xiang, Y.; Luken, B.M.; Lane, D.A. Unraveling the scissile bond: How ADAMTS13 recognizes and cleaves von Willebrand factor. *Blood* **2011**, *118*, 3212–3221. [CrossRef]
58. Shim, K.; Anderson, P.J.; Tuley, E.A.; Wiswall, E.; Sadler, J.E. Platelet-VWF complexes are preferred substrates of ADAMTS13 under fluid shear stress. *Blood* **2008**, *111*, 651–657. [CrossRef]
59. Chandraratne, S.; von Bruehl, M.L.; Pagel, J.I.; Stark, K.; Kleinert, E.; Konrad, I.; Farschtschi, S.; Coletti, R.; Gartner, F.; Chillo, O.; et al. Critical role of platelet glycoprotein ibalpha in arterial remodeling. *Arterioscler. Thromb. Vasc. Biol.* **2015**, *35*, 589–597. [CrossRef]
60. Chillo, O.; Kleinert, E.C.; Lautz, T.; Lasch, M.; Pagel, J.I.; Heun, Y.; Troidl, K.; Fischer, S.; Caballero-Martinez, A.; Mauer, A.; et al. Perivascular Mast Cells Govern Shear Stress-Induced Arteriogenesis by Orchestrating Leukocyte Function. *Cell Rep.* **2016**, *16*, 2197–2207. [CrossRef]
61. Page, C.; Pitchford, S. Neutrophil and platelet complexes and their relevance to neutrophil recruitment and activation. *Int. Immunopharmacol.* **2013**, *17*, 1176–1184. [CrossRef] [PubMed]
62. Deindl, E.; Ziegelhoffer, T.; Kanse, S.M.; Fernandez, B.; Neubauer, E.; Carmeliet, P.; Preissner, K.T.; Schaper, W. Receptor-independent role of the urokinase-type plasminogen activator during arteriogenesis. *FASEB J.* **2003**, *17*, 1174–1176. [CrossRef] [PubMed]
63. Brinkmann, V.; Reichard, U.; Goosmann, C.; Fauler, B.; Uhlemann, Y.; Weiss, D.S.; Weinrauch, Y.; Zychlinsky, A. Neutrophil Extracellular Traps Kill Bacteria. *Science* **2004**, *303*, 1532–1535. [CrossRef] [PubMed]
64. Sadler, J.E. Contact—How platelets touch von Willebrand factor. *Science* **2002**, *297*, 1128–1129. [CrossRef] [PubMed]
65. Andrews, R.K.; Gardiner, E.E.; Shen, Y.; Whisstock, J.C.; Berndt, M.C. Glycoprotein Ib-IX-V. *Int. J. Biochem. Cell Biol.* **2003**, *35*, 1170–1174. [CrossRef]
66. Savage, B.; Saldivar, E.; Ruggeri, Z.M. Initiation of platelet adhesion by arrest onto fibrinogen or translocation on von Willebrand factor. *Cell* **1996**, *84*, 289–297. [CrossRef]
67. Goto, S.; Ichikawa, N.; Lee, M.; Goto, M.; Sakai, H.; Kim, J.J.; Yoshida, M.; Handa, M.; Ikeda, Y.; Handa, S. Platelet surface P-selectin molecules increased after exposing platelet to a high shear flow. *Int. Angiol.* **2000**, *19*, 147–151.

68. Moore, K.L.; Patel, K.D.; Bruehl, R.E.; Li, F.; Johnson, D.A.; Lichenstein, H.S.; Cummings, R.D.; Bainton, D.F.; McEver, R.P. P-selectin glycoprotein ligand-1 mediates rolling of human neutrophils on P-selectin. *J. Cell Biol.* **1995**, *128*, 661–671. [CrossRef]
69. Xiao, Z.; Goldsmith, H.L.; McIntosh, F.A.; Shankaran, H.; Neelamegham, S. Biomechanics of P-selectin PSGL-1 bonds: Shear threshold and integrin-independent cell adhesion. *Biophys. J.* **2006**, *90*, 2221–2234. [CrossRef]
70. Dole, V.S.; Bergmeier, W.; Mitchell, H.A.; Eichenberger, S.C.; Wagner, D.D. Activated platelets induce Weibel-Palade-body secretion and leukocyte rolling in vivo: Role of P-selectin. *Blood* **2005**, *106*, 2334–2339. [CrossRef]
71. De Wit, T.R.; van Mourik, J.A. Biosynthesis, processing and secretion of von Willebrand factor: Biological implications. *Best Pract. Res. Clin. Haematol.* **2001**, *14*, 241–255. [CrossRef] [PubMed]
72. Levy, G.G.; Nichols, W.C.; Lian, E.C.; Foroud, T.; McClintick, J.N.; McGee, B.M.; Yang, A.Y.; Siemieniak, D.R.; Stark, K.R.; Gruppo, R.; et al. Mutations in a member of the ADAMTS gene family cause thrombotic thrombocytopenic purpura. *Nature* **2001**, *413*, 488–494. [CrossRef] [PubMed]
73. Feys, H.B.; Anderson, P.J.; Sadler, J.E. Binding of ADAMTS13 to Von Willebrand Factor Under Static Conditions and Under Fluid Shear Stress. *Blood* **2008**, *112*, 258. [CrossRef]
74. Chauhan, A.K.; Motto, D.G.; Lamb, C.B.; Bergmeier, W.; Dockal, M.; Plaimauer, B.; Scheiflinger, F.; Ginsburg, D.; Wagner, D.D. Systemic antithrombotic effects of ADAMTS13. *J. Exp. Med.* **2006**, *203*, 767–776. [CrossRef] [PubMed]
75. Xu, H.; Cao, Y.; Yang, X.; Cai, P.; Kang, L.; Zhu, X.; Luo, H.; Lu, L.; Wei, L.; Bai, X.; et al. ADAMTS13 controls vascular remodeling by modifying VWF reactivity during stroke recovery. *Blood* **2017**, *130*, 11–22. [CrossRef]
76. Lee, M.; Keener, J.; Xiao, J.; Long Zheng, X.; Rodgers, G.M. ADAMTS13 and its variants promote angiogenesis via upregulation of VEGF and VEGFR2. *Cell. Mol. Life Sci.* **2015**, *72*, 349–356. [CrossRef]
77. Tang, H.; Lee, M.; Kim, E.H.; Bishop, D.; Rodgers, G.M. siRNA-knockdown of ADAMTS-13 modulates endothelial cell angiogenesis. *Microvasc. Res.* **2017**, *113*, 65–70. [CrossRef]
78. Wheway, J.; Latham, S.L.; Combes, V.; Grau, G.E. Endothelial microparticles interact with and support the proliferation of T cells. *J.Immunol.* **2014**, *193*, 3378–3387. [CrossRef]
79. Mesri, M.; Altieri, D.C. Endothelial cell activation by leukocyte microparticles. *J. Immunol.* **1998**, *161*, 4382–4387.
80. Baj-Krzyworzeka, M.; Majka, M.; Pratico, D.; Ratajczak, J.; Vilaire, G.; Kijowski, J.; Reca, R.; Janowska-Wieczorek, A.; Ratajczak, M.Z. Platelet-derived microparticles stimulate proliferation, survival, adhesion, and chemotaxis of hematopoietic cells. *Exp. Hematol.* **2002**, *30*, 450–459. [CrossRef]
81. Kunder, C.A.; St John, A.L.; Li, G.; Leong, K.W.; Berwin, B.; Staats, H.F.; Abraham, S.N. Mast cell-derived particles deliver peripheral signals to remote lymph nodes. *J. Exp. Med.* **2009**, *206*, 2455–2467. [CrossRef] [PubMed]
82. Van der Pol, E.; Boing, A.N.; Harrison, P.; Sturk, A.; Nieuwland, R. Classification, functions, and clinical relevance of extracellular vesicles. *Pharmacol. Rev.* **2012**, *64*, 676–705. [CrossRef] [PubMed]
83. Shai, E.; Varon, D. Development, cell differentiation, angiogenesis–microparticles and their roles in angiogenesis. *Arterioscler. Thromb. Vasc. Biol.* **2011**, *31*, 10–14. [CrossRef] [PubMed]
84. Skog, J.; Wurdinger, T.; van Rijn, S.; Meijer, D.H.; Gainche, L.; Sena-Esteves, M.; Curry, W.T., Jr.; Carter, B.S.; Krichevsky, A.M.; Breakefield, X.O. Glioblastoma microvesicles transport RNA and proteins that promote tumour growth and provide diagnostic biomarkers. *Nat. Cell Biol.* **2008**, *10*, 1470–1476. [CrossRef] [PubMed]
85. Bradley, J.R. TNF-mediated inflammatory disease. *J. Pathol.* **2008**, *214*, 149–160. [CrossRef] [PubMed]
86. Bowers, E.; Slaughter, A.; Frenette, P.S.; Kuick, R.; Pello, O.M.; Lucas, D. Granulocyte-derived TNFalpha promotes vascular and hematopoietic regeneration in the bone marrow. *Nat. Med.* **2018**, *24*, 95–102. [CrossRef]
87. Tanaka, H.; Sukhova, G.; Schwartz, D.; Libby, P. Proliferating arterial smooth muscle cells after balloon injury express TNF-alpha but not interleukin-1 or basic fibroblast growth factor. *Arterioscler. Thromb. Vasc. Biol.* **1996**, *16*, 12–18. [CrossRef]
88. Buschmann, I.R.; Hoefer, I.E.; van Royen, N.; Katzer, E.; Braun-Dulleaus, R.; Heil, M.; Kostin, S.; Bode, C.; Schaper, W. GM-CSF: A strong arteriogenic factor acting by amplification of monocyte function. *Atherosclerosis* **2001**, *159*, 343–356. [CrossRef]

89. Griffin, G.K.; Newton, G.; Tarrio, M.L.; Bu, D.X.; Maganto-Garcia, E.; Azcutia, V.; Alcaide, P.; Grabie, N.; Luscinskas, F.W.; Croce, K.J.; et al. IL-17 and TNF-alpha sustain neutrophil recruitment during inflammation through synergistic effects on endothelial activation. *J. Immunol.* **2012**, *188*, 6287–6299. [CrossRef]
90. Stabile, E.; Burnett, M.S.; Watkins, C.; Kinnaird, T.; Bachis, A.; la Sala, A.; Miller, J.M.; Shou, M.; Epstein, S.E.; Fuchs, S. Impaired arteriogenic response to acute hindlimb ischemia in CD4-knockout mice. *Circulation* **2003**, *108*, 205–210. [CrossRef]
91. Stabile, E.; Kinnaird, T.; la Sala, A.; Hanson, S.K.; Watkins, C.; Campia, U.; Shou, M.; Zbinden, S.; Fuchs, S.; Kornfeld, H.; et al. $CD8^+$ T lymphocytes regulate the arteriogenic response to ischemia by infiltrating the site of collateral vessel development and recruiting CD4+ mononuclear cells through the expression of interleukin-16. *Circulation* **2006**, *113*, 118–124. [CrossRef] [PubMed]
92. Hoefer, I.E.; van Royen, N.; Rectenwald, J.E.; Bray, E.J.; Abouhamze, Z.; Moldawer, L.L.; Voskuil, M.; Piek, J.J.; Buschmann, I.R.; Ozaki, C.K. Direct evidence for tumor necrosis factor-alpha signaling in arteriogenesis. *Circulation* **2002**, *105*, 1639–1641. [CrossRef] [PubMed]
93. Grundmann, S.; Hoefer, I.; Ulusans, S.; van Royen, N.; Schirmer, S.H.; Ozaki, C.K.; Bode, C.; Piek, J.J.; Buschmann, I. Anti-tumor necrosis factor-{alpha} therapies attenuate adaptive arteriogenesis in the rabbit. *Am. J. Physiol. Heart Circ. Physiol.* **2005**, *289*, H1497–H1505. [CrossRef] [PubMed]
94. Schirmer, S.H.; Buschmann, I.R.; Jost, M.M.; Hoefer, I.E.; Grundmann, S.; Andert, J.P.; Ulusans, S.; Bode, C.; Piek, J.J.; van Royen, N. Differential effects of MCP-1 and leptin on collateral flow and arteriogenesis. *Cardiovasc. Res.* **2004**, *64*, 356–364. [CrossRef] [PubMed]
95. Ito, W.D.; Arras, M.; Winkler, B.; Scholz, D.; Schaper, J.; Schaper, W. Monocyte chemotactic protein-1 increases collateral and peripheral conductance after femoral artery occlusion. *Circ. Res.* **1997**, *80*, 829–837. [CrossRef] [PubMed]
96. Hoefer, I.E.; van Royen, N.; Buschmann, I.R.; Piek, J.J.; Schaper, W. Time course of arteriogenesis following femoral artery occlusion in the rabbit. *Cardiovasc. Res.* **2001**, *49*, 609–617. [CrossRef]
97. Gunn, M.D.; Nelken, N.A.; Liao, X.; Williams, L.T. Monocyte chemoattractant protein-1 is sufficient for the chemotaxis of monocytes and lymphocytes in transgenic mice but requires an additional stimulus for inflammatory activation. *J. Immunol.* **1997**, *158*, 376–383.
98. Deshmane, S.L.; Kremlev, S.; Amini, S.; Sawaya, B.E. Monocyte chemoattractant protein-1 (MCP-1): An overview. *J. Interferon Cytokine Res.* **2009**, *29*, 313–326. [CrossRef]
99. Kinoshita, M.; Okada, M.; Hara, M.; Furukawa, Y.; Matsumori, A. Mast cell tryptase in mast cell granules enhances MCP-1 and interleukin-8 production in human endothelial cells. *Arterioscler. Thromb. Vasc. Biol.* **2005**, *25*, 1858–1863. [CrossRef]
100. Cushing, S.D.; Berliner, J.A.; Valente, A.J.; Territo, M.C.; Navab, M.; Parhami, F.; Gerrity, R.; Schwartz, C.J.; Fogelman, A.M. Minimally modified low density lipoprotein induces monocyte chemotactic protein 1 in human endothelial cells and smooth muscle cells. *Proc. Natl. Acad. Sci. USA* **1990**, *87*, 5134–5138. [CrossRef]
101. Black, R.A.; Rauch, C.T.; Kozlosky, C.J.; Peschon, J.J.; Slack, J.L.; Wolfson, M.F.; Castner, B.J.; Stocking, K.L.; Reddy, P.; Srinivasan, S.; et al. A metalloproteinase disintegrin that releases tumour-necrosis factor-alpha from cells. *Nature* **1997**, *385*, 729–733. [CrossRef] [PubMed]
102. Fischer, S.; Gesierich, S.; Griemert, B.; Schanzer, A.; Acker, T.; Augustin, H.G.; Olsson, A.K.; Preissner, K.T. Extracellular RNA liberates tumor necrosis factor-alpha to promote tumor cell trafficking and progression. *Cancer Res.* **2013**, *73*, 5080–5089. [CrossRef] [PubMed]
103. Abraham, E. NF-kappaB activation. *Crit. Care Med.* **2000**, *28*, N100–N104. [CrossRef] [PubMed]
104. Cabrera-Fuentes, H.A.; Lopez, M.L.; McCurdy, S.; Fischer, S.; Meiler, S.; Baumer, Y.; Galuska, S.P.; Preissner, K.T.; Boisvert, W.A. Regulation of monocyte/macrophage polarisation by extracellular RNA. *Thromb. Haemost.* **2015**, *113*, 473–481. [CrossRef] [PubMed]
105. Troidl, C.; Jung, G.; Troidl, K.; Hoffmann, J.; Mollmann, H.; Nef, H.; Schaper, W.; Hamm, C.W.; Schmitz-Rixen, T. The temporal and spatial distribution of macrophage subpopulations during arteriogenesis. *Curr. Vasc. Pharmacol.* **2013**, *11*, 5–12. [CrossRef] [PubMed]
106. Sharifpanah, F.; De Silva, S.; Bekhite, M.M.; Hurtado-Oliveros, J.; Preissner, K.T.; Wartenberg, M.; Sauer, H. Stimulation of vasculogenesis and leukopoiesis of embryonic stem cells by extracellular transfer RNA and ribosomal RNA. *Free Radic. Biol. Med.* **2015**, *89*, 1203–1217. [CrossRef] [PubMed]

107. Bekhite, M.M.; Finkensieper, A.; Binas, S.; Muller, J.; Wetzker, R.; Figulla, H.R.; Sauer, H.; Wartenberg, M. VEGF-mediated PI3K class IA and PKC signaling in cardiomyogenesis and vasculogenesis of mouse embryonic stem cells. *J. Cell Sci.* **2011**, *124*, 1819–1830. [CrossRef]
108. Ushio-Fukai, M.; Urao, N. Novel role of NADPH oxidase in angiogenesis and stem/progenitor cell function. *Antioxid. Redox Signal.* **2009**, *11*, 2517–2533. [CrossRef]
109. Lu, L.; Li, J.; Moussaoui, M.; Boix, E. Immune Modulation by Human Secreted RNases at the Extracellular Space. *Front. Immunol.* **2018**, *9*, 1012. [CrossRef]
110. Fett, J.W.; Strydom, D.J.; Lobb, R.R.; Alderman, E.M.; Bethune, J.L.; Riordan, J.F.; Vallee, B.L. Isolation and characterization of angiogenin, an angiogenic protein from human carcinoma cells. *Biochemistry* **1985**, *24*, 5480–5486. [CrossRef]

11

VEGF-A-Cleavage by FSAP and Inhibition of Neo-Vascularization

Özgür Uslu [1], Joerg Herold [2] and Sandip M. Kanse [3,*]

1 Institute for Biochemistry, Justus-Liebig-University Giessen, 35392 Giessen, Germany; Oezguer1975@gmx.de
2 Department of Angiology, Clinic for Vascular Medicine, Klinikum Darmstadt, 64283 Darmstadt, Germany; joerg_herold@hotmail.com
3 Institute for Basic Medical Sciences, University of Oslo, Sognvannsveien 9, 0372 Oslo, Norway
* Correspondence: Sandip.kanse@medisin.uio.no

Abstract: Alternative splicing leads to the secretion of multiple forms of vascular endothelial growth factor-A (VEGF-A) that differ in their activity profiles with respect to neovascularization. FSAP (factor VII activating protease) is the zymogen form of a plasma protease that is activated (FSAPa) upon tissue injury via the release of histones. The purpose of the study was to determine if FSAPa regulates VEGF-A activity in vitro and in vivo. FSAP bound to $VEGF_{165}$, but not $VEGF_{121}$, and $VEGF_{165}$ was cleaved in its neuropilin/proteoglycan binding domain. $VEGF_{165}$ cleavage did not alter its binding to VEGF receptors but diminished its binding to neuropilin. The stimulatory effects of $VEGF_{165}$ on endothelial cell proliferation, migration, and signal transduction were not altered by FSAP. Similarly, proliferation of VEGF receptor-expressing BAF3 cells, in response to $VEGF_{165}$, was not modulated by FSAP. In the mouse matrigel model of angiogenesis, FSAP decreased the ability of $VEGF_{165}$, basic fibroblast growth factor (bFGF), and their combination, to induce neovascularization. Lack of endogenous FSAP in mice did not influence neovascularization. Thus, FSAP inhibited $VEGF_{165}$-mediated angiogenesis in the matrigel model in vivo, where VEGF's interaction with the matrix and its diffusion are important.

Keywords: factor VII activating protease; HABP2; VEGF; matrigel; neo-vascularization; hind limb ischemia

---

1. Introduction

FSAP (factor VII activating protease) is a serine protease that circulates in plasma as an inactive zymogen. It belongs to the family of proteases that also includes the urokinase-plasminogen activator (uPA), tissue-PA (tPA), as well as hepatocyte growth factor activator (HGFA). Although a number of charged molecules can activate FSAP into the active protease (FSAPa), histones are the only endogenous molecules identified so far that can activate the zymogen form into FSAPa in plasma and in vivo [1]. In situations such as tissue injury [2], apoptosis, or necrosis [3], as well as when neutrophils undergo NETosis [4], the DNase activity in blood [5] is likely to release histones. FSAPa in turn can cleave and degrade histones and decrease their toxicity towards cells [3,4]. A single nucleotide polymorphism (SNP) in the FSAP gene, Marburg I (MI, G534E) is associated with a weak proteolytic activity [6] and an increased risk of carotid stenosis [7], stroke [8], venous thrombosis [9,10], liver fibrosis [11], and thyroid cancer [12]. The relationship to venous thrombosis [13] and thyroid cancer [14] was not replicated in a number of subsequent studies.

This relationship between the loss of FSAP activity and diseases is also replicated in FSAP-deficient (*Habp2*$^{-/-}$) mice. *Habp2*$^{-/-}$ mice show no explicit characteristics when maintained under standard pathogen-free laboratory conditions and do not exhibit any developmental abnormalities. These mice have been studied in two different models of vascular remodeling. In the wire-induced injury model of neointima formation, *Habp2*$^{-/-}$ mice formed a bigger neointima than wildtype (WT mice) [15]. In the model of hind limb ischemia, arteriogenesis in the adductor muscle was enhanced in *Habp2*$^{-/-}$ mice, whereas neovascularization was unchanged in the gastrocnemius muscle [16]. Thus, the lack of *Habp2* gene in mice promotes a more exacerbated repair response that is related to enhanced inflammation and increased activity of the pericellular proteolysis system [15,16].

The effects of FSAP in relation to human diseases and mouse models is likely to be related to proteolysis of different substrates. Although a number of substrates for FSAP have been identified [17] we will focus here only on pathways that are linked to vascular remodeling. Growth factors are cleaved by FSAP, which in some cases leads to a loss of activity, such as platelet derived growth factor-BB (PDGF-BB) [18]. PDGF-BB cleavage leads to an inhibition of vascular smooth muscle cells (VSMC) migration and proliferation, as well as neointima formation. FSAP inhibits basic fibroblast growth factor (bFGF)-mediated endothelial cell proliferation by binding to and/or slowly degrading the growth factor [19] and can also activate bFGF by releasing it from the matrix [20]. Activation of bone morphogenetic protein (BMP)-2 and the conversion of pro-BMP-2 into the active form of cytokine is also a function of FSAP that leads to differentiation of cells [21]. FSAP also cleaves protease activated receptors (PARs)-1 and -3 and influences vascular permeability in combination with hyaluronic fragments of different molecular weights [22]. PAR-1 was identified as a receptor on astrocytes and neurons that mediate the anti-apoptotic effects of FSAP in the context of stroke [23]. Stimulation of VSMC and endothelial cells by FSAP leads to an increased expression of proinflammatory genes in both cells types. Whereas the effect of FSAP could be clearly ascribed to PAR-1 on VSMC, this was clearly not the case for endothelial cells.

Vascular endothelial growth factor (VEGF) is a key factor for determining endothelial lineage, endothelial cell proliferation and migration, as well as recruitment of pericytes and vessel assembly [24]. It belongs to the cysteine knot family of growth factors that include the four genes of the PDGF family as well as placental growth factor (PLGF). Of the four genes encoding for VEGF, denoted A, B, C, and D, VEGF-A is considered to be the most important for hypoxia-driven angiogenesis and is secreted in multiple forms, such as $VEGF_{121}$, $VEGF_{165}$, and $VEGF_{189}$, by alternative splicing [25]. These isoforms have a common N-terminal region for receptor binding, whereas the C-terminal part that mediates binding to co-receptors such as neuropilin and cell- and matrix-associated proteoglycans (ECM) [26] is progressively longer. This C-terminal region has a cluster of negatively charged amino acids and has cleavage sites for uPA, plasmin, and matrix metalloproteinases [27], which regulate VEGF's association with the matrix and co-receptors and results in a different pattern of neovascularization.

With the knowledge that FSAP can cleave proteins at clusters of basic amino acids [17] and that it cleaves PDGF-BB [18], we hypothesized that the homologous protein VEGF-A is also cleaved, and its activity regulated by FSAP. We performed binding and cleavage studies with purified proteins to show that FSAP can indeed cleave long forms of VEGF in their heparin/neuropilin-binding domain and that, as expected, this disturbs their binding properties. However, no modulation of $VEGF_{165}$ activity in vitro on cellular functions was observed. An inhibiting effect of FSAP in the in vivo matrigel model of neovascularization model was observed, which supports the notion that this effect of FSAP may operate in vivo where matrix association, sequestration, and release of VEGF are decisive.

2. Material and Methods

FSAP preparations: The isolation of wild type-FSAP as well as the MI-SNP (G534E isoform) from human plasma, along with the preparation of enzymatically inactivated Phe-Pro-Arg-chloromethylketone (PPACK)-FSAP has been described before [18,28]. The buffer for storage of FSAP was 0.2 M arginine, 0.2 M lysine, 5 mM citrate, pH 4.5, and was also used at the appropriate dilution to exclude any influence of the vehicle. Because of the rapid auto-activation of the zymogen form of FSAP into FSAPa, under the experimental conditions used in this study, the term FSAP is synonymous for FSAPa.

Specific cleavage of VEGF isoforms: $VEGF_{165}$ or $VEGF_{121}$ (R & D Systems, Wiesbaden, Germany) (2 μg/mL) was incubated with FSAP (12 μg/mL) in Tris pH 7.4, 100 mM NaCl, 2 mM $CaCl_2$ for 1 h at 37 °C in the absence or presence of heparin (10 μg/mL) or aprotinin (15 μg/mL), and the reaction was stopped with SDS sample buffer. Western blots were performed under non-reducing and reducing conditions (β-mercaptoethanol; 10%, vol/vol) and VEGF was detected with a polyclonal goat antibody from R & D Systems. Cleaved VEGF was subjected to amino terminal sequencing using the automated Edman degradation procedure with an online phenylthiohydantoin derivative analyzer (Applied Biosystems, Darmstadt, Germany).

Binding interactions between FSAP, VEGFR2, VEGF, and neuropilin: $VEGF_{121}$ or $VEGF_{165}$ was immobilized in a Maxisorp microtiter 96-well plate (Nunc, Roskilde, Denmark) at a concentration of 1 μg/mL (50 mL) overnight at 4 °C in 50 mM $NaHCO_3$ buffer, pH 9.6. The plate was blocked with 3% (wt/vol) BSA in Tris pH 7.4, 100 mM NaCl. FSAP (0–2 μg/mL) was added to the wells with 0.3% (wt/vol) BSA for 2 h at 22 °C. After extensive washing, bound FSAP was detected with an antibody followed by peroxidase-linked secondary antibody. The binding of ligands to BSA-coated wells was used as a blank in all the experiments and was subtracted to obtain specific binding. Similarly, either neuropilin-1-Fc or VEGFR2-Fc (R & D Systems) were immobilized to study the binding of FSAP or VEGF.

Cellular assays: Human umbilical vein endothelial cells (HUVEC) were cultivated in ECBM medium (modified MCDB-151) containing 5% (vol/vol) FCS (Promocell, Heidelberg, Germany) on fibronectin-coated dishes. For regular growth of these cells, the medium was supplemented with amphotericin B (50 ng/mL), gentamicin (50 ng/mL), epidermal growth factor (0.1 ng/mL), and bFGF (1.0 ng/mL), as described by the manufacturer. Growth factors were preincubated with FSAP for 60 min at 37 °C before stimulation of serum starved cells, as described previously [18]. DNA synthesis was determined using the BrdU incorporation kit from Roche Diagnostics (Mannheim, Germany). Migration was tested in a Boyden chamber on a collagen type I coated membrane with 8 μm pores. Growth factors were preincubated with FSAP for 60 min at 37 °C before cell stimulation. Cells were incubated in medium containing 0.1% (vol/vol) FCS in the upper chamber, whereas the lower chamber received the same medium with different additives, as indicated. After an incubation period of 5 h at 37 °C, the upper side of the membrane was scraped to remove all cells. Thereafter, the membrane was fixed, stained, and the optical density of each well was measured to quantify cell migration. Cells were lysed in SDS-sample buffer and applied onto SDS-PAGE followed by western blotting and detection of phosphorylated ERK with a phospho-specific antibody with total ERK as a loading control (both from Cell Signaling Technology, Leiden, The Netherlands).

BAF3-VEGFR2 cells were obtained from Steven Stacker and Marc Achen (Ludwig Cancer Research Institute, Melbourne Branch, Australia) and BAF3-VEGFR1 cells were provided by Kari Alitalo (Ludwig Cancer Research Institute, Helsinki, Finland) and were cultured in RPMI-1640 medium containing murine interleukin (IL)-3 (Strathman Biotech, Hannover, Germany). Cell number was determined by the WST-1 assay (Roche Diagnostics).

Western blotting analysis: HUVEC were starved for 4 h in serum-free medium and then stimulated for 15 min with the appropriate agonist. Cells were pre-incubated with inhibitors for 30 min before induction with agonist. The experiments were stopped by adding SDS sample buffer containing 10 mM NaF, 1 mM orthovanadate, and 1 mM pyrophosphate, and the samples were processed for western blotting. SDS-PAGE was performed and proteins were transferred to Hybond nitrocellulose membranes (GE Healthcare, Freiberg, Germany). For analysis of western blotting, ECL prime chemiluminescence (GE Healthcare) was used. Tissue pieces were homogenized in a glass homogenizer in TBS (50 mM Tris, pH 7.4, containing 100 mM NaCl) with 1% (w/v) SDS. After centrifugation, the extracts were frozen at −80 °C until further analysis. Densitometric analysis was performed to calculate relative expression using ImageJ (NIH, Bethesda, Maryland, USA).

Matrigel model of in vivo *angiogenesis*: The matrigel model was performed essentially as described previously [29] and there were 7–8 mice per group. Growth factor-reduced matrigel (BD Biosciences) was supplemented with heparin (200 μg/mL), $VEGF_{165}$, and bFGF (200 ng/mL each), FSAP, MI-FSAP, or PPACK-FSAP (12 μg/mL), as well as the appropriate volume of buffer control. Without the presence of heparin, the neovascularization response is very weak in this model system. The concentration of each growth factor was halved when used in combination. Matrigel was applied subcutaneously into the right and left underside flank of 8–12 week old female C57/BL6 mice. The mice were sacrificed after 7 days and the matrigel plugs were removed, fixed with formaldehyde, and embedded in paraffin. Then, 7 μm serial sections were cut and mounted on slides, deparaffinized in xylene, and rehydrated through graded ethanol washes. After antigen retrieval with Tris-EDTA buffer (pH 9.0), the sections were stained with endothelial-specific lectin called bandeirea simplificifolia-1 (BS-1, FITC labelled) [30] and Cy3 labelled anti-α-SMA (α smooth muscle specific-actin) (Sigma) and DAPI. The number of red/green positive vessels counted per section from three different levels of the matrigel plugs and vascular density was expressed as number of vessels per mm^2. Percentage area of anti-α SMA, BS-1, and DAPI staining was also quantified using ImageJ. All three parameters essentially gave qualitatively very similar results, and only bona-fide vessel density results are presented here. We also localized von Willebrand factor (vWF), an alternative marker for endothelial cells (rabbit polyclonal, DAKO, Glostrup, Denmark), in some staining experiments. Both methods of endothelial cell quantification gave similar results.

Hind limb ischemia model and western blotting of VEGF-A: The model of hind limb ischemia and the resulting changes in arteriogenesis and angiogenesis have been described in detail in our earlier manuscript [16]. Western blotting with anti-VEGF-A and anti-COX IV was performed to adjust for differences in protein concentrations. Band density was measured using the image analysis system Quantity One system (Biorad, Munich, Germany). Experiments were performed in four mice per group.

Statistics and reproducibility: All biochemical and cellular experiments were performed in 3-5 independent experiments. Statistical significance was tested by using analysis of variance (ANOVA) with Bonferroni post-hoc test using the programme Graphpad Prism Biostatistics Software (Graphpad, San Diego, CA). A p-value < 0.05 was considered to be significant.

Study approval: All procedures involving experimental animals were approved by the local government animal care committee (GI 20/10-No. 66/2012) and complied with the Directive 2010/63/EU of the European Parliament.

3. Results

Binding and cleavage of VEGF-A by FSAP: In solid phase binding assays, FSAP bound to immobilized $VEGF_{165}$, but not to $VEGF_{121}$, in the presence of heparin (Figure 1A,B). Under non-reducing conditions, there was no change in the intensity or size of the $VEGF_{165}$ upon incubation with FSAP (Figure 1C,D); however, under reducing conditions, there was a decrease in VEGF immunoreactivity (Figure 1C,D). Cleavage was enhanced by heparin, which often functions as a co-factor for FSAP activity. Inhibition of FSAP by aprotinin reduced this cleavage. The enzymatically inactive PPACK-FSAP had no effect (Figure 1C). Cleavage of $VEGF_{165}$ was time-dependent (Figure 1D), but $VEGF_{121}$ was not cleaved at all (Supplementary Figure S1). The cleavage site was identified by amino acid sequencing and was found to be in the neuropilin/heparin-binding domain at position 124/125, which was distinct from the plasmin cleavage site at 110/111 (Figure 2). The cleavage site for plasmin and FSAP in relation to the disulphide bridges [31] is shown in Figure 2. Thus, FSAP cleaves $VEGF_{165}$ in the heparin/neuropilin-binding region.

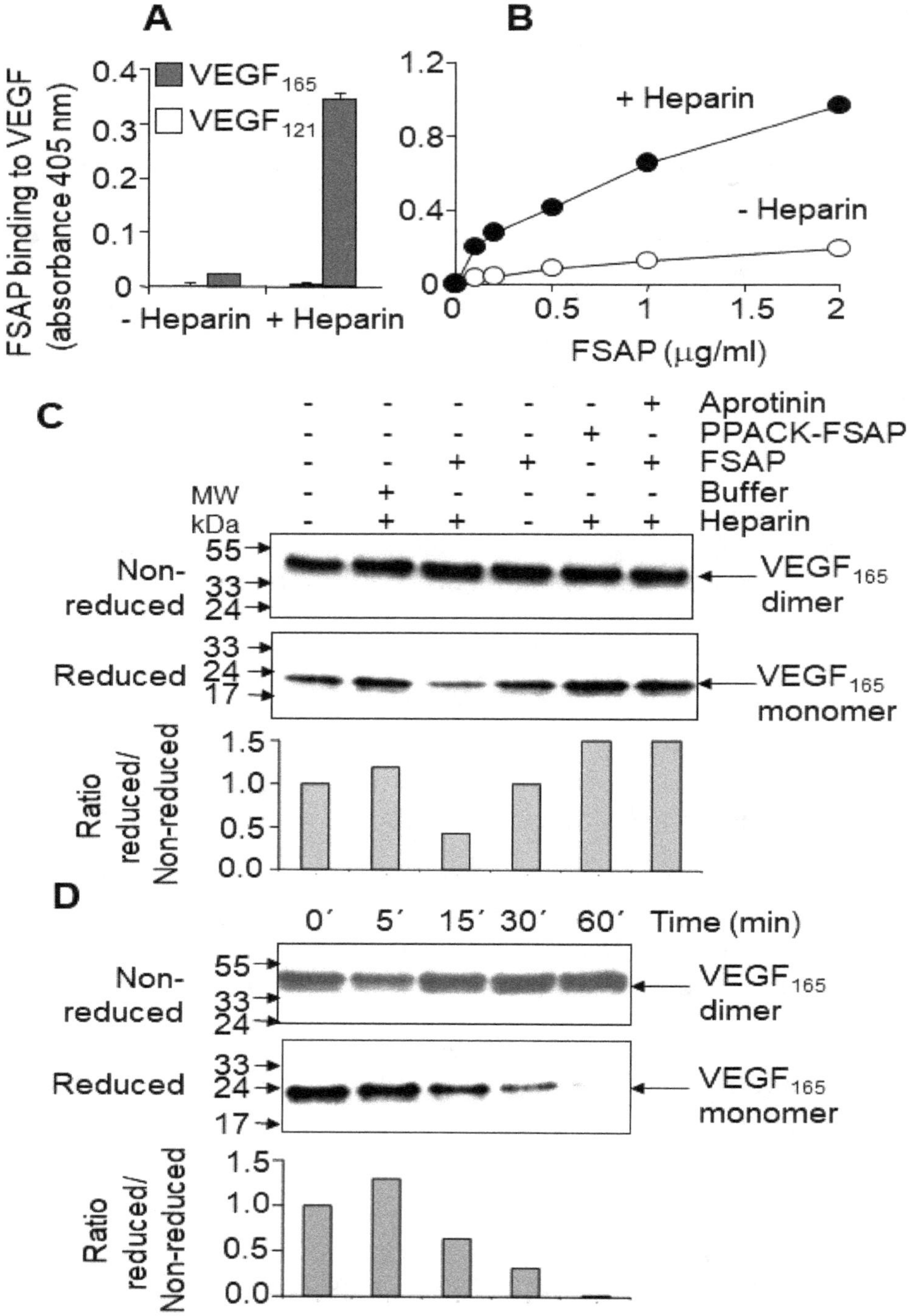

Figure 1. Binding of FSAP (factor VII activating protease) to VEGF (vascular endothelial growth factor) and its specific proteolytic cleavage: (**A**) $VEGF_{121}$ (open bars) or $VEGF_{165}$ (grey bars) was immobilized, and the binding of FSAP, in the absence or presence of heparin, was detected with an anti-FSAP antibody (mean ± SD of triplicate wells); (**B**) $VEGF_{165}$ was immobilized, and the binding of increasing concentrations of FSAP in the absence (open circles) or presence (filled circles) of heparin was determined. Error bars are smaller than the size of the symbols; (**C**) Mixtures of FSAP (or Phe-Pro-Arg-chloromethylketone (PPACK)-FSAP), buffer, heparin, $VEGF_{165}$, and aprotinin, as indicated, were incubated, and the reaction was analyzed by western blotting with an anti-VEGF antibody under reducing or non-reducing conditions; (**D**) FSAP, $VEGF_{165}$, and heparin were incubated for the indicated time intervals and the samples were analyzed for VEGF, as above. Densiometric analysis was performed to calculate the ratio of VEGF under reduced and non-reduced conditions.

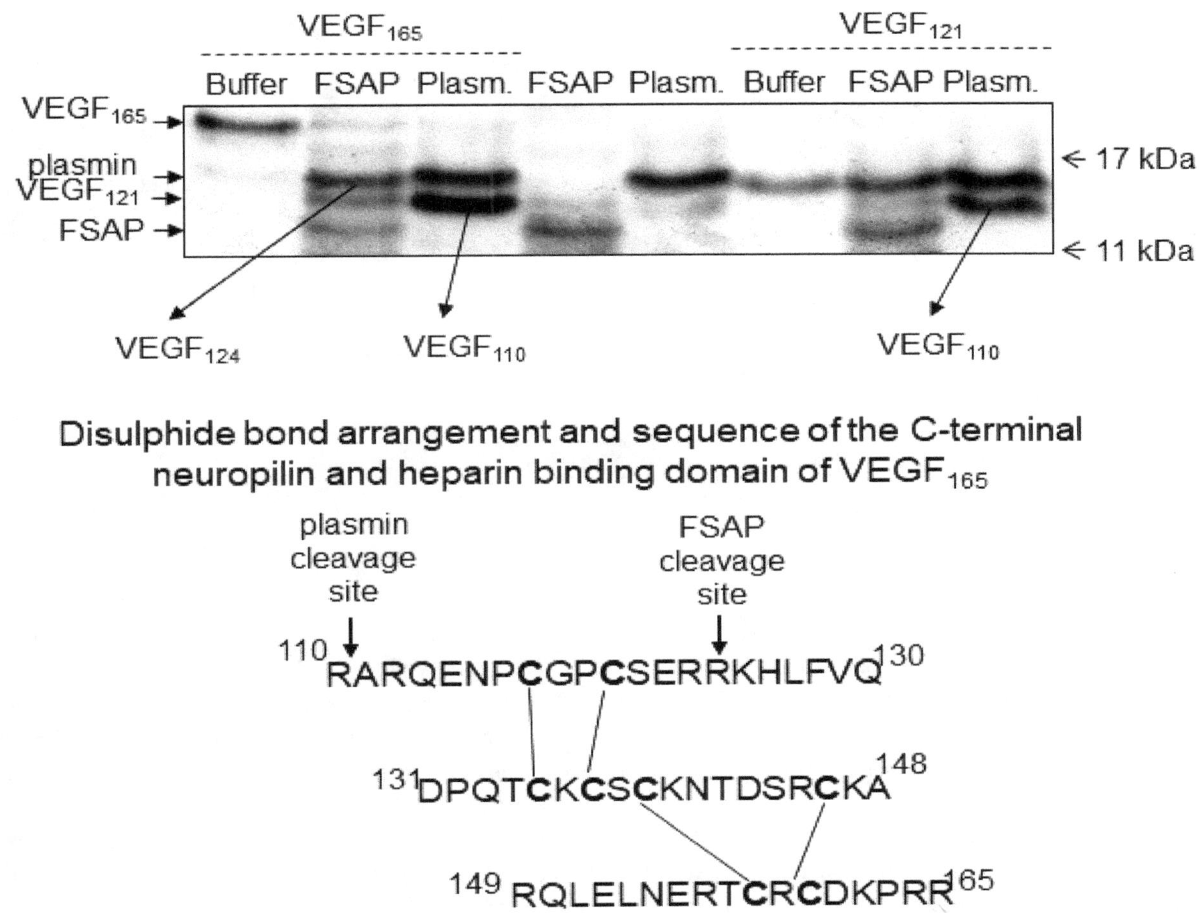

Figure 2. Sequencing of proteolytically cleaved VEGF: $VEGF_{165}$ or $VEGF_{121}$ (20 μg/mL) was incubated with FSAP (200 μg/mL) or plasmin (200 μg/mL) in the presence of heparin (10 μg/mL) for 2 h at 37 °C. The mixture was separated by SDS-PAGE under reducing conditions and processed for N-terminal sequencing. The FSAP and plasmin cleavage sites, as well as the disulphide bond assignments in the heparin/neuropilin-binding domain [31] sequence of $VEGF_{165}$ are indicated.

Interaction of FSAP with neuropilin and VEGFR-2: Neuropilins are co-receptors that bind to larger VEGF isoforms, such as $VEGF_{165}$, in a heparin-dependent manner, and regulate the activity of long forms of VEGF. Thus, the binding interactions between FSAP, $VEGF_{165}$, VEGFR, and neuropilin were investigated. FSAP bound strongly to neuropilin-1-Fc in a heparin-dependent manner, but there was no binding to VEGFR-2-Fc (Figure 3A). There was no difference in the binding of PPACK-FSAP, the MI-SNP of FSAP, or WT-FSAP (Figure 3A,B), indicating that the enzymatic activity of FSAP was not involved in the binding to neuropilin. $VEGF_{165}$ bound to both neuropilin and VEGFR2 in a heparin-dependent manner (Figure 3C). $VEGF_{165}$ binding to neuropilin-1-Fc was partially inhibited by FSAP in the absence or presence of heparin, but FSAP had no influence on binding of $VEGF_{165}$ to VEGFR-2-Fc (Figure 3C,D). Hence, FSAP binds to neuropilin, thereby cleaving $VEGF_{165}$ that, in turn, partially decreases its interactions with neuropilin but not VEGFR2.

Effect of FSAP on proliferation and migration of HUVEC or VEGFR-transfected BAF3 cells: Because FSAP can cleave $VEGF_{165}$ and inhibits its binding to neuropilin, the effect of FSAP-treated $VEGF_{165}$ on the activation of HUVEC was investigated in the absence or presence of heparin. FSAP did not influence bFGF- or $VEGF_{165}$-induced DNA synthesis or cell migration (Figure 4A,B). Phosphorylation of ERK in HUVEC with bFGF or VEGF pretreated with FSAP was not altered (Figure 5).

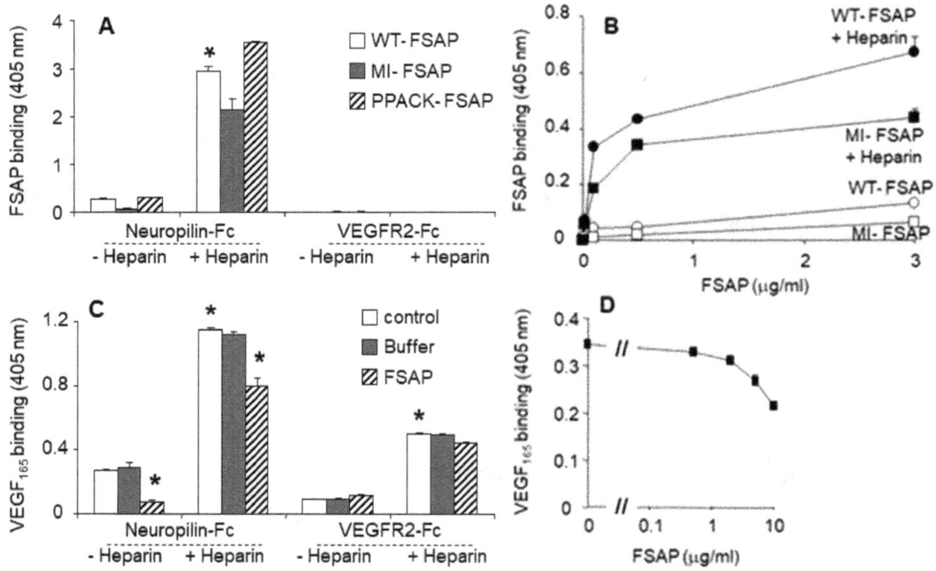

Figure 3. Interactions between FSAP, neuropilin, VEGFR2, and $VEGF_{165}$: (**A**) Neuropilin-1-Fc or VEGFR2-Fc was immobilized and the binding of wild type (WT)-FSAP (open bars), Marburg I (MI)-FSAP (G534E-SNP) (grey bars), or PPACK-FSAP (hatched bars) was determined in the absence or presence of heparin; (**B**) To immobilized neuropilin-1-Fc, increasing concentrations of WT-FSAP (circles) or MI-FSAP (squares) in the absence (open symbols) or presence (closed symbols) of heparin (filled circles) was added, and FSAP binding was determined; (**C**) Neuropilin-1-Fc or VEGFR2-Fc was immobilized, and the binding of $VEGF_{165}$ was determined in the absence or presence of heparin (open bars), buffer (grey bars), or FSAP (hatched bars); (**D**) Neuropilin-1-Fc was immobilized and the binding of $VEGF_{165}$ was determined in the presence of heparin and increasing concentrations of FSAP, as indicated. Results are shown as absorbance (mean + SD of triplicate wells). Error bars in 2B and 2D are smaller than the size of the symbols. * $p < 0.05$.

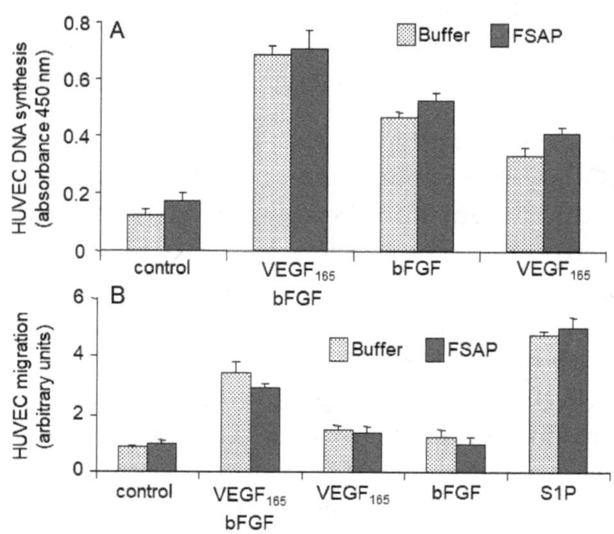

Figure 4. Effect of FSAP on proliferation and migration of human umbilical vein endothelial cells (HUVEC): basic fibroblast growth factor (bFGF) (40 ng/mL) and/or $VEGF_{165}$ (20 ng/mL) in the presence of FSAP (12 μg/mL) (dark bars) or buffer control (dotted bars), as well as heparin (10 μg/mL) was preincubated for 60 min at 37 °C, and the mixtures were used to stimulate serum-starved HUVEC. (**A**) DNA synthesis was determined using the BrdU incorporation kit; (**B**) Migration was tested in a Boyden chamber. Sphingosine-1-phosphate (S1P) was used a positive control and its concentration was 200 nM. Data are mean + SD of triplicate wells.

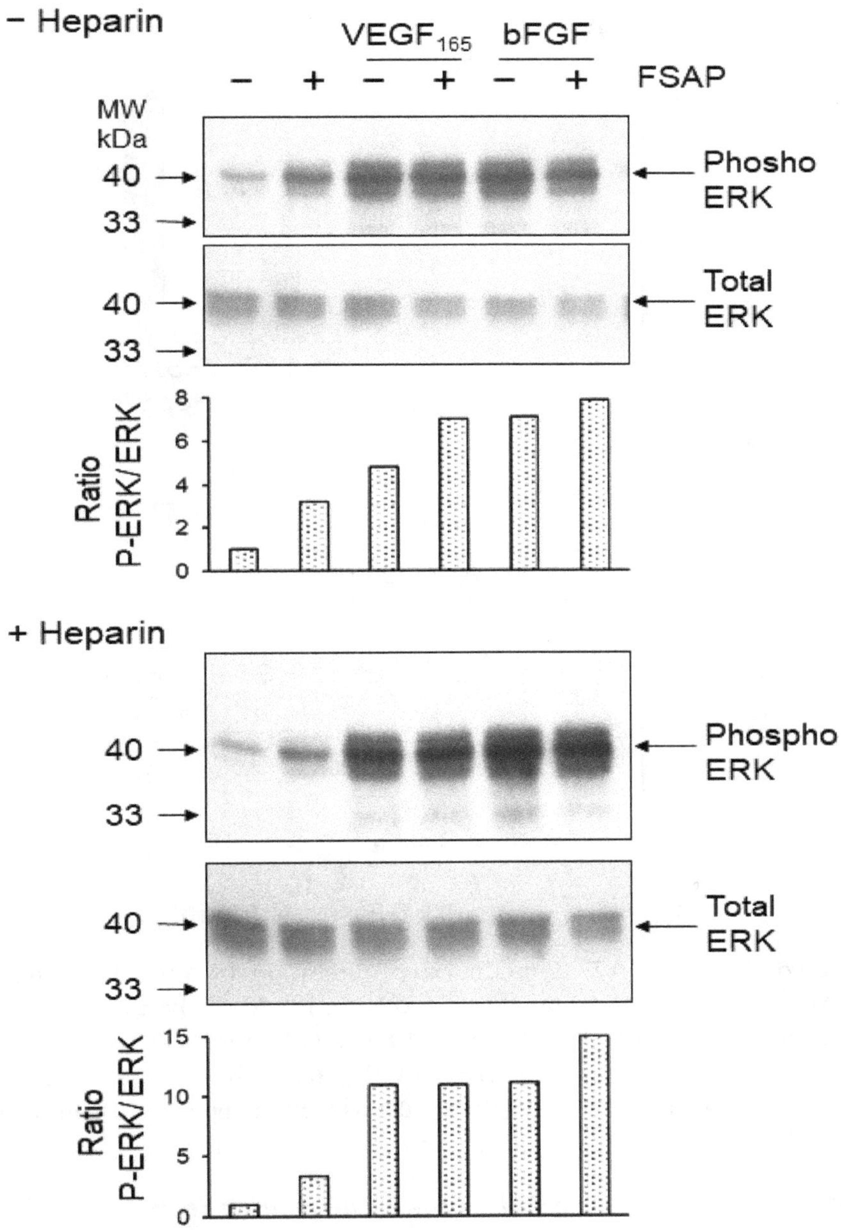

Figure 5. Effect of FSAP on ERK phosphorylation in HUVEC: Mixtures of FSAP (12 μg/mL), buffer, heparin (10 μg/mL), $VEGF_{165}$ (20 ng/mL), and/or (bFGF 50 ng/mL) were preincubated for 1 h at 37 °C in serum-free medium and then added to cells for 15 min. Cells extracts were analyzed by Western blotting for phosphorylated ERK. Analysis of total ERK was performed to confirm equal loading of gel with lysates. Relative phospho ERK levels were determined by densiometric analysis.

In order to further characterize this result, we also tested the activation of VEGFR-transfected BAF3 cells that are very sensitive to the effects of VEGF. Even in this very sensitive cellular system, FSAP did not inhibit $VEGF_{165}$- or $VEGF_{121}$-induced proliferation of BAF-3 cells transfected with VEGFR1 or VEGFR2 (Figure 6A,B). FSAP did not inhibit the effect of bFGF on HUVEC, which is in accordance with our previous results on VSMC [18], but is in contrast to earlier studies on HUVEC [19,20,32]. Expression of neuropilin-1 was observed on both cell types by flow cytometry (data not shown). Thus, in different cellular test systems, FSAP-mediated cleavage of $VEGF_{165}$ did not alter its ability to activate cellular functions.

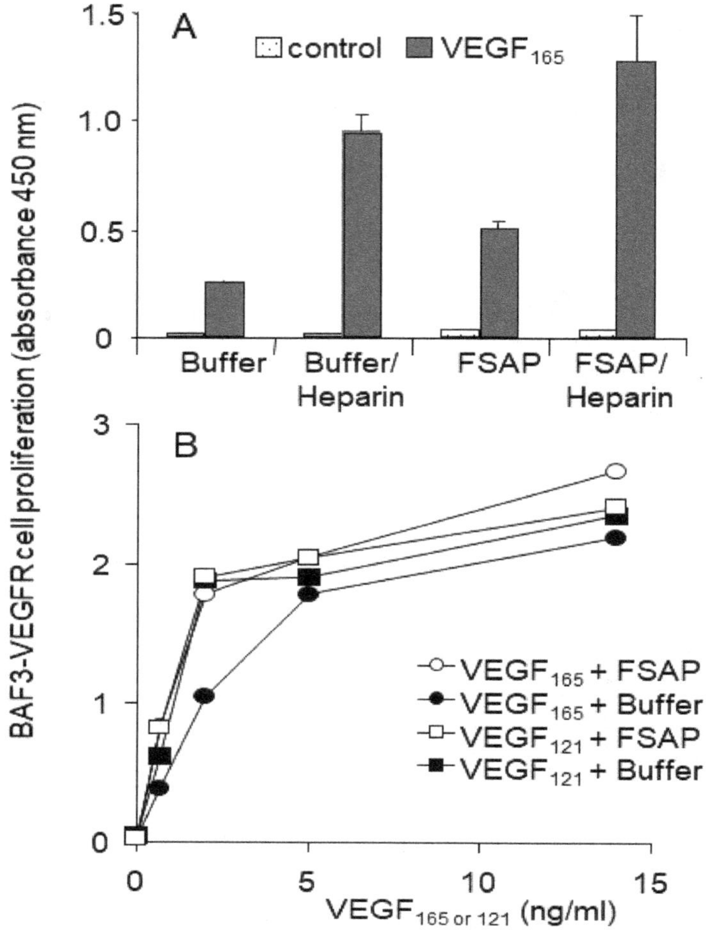

Figure 6. Effect of FSAP on VEGF-mediated proliferation of VEGFR expressing BAF3 cells: (**A**) VEGFR2-BAF3 cells were stimulated for 4 days with (dark bars) or without $VEGF_{165}$ (10 ng/mL) (dotted bars) in the absence or presence of FSAP (12 μg/mL), as well as heparin (10 μg/mL); (**B**) VEGFR1-BAF3 cells were stimulated with $VEGF_{165}$ (circles) or with $VEGF_{121}$ (squares) in the absence (filled) or presence (open) of FSAP (12 μg/mL), as well as heparin (10 μg/mL). Cell number was determined by the WST-1 assay. Mean + SD of triplicate wells is shown.

Effect of FSAP on growth factor-mediated neo-vascularization in matrigel plugs in vivo: We then tested the effect of FSAP in a model system where $VEGF_{165}$ interaction with the matrix is important. This model was based on measuring neovascularization in vivo into matrigel plugs that is essentially an extract of tumor extracellular matrix. $VEGF_{165}$ or bFGF, alone or in combination in the presence of heparin, stimulated the development of new vessels in matrigel, as determined by immunostaining for endothelial and smooth muscle cell markers (Figure 7A; endothelial-specific BS-1 (green) and α-SMA (α smooth muscle specific-actin) (red)). Quantification of the staining showed that the concomitant presence of FSAP reduced neovascularization induced by growth factors (Figure 7B). Enzymatically inactivated PPACK-FSAP did not inhibit growth factor-mediated neo-vascularization (Figure 7A,B), indicating the importance of the FSAP proteolytic activity for this effect. Similarly, the enzymatically inactive MI-isoform of FSAP did not inhibit $VEGF_{165}$/bFGF-mediated neo-vascularization (Supplementary Figure S2). The effect of $VEGF_{121}$-mediated neo-vascularization was not inhibited by FSAP (Supplementary Figure S2). Thus, exogenously applied FSAP could inhibit the effects of $VEGF_{165}$, bFGF, and their combination on neovascularization in matrigel plugs in vivo. Preliminary experiments showed that the neovascularization into matrigel in response to growth factors, in the absence of endogenous FSAP (*Habp2*$^{-/-}$ mice), was similar as in WT mice (data not shown).

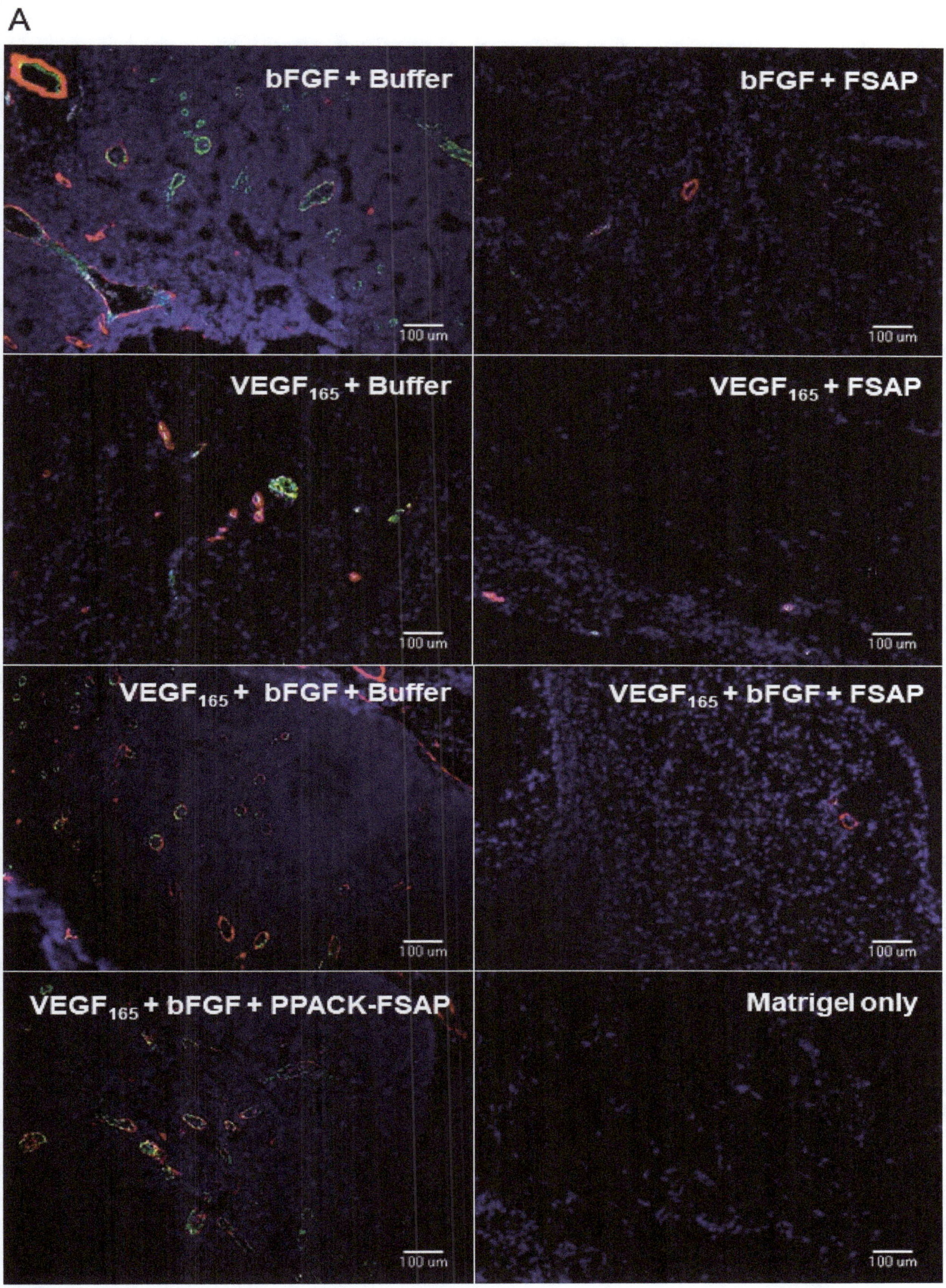

Figure 7. *Cont.*

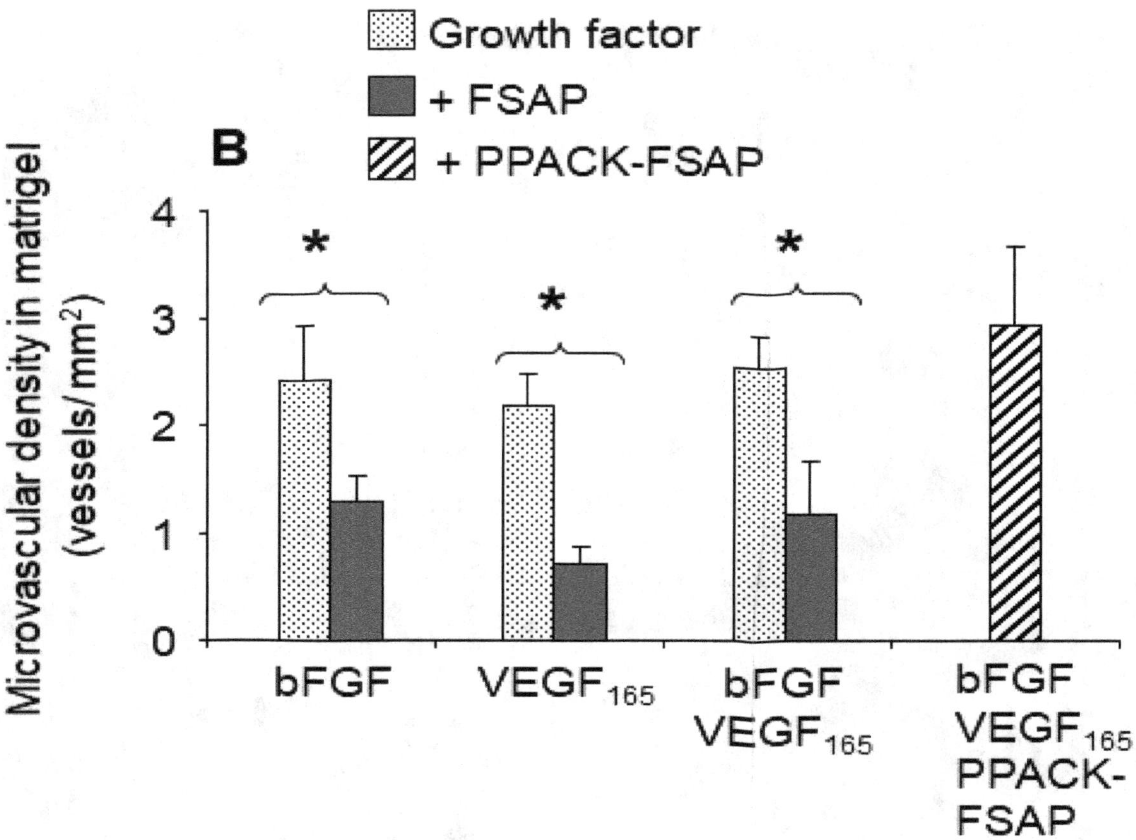

Figure 7. Effect of FSAP on microvascular density in matrigel plugs in vivo: (**A**) Photomicrographs of matrigel plugs after 7 days and stained for BS-1 (FITC, green), α-SMA (α smooth muscle specific-actin) (Cy3, red), and nuclei (DAPI, blue); (**B**) Microvascular density of plugs was determined, bars are means ± SEM (n = 7–8), * $p < 0.05$. Matrigel was supplemented with heparin and with either buffer (dotted bars), FSAP (black bars), or PPACK-FSAP (striped bars), as well as $VEGF_{165}$ or bFGF, as indicated.

VEGF expression in the Habp2$^{-/-}$ mice subjected to hind limb ischemia: We then examined whether the levels of the long forms of VEGF were higher in mice in the absence of endogenous FSAP (*Habp2$^{-/-}$* mice). For this, we used the hind limb ischemia model where angiogenesis is induced in the gastrocnemius muscle after femoral artery ligation [16]. Although, collateral growth in the adductor muscle was enhanced in *Habp2$^{-/-}$* mice, capillary density in the gastrocnemius muscle was not altered at 21 days. Western blotting showed that, at an earlier time point of day 3 after ligation, VEGF-A protein was significantly upregulated in the gastrocnemius muscle of *Habp2$^{-/-}$* mice compared to WT mice, whereas no increase was observed in the adductor muscle (Figure 8). At day 7, after ligation, this effect on VEGF-A protein was no longer evident. The VEGF-A isoform detected was largely the $VEGF_{121}$ dimer (30 kDa), and longer forms seemed not to be produced in this tissue. It was also possible that longer forms were produced and then cleaved to smaller forms. No change in VEGF-A mRNA was detected at the day 3 time point (Supplementary Figure S3). Thus, it was not possible to establish a causal link between the absence of endogenous FSAP and the increased presence of longer forms of VEGF in this experimental system.

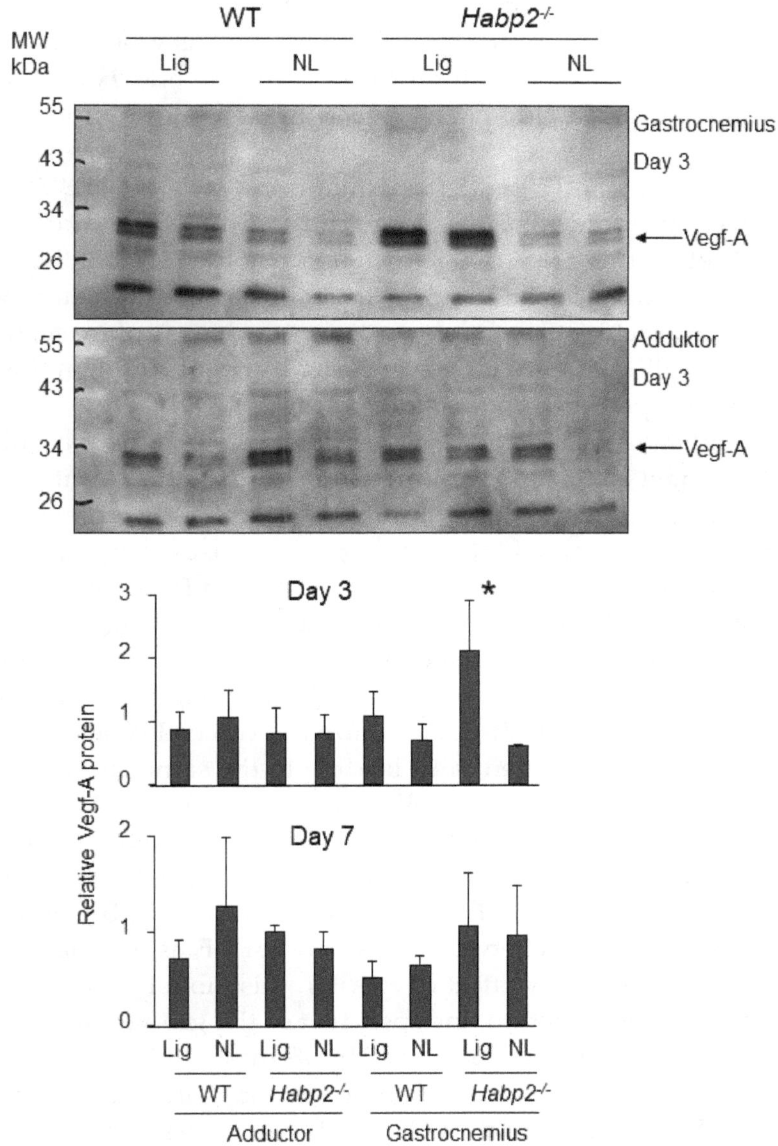

Figure 8. Changes in VEGF protein levels in the *Habp2*$^{-/-}$ mice after hind limb ischemia: In the hind limb muscles of WT- and *Habp2*$^{-/-}$ mice, VEGF-A protein was detected by western blotting at day 3 in the gastrocnemius muscle (top panel) and adductor muscles (bottom panel). VEGF-A was normalized to the expression of cytochrome C oxidase, as measured by western blotting on stripped blots. Relative VEGF-A levels were quantified by densitometry (means + SEM, $n = 4$, * $p < 0.05$).

4. Discussion

$VEGF_{165}$ was cleaved at position 124/125 in the heparin/neuropilin-binding region that resembles a classic, multi-basic, FSAP cleavage site. Because the disulphide bonds in this region were still intact, there was no difference in mobility of the protein under non-reducing conditions, only under reducing conditions. Only the larger forms of VEGF, 165 but not 121, bound to FSAP, thus conferring specificity to the process. FSAP also bound to neuropilin but not to VEGF-R2, and partially inhibited $VEGF_{165}$ binding to neuropilin. The binding and cleavage by FSAP was more pronounced in the presence of heparin, which is cofactor for FSAP. As previously reported, plasmin cleaved VEGF after position 110, thereby completely separating the receptor-binding domain from the heparin/neuropilin-binding domain [33,34]. Cleavage in the C-terminal region of $VEGF_{165}$ occurs naturally in vivo, and such cleaved forms have been observed in tumor ascites [35] as well as wound fluids [34]. Such cleavage is likely to reduce the association of VEGF long forms with the matrix and increase their mobility, thus raising the possibility of activating VEGF receptor as well as modulating their binding to co-receptors [27].

In proliferation, migration, and signal transduction assays on HUVEC, no consequence of the $VEGF_{165}$ cleavage was observed. This cleavage did not affect the induction of proliferation of VEGFR-transfected BAF3 cells either. This can be explained by the fact that the position of the cleavage in $VEGF_{165}$, in relation to the disulphide bond, was such that the molecule was still held together and preserved some of its characteristics. Other proteases such as urokinase, matrix metalloprotease (MMP), elastase, and tissue kallikrein also cleave the long forms of VEGF in this region and modulate its activity in different ways depending on the site of cleavage.

Matrigel-embedded growth factors provide a model to study neovascularization in vivo [29]. Growth factor-reduced matrigel is the matrix of mouse sarcoma, which contains 1851 unique proteins including classical matrix proteins such as laminin, collagen IV, entactin/nidogen, fibronectin, and heparan sulphate proteoglycans [36]. Heparin increases angiogenesis in this model by multiple mechanisms that probably include modifying growth factor's presentation to the cellular receptors [37]. In this model, FSAP inhibited the activity of $VEGF_{165}$, bFGF, and a combination of both, and microvascular density was decreased. We used BS1 and vWF as markers for endothelial cells and α-SMC actin as a marker for pericytes/VSMC. Individually, the staining of each marker was reduced by FSAP, indicating that FSAP directly inhibited both cell types. FSAP may also influence paracrine interactions between them, potentially, leading to the same end result. In this model, bFGF and $VEGF_{165}$ were known to upregulate PDGF-BB, and this in turn may have been responsible for the recruitment of the smooth muscle cells [38]. Smooth muscle cells and pericytes can indirectly contribute to the regulation of neo-vascularization through various paracrine/juxtacrine mechanisms [39], and we have previously shown that FSAP can inhibit PDGF-BB [18]. The inhibitory effect of FSAP on bFGF may be related to a complex interaction between FSAP and bFGF, as described before [19]. This result also illustrates the fact that the inhibitory effect of FSAP in this model was not limited to $VEGF_{165}$, and a completely different mechanism of action, independent of the growth factor, cannot be excluded.

In view of the lack of the effect of FSAP on VEGF-mediated proliferation and migration of endothelial cells in vitro, the strong reduction of angiogenesis in the matrigel model was remarkable. Because FSAP cleavage of $VEGF_{165}$ led to a $VEGF_{121}$-like molecule, the difference in the in vitro and in vivo results must be related to the difference between the two isoforms. It was possible that in the matrigel model, the VEGF was presented to the cells in a form that was bound to the matrix, and that the haptotaxis-effect was altered by FSAP. Evidence for proteolysis-mediated modulation of haptotaxis of matrix-anchored VEGF has been demonstrated before [40]. The cleavage of VEGF by FSAP may also alter the sequestration of the growth factor by the matrix or its spatial complexity, both of which are known to be important for VEGF activity [41]. VEGF can also activate leukocytes and other VEGFR-bearing cells, which may indirectly mediate the inhibition of angiogenesis by FSAP. An effect of VEGF in the matrigel model through changes in vascular permeability was also a possibility. The time course of the in vitro experiments, ranging from minutes to 24 h, were different from the in vivo matrigel experiments that lasted a few days, and this could also account for the differences in the results.

The induction of ischemia led to angiogenesis in the gastrocnemius muscle in the hind limb ischemia model. Mice without endogenous FSAP showed no changes in their angiogenesis response in this model, indicating that endogenous FSAP was not involved in this process [16]. However, collateral vessel growth was increased in the adductor muscle. Application of exogenous FSAP, directly into the adductor muscle, decreased collateral growth there, but increased angiogenesis in the gastrocnemius muscle. This was most likely a response to the decreased collateral growth in the vessels feeding the gastrocnemius muscle [16]. In the neointimal growth model, exogenous FSAP decreased neointima formation [15] and a lack of endogenous FSAP increased it [18]. Thus, in two independent models of vascular growth and repair, FSAP seemed to be involved in regulating vascular remodeling but not angiogenesis. This also fits with the lack of difference in neovascularization in *Habp2*$^{-/-}$ mice in the matrigel model (see Table 1 for an overview).

Table 1. Summary of the effects of FSAP on vascular growth and repair processes.

	***Habp2*$^{-/-}$ Mice: Lack of Endogenous FSAP**	**Local Application of Exogenous Purified FSAP**
Neointima formation in response to intraluminal injury in the femoral artery	Increased [15]	Decreased [18]
Femoral artery ligation and stimulation of collateral development in the adductor muscle	Increased [16]	Decreased [16]
Femoral artery ligation and stimulation of angiogenesis in the gastrocnemius muscle	No change [16]	Increased, probably as a consequence of decreased collateral growth [16]
Matrigel/growth factor model of angiogenesis	No change (this study)	Decreased (this study)

We chose to study the hind limb ischemia model to investigate processing of long forms of VEGF because we have performed studies using this model in FSAP-deficient mice [16]. However, we did not detect any $VEGF_{165}$ in this tissue and it was not possible to find any direct evidence for changes in cleavage of this VEGF isoform. However, we did observe an increase in $VEGF_{121}$ in *Habp2*$^{-/-}$ in the absence of any increase in mRNA. Further experiments would be required to study VEGF isoform-specific mRNA and protein to provide compelling evidence for this hypothesis. In this model system there was an upregulation of uPA and MMP-9 at the mRNA and protein level in the gastrocnemius muscle, which could also account for the fact that only the short form of VEGF was detected [16]. Such experiments would be more conclusive in performed in relation to angiogenesis in the eye or the brain because they display the sharpest concentration gradients of $VEGF_{165}$ [27].

Although endogenous FSAP did not regulate angiogenesis and neovascularization, it did influence remodeling of vessels in general. $VEGF_{165}$ cleavage, binding properties towards neuropilin, and angiogenesis in matrigel were inhibited by exogenous FSAP. Thus, FSAP has the potential to modulate $VEGF_{165}$-mediated angiogenesis that may be relevant in some pathophysiological conditions.

Author Contributions: Ö.U. and J.H. performed experiments, analyzed the data, and edited the manuscript. S.M.K. designed the research, obtained the funding, analyzed data, and drafted the manuscript.

Acknowledgments: We would like to thank Lars Muhl, Susanne Tannert-Otto, Thomas Schmidt Wöll, and Baerbel Fuehler for their excellent technical assistance. The gift of VEGFR cells from Steven Stacker and Marc Achen (Ludwig Cancer Research Institute, Melbourne Branch, Australia) and Kari Alitalo (Helsinki Branch, Finland) is greatly appreciated. This study was done as part of the MD/PhD thesis of Özgür Uslu at the Justus Liebig University, Giessen, Germany.

References

1. Yamamichi, S.; Fujiwara, Y.; Kikuchi, T.; Nishitani, M.; Matsushita, Y.; Hasumi, K. Extracellular histone induces plasma hyaluronan-binding protein (factor VII activating protease) activation in vivo. *Biochem. Biophys. Res. Commun.* **2011**, *409*, 483–488. [CrossRef] [PubMed]
2. Kanse, S.M.; Gallenmueller, A.; Zeerleder, S.; Stephan, F.; Rannou, O.; Denk, S.; Etscheid, M.; Lochnit, G.; Krueger, M.; Huber-Lang, M. Factor VII-activating protease is activated in multiple trauma patients and generates anaphylatoxin C5a. *J. Immunol.* **2012**, *188*, 2858–2865. [CrossRef] [PubMed]

3. Marsman, G.; von Richthofen, H.; Bulder, I.; Lupu, F.; Hazelzet, J.; Luken, B.M.; Zeerleder, S. DNA and factor VII-activating protease protect against the cytotoxicity of histones. *Blood Adv.* **2017**, *1*, 2491–2502. [CrossRef] [PubMed]
4. Grasso, S.; Neumann, A.; Lang, I.M.; Etscheid, M.; von Kockritz-Blickwede, M.; Kanse, S.M. Interaction of factor VII activating protease (FSAP) with neutrophil extracellular traps (NETs). *Thromb. Res.* **2018**, *161*, 36–42. [CrossRef] [PubMed]
5. Serpas, L.; Chan, R.W.Y.; Jiang, P.; Ni, M.; Sun, K.; Rashidfarrokhi, A.; Soni, C.; Sisirak, V.; Lee, W.S.; Cheng, S.H.; et al. Dnase1l3 deletion causes aberrations in length and end-motif frequencies in plasma DNA. *Proc. Natl. Acad. Sci. USA* **2019**, *116*, 641–649. [CrossRef]
6. Etscheid, M.; Muhl, L.; Pons, D.; Jukema, J.W.; Koenig, H.; Kanse, S.M. The Marburg I polymorphism of factor VII activating protease is associated with low proteolytic and low pro-coagulant activity. *Thromb. Res.* **2012**, *130*, 935–941. [CrossRef]
7. Willeit, J.; Kiechl, S.; Weimer, T.; Mair, A.; Santer, P.; Wiedermann, C.J.; Roemisch, J. Marburg I polymorphism of factor VII—Activating protease: A prominent risk predictor of carotid stenosis. *Circulation* **2003**, *107*, 667–670. [CrossRef]
8. Trompet, S.; Pons, D.; Kanse, S.M.; de Craen, A.J.; Ikram, M.A.; Verschuren, J.J.; Zwinderman, A.H.; Doevendans, P.A.; Tio, R.A.; de Winter, R.J.; et al. Factor VII Activating Protease Polymorphism (G534E) Is Associated with Increased Risk for Stroke and Mortality. *Stroke Res. Treat.* **2011**, *2011*, 424759. [CrossRef]
9. Ahmad-Nejad, P.; Dempfle, C.E.; Weiss, C.; Bugert, P.; Borggrefe, M.; Neumaier, M. The G534E-polymorphism of the gene encoding the factor VII-activating protease is a risk factor for venous thrombosis and recurrent events. *Thromb. Res.* **2012**, *130*, 441–444. [CrossRef]
10. Hoppe, B.; Tolou, F.; Dorner, T.; Kiesewetter, H.; Salama, A. Gene polymorphisms implicated in influencing susceptibility to venous and arterial thromboembolism: Frequency distribution in a healthy German population. *Thromb. Haemost.* **2006**, *96*, 465–470.
11. Wasmuth, H.E.; Tag, C.G.; Van de Leur, E.; Hellerbrand, C.; Mueller, T.; Berg, T.; Puhl, G.; Neuhaus, P.; Samuel, D.; Trautwein, C.; et al. The Marburg I variant (G534E) of the factor VII-activating protease determines liver fibrosis in hepatitis C infection by reduced proteolysis of platelet-derived growth factor BB. *Hepatology* **2009**, *49*, 775–780. [CrossRef] [PubMed]
12. Gara, S.K.; Jia, L.; Merino, M.J.; Agarwal, S.K.; Zhang, L.; Cam, M.; Patel, D.; Kebebew, E. Germline HABP2 Mutation Causing Familial Nonmedullary Thyroid Cancer. *N. Engl. J. Med.* **2015**, *373*, 448–455. [CrossRef] [PubMed]
13. Reiner, A.P.; Lange, L.A.; Smith, N.L.; Zakai, N.A.; Cushman, M.; Folsom, A.R. Common hemostasis and inflammation gene variants and venous thrombosis in older adults from the Cardiovascular Health Study. *J. Thromb. Haemost. JTH* **2009**, *7*, 1499–1505. [CrossRef] [PubMed]
14. Ngeow, J.; Eng, C. HABP2 in Familial Non-medullary Thyroid Cancer: Will the Real Mutation Please Stand Up? *J. Natl. Cancer Inst.* **2016**, *108*. [CrossRef] [PubMed]
15. Daniel, J.M.; Reichel, C.A.; Schmidt-Woell, T.; Dutzmann, J.; Zuchtriegel, G.; Krombach, F.; Herold, J.; Bauersachs, J.; Sedding, D.G.; Kanse, S.M. Factor VII-activating protease deficiency promotes neointima formation by enhancing leukocyte accumulation. *J. Thromb. Haemost. JTH* **2016**, *14*, 2058–2067. [CrossRef] [PubMed]
16. Herold, J.; Nowak, S.; Kostin, S.; Daniel, J.M.; Francke, A.; Subramaniam, S.; Braun-Dullaeus, R.C.; Kanse, S.M. Factor VII activating protease (FSAP) influences vascular remodeling in the mouse hind limb ischemia model. *Am. J. Transl. Res.* **2017**, *9*, 3084–3095.
17. Kara, E.; Manna, D.; Loset, G.A.; Schneider, E.L.; Craik, C.S.; Kanse, S. Analysis of the substrate specificity of Factor VII activating protease (FSAP) and design of specific and sensitive peptide substrates. *Thromb. Haemost.* **2017**, *117*, 1750–1760. [CrossRef]
18. Sedding, D.; Daniel, J.M.; Muhl, L.; Hersemeyer, K.; Brunsch, H.; Kemkes-Matthes, B.; Braun-Dullaeus, R.C.; Tillmanns, H.; Weimer, T.; Preissner, K.T.; et al. The G534E polymorphism of the gene encoding the factor VII-activating protease is associated with cardiovascular risk due to increased neointima formation. *J. Exp. Med.* **2006**, *203*, 2801–2807. [CrossRef]

19. Etscheid, M.; Beer, N.; Kress, J.A.; Seitz, R.; Dodt, J. Inhibition of bFGF/EGF-dependent endothelial cell proliferation by the hyaluronan-binding protease from human plasma. *Eur. J. Cell. Biol.* **2004**, *82*, 597–604. [CrossRef]
20. Kress, J.A.; Seitz, R.; Dodt, J.; Etscheid, M. Induction of intracellular signalling in human endothelial cells by the hyaluronan-binding protease involves two distinct pathways. *Biol. Chem.* **2006**, *387*, 1275–1283. [CrossRef]
21. Roedel, E.K.; Schwarz, E.; Kanse, S.M. The Factor VII-activating protease (FSAP) enhances the activity of bone morphogenetic protein-2 (BMP-2). *J. Biol. Chem.* **2013**, *288*, 7193–7202. [CrossRef] [PubMed]
22. Mambetsariev, N.; Mirzapoiazova, T.; Mambetsariev, B.; Sammani, S.; Lennon, F.E.; Garcia, J.G.; Singleton, P.A. Hyaluronic Acid binding protein 2 is a novel regulator of vascular integrity. *Arterioscler. Thromb. Vasc. Biol.* **2010**, *30*, 483–490. [CrossRef] [PubMed]
23. Joshi, A.U.; Orset, C.; Engelhardt, B.; Baumgart-Vogt, E.; Gerriets, T.; Vivien, D.; Kanse, S.M. Deficiency of Factor VII activating protease alters the outcome of ischemic stroke in mice. *Eur. J. Neurosci.* **2015**, *41*, 965–975. [CrossRef] [PubMed]
24. Apte, R.S.; Chen, D.S.; Ferrara, N. VEGF in Signaling and Disease: Beyond Discovery and Development. *Cell* **2019**, *176*, 1248–1264. [CrossRef]
25. Holmes, D.I.; Zachary, I. The vascular endothelial growth factor (VEGF) family: Angiogenic factors in health and disease. *Genome Biol.* **2005**, *6*, 209. [CrossRef]
26. Peng, K.; Bai, Y.; Zhu, Q.; Hu, B.; Xu, Y. Targeting VEGF-neuropilin interactions: A promising antitumor strategy. *Drug Discov. Today* **2019**, *24*, 656–664. [CrossRef]
27. Vempati, P.; Popel, A.S.; Mac Gabhann, F. Extracellular regulation of VEGF: Isoforms, proteolysis, and vascular patterning. *Cytokine Growth Factor Rev.* **2014**, *25*, 1–19. [CrossRef]
28. Kannemeier, C.; Al-Fakhri, N.; Preissner, K.T.; Kanse, S.M. Factor VII activating protease (FSAP) inhibits growth factor-mediated cell proliferation and migration of vascular smooth muscle cells. *FASEB J.* **2004**, *18*, 728–730. [CrossRef]
29. Pauly, R.R.; Passaniti, A.; Crow, M.; Kinsella, J.L.; Papadopoulos, N.; Monticone, R.; Lakatta, E.G.; Martin, G.R. Experimental models that mimic the differentiation and dedifferentiation of vascular cells. *Circulation* **1992**, *86*, III68-73.
30. Magee, J.C.; Stone, A.E.; Oldham, K.T.; Guice, K.S. Isolation, culture, and characterization of rat lung microvascular endothelial cells. *Am. J. Physiol.* **1994**, *267*, L433–L441. [CrossRef]
31. Keck, R.G.; Berleau, L.; Harris, R.; Keyt, B.A. Disulfide structure of the heparin binding domain in vascular endothelial growth factor: Characterization of posttranslational modifications in VEGF. *Arch. Biochem. Biophys.* **1997**, *344*, 103–113. [CrossRef] [PubMed]
32. Jeon, J.W.; Song, H.S.; Moon, E.J.; Park, S.Y.; Son, M.J.; Jung, S.Y.; Kim, J.T.; Nam, D.H.; Choi-Miura, N.H.; Kim, K.W.; et al. Anti-angiogenic action of plasma hyaluronan binding protein in human umbilical vein endothelial cells. *Int. J. Oncol.* **2006**, *29*, 209–215. [CrossRef] [PubMed]
33. Keyt, B.A.; Berleau, L.T.; Nguyen, H.V.; Chen, H.; Heinsohn, H.; Vandlen, R.; Ferrara, N. The carboxyl-terminal domain (111–165) of vascular endothelial growth factor is critical for its mitogenic potency. *J. Biol. Chem.* **1996**, *271*, 7788–7795. [CrossRef]
34. Roth, D.; Piekarek, M.; Paulsson, M.; Christ, H.; Krieg, T.; Bloch, W.; Davidson, J.M.; Eming, S.A. Plasmin modulates vascular endothelial growth factor-A-mediated angiogenesis during wound repair. *Am. J. Pathol.* **2006**, *168*, 670–684. [CrossRef] [PubMed]
35. Lee, S.; Jilani, S.M.; Nikolova, G.V.; Carpizo, D.; Iruela-Arispe, M.L. Processing of VEGF-A by matrix metalloproteinases regulates bioavailability and vascular patterning in tumors. *J. Cell. Biol.* **2005**, *169*, 681–691. [CrossRef] [PubMed]
36. Hughes, C.S.; Postovit, L.M.; Lajoie, G.A. Matrigel: A complex protein mixture required for optimal growth of cell culture. *Proteomics* **2010**, *10*, 1886–1890. [CrossRef]
37. Wake, H.; Mori, S.; Liu, K.; Takahashi, H.K.; Nishibori, M. Histidine-rich glycoprotein inhibited high mobility group box 1 in complex with heparin-induced angiogenesis in matrigel plug assay. *Eur. J. Pharmacol.* **2009**, *623*, 89–95. [CrossRef]
38. Kano, M.R.; Morishita, Y.; Iwata, C.; Iwasaka, S.; Watabe, T.; Ouchi, Y.; Miyazono, K.; Miyazawa, K. VEGF-A and FGF-2 synergistically promote neoangiogenesis through enhancement of endogenous PDGF-B-PDGFRβ signaling. *J. Cell. Sci.* **2005**, *118*, 3759–3768. [CrossRef]

39. Armulik, A.; Abramsson, A.; Betsholtz, C. Endothelial/pericyte interactions. *Circ. Res.* **2005**, *97*, 512–523. [CrossRef]
40. Chen, T.T.; Luque, A.; Lee, S.; Anderson, S.M.; Segura, T.; Iruela-Arispe, M.L. Anchorage of VEGF to the extracellular matrix conveys differential signaling responses to endothelial cells. *J. Cell. Biol.* **2010**, *188*, 595–609. [CrossRef]
41. Ekker, S.C.; Bedell, V.M. The ins and outs of VEGF signaling. *Blood* **2009**, *113*, 2123–2124. [CrossRef] [PubMed]

12

Development of an Exercise Training Protocol to Investigate Arteriogenesis in a Murine Model of Peripheral Artery Disease

Ayko Bresler [1], Johanna Vogel [2], Daniel Niederer [2], Daphne Gray [1], Thomas Schmitz-Rixen [1] and Kerstin Troidl [1,3,*]

1 Department of Vascular and Endovascular Surgery, University Hospital Frankfurt, Theodor-Stern-Kai 7, 60590 Frankfurt, Germany
2 Department of Sports Medicine, Institute of Sport Sciences, Goethe University, Ginnheimer Landstraße 39, 60487 Frankfurt, Germany
3 Department of Pharmacology, Max-Planck-Institute for Heart and Lung Research, Ludwigstr. 43, 61231 Bad Nauheim, Germany
* Correspondence: Kerstin.troidl@mpi-bn.mpg.de

Abstract: Exercise is a treatment option in peripheral artery disease (PAD) patients to improve their clinical trajectory, at least in part induced by collateral growth. The ligation of the femoral artery (FAL) in mice is an established model to induce arteriogenesis. We intended to develop an animal model to stimulate collateral growth in mice through exercise. The training intensity assessment consisted of comparing two different training regimens in C57BL/6 mice, a treadmill implementing forced exercise and a free-to-access voluntary running wheel. The mice in the latter group covered a much greater distance than the former pre- and postoperatively. C57BL/6 mice and hypercholesterolemic ApoE-deficient ($ApoE^{-/-}$) mice were subjected to FAL and had either access to a running wheel or were kept in motion-restricting cages (control) and hind limb perfusion was measured pre- and postoperatively at various times. Perfusion recovery in C57BL/6 mice was similar between the groups. In contrast, $ApoE^{-/-}$ mice showed significant differences between training and control 7 d postoperatively with a significant increase in pericollateral macrophages while the collateral diameter did not differ between training and control groups 21 d after surgery. $ApoE^{-/-}$ mice with running wheel training is a suitable model to simulate exercise induced collateral growth in PAD. This experimental set-up may provide a model for investigating molecular training effects.

Keywords: arteriogenesis; exercise training; mouse model; femoral artery ligation; running wheel; voluntary training; peripheral artery disease

1. Introduction

Patients with peripheral arterial disease (PAD) often suffer from intermittent claudication, leading to a significant walking impairment. According to the 2017 guidelines of the European Society of Vascular Surgery (ESVS), supervised exercise training is a Class I, Level A recommendation in patients presenting intermittent claudication, whereas unsupervised training is a Class I, Level C recommendation. Walking has thus been shown to be a safe and effective treatment for patients with PAD [1,2]. In particular, walking performance, cardiovascular parameters, and quality of life can be improved by exercise.

Some potential exercise effects and scheduling modifiers are still unclear, in particular, risk factors such as smoking, dyslipidemia, diabetes mellitus, obesity, and arterial hypertension as major comorbidities of PAD are only considered infrequently [3–6]. Physical activity has suppressive effects on inflammation [7] and proinflammatory immune cells [8,9], as well as beneficial effects on endothelial function [10]. Additionally, physical training has the potential to promote an additional vascularization in hypoxic/ischemic tissues, such as the myocardium or peripheral limb [11]. Arteriogenesis, can be induced by exercise in human [12–14] and in animal studies [15]. The driving force of arteriogenesis is altered fluid shear stress (FSS) in the preformed collateral arteries due to increased blood flow [16]. The increased blood flow initiates vascular remodeling and diameter growth [17] and alters the miRNA profile [18].

Nevertheless, the physiological pathways of how exercise affects collateral growth at the molecular level are still not finally delineated.

Arteriogenesis is the process that results in growth of pre-existing collateral arterioles into functional collateral arteries, triggered by a hemodynamically relevant stenosis of supplying blood vessels. These bypassing vessels can sometimes be remarkably efficient and nearly completely replace the occluded arteries [19]. This formation is stimulated by an increase of shear stress on the endothelium [20]. An increase of blood flow can be achieved by a high demand and walking exercise gives the best possibility to maximize the flow physiologically [6].

In past decades various models have been developed that help in understanding the mechanisms of arteriogenesis. The ligation of the femoral artery (FAL) in mammals, especially the mouse, has become a well-established model for the induction of arteriogenesis [3,21,22]. Exercise stress tests are widely used for a variety of training protocols [23–25]. In most of the mice models, the training is voluntary (treadmill or running wheel), only a minor share of the protocols is forced. As exercise characteristics like frequency, intensity, type, and time cannot be controlled, a forced protocol may be appropriate. On the other hand, forced exercise is, unlike voluntary exercise, affected by distress [25–27].

The aim of this study was to find a suitable mouse model for simulating PAD as well as to establish a training protocol that would be accepted by cardiovascular-diseased animals and stimulate arteriogenesis. Such a protocol could provide the basis to methodically investigate effects of training on PAD at the molecular level in an experimental setup.

2. Results

2.1. Evaluation of a Training Regime in C57BL/6

In order to maximize training intensity, we compared two training regimens: A treadmill to implement forced exercise and a free-to-access voluntary running wheel. During the treadmill protocol the mice were trained using an incremental protocol: initial running speed was 0.2 m/s, increased daily to the maximal speed of 0.3 m/s at day 7. The training frequency was twice per day, and each training lasted 30 min. A maximum distance of 1.08 km was covered each day. Distances traveled and running wheel speeds were recorded continuously. After an adaptation period a running distance of 4.36 ± 0.41 km/d with an average speed of 0.5 m/s of was recorded. We observed increased speed and distance values for the voluntary exercise mice when compared to those forced to exercise in a treadmill throughout the observation period (Figure 1a,b).

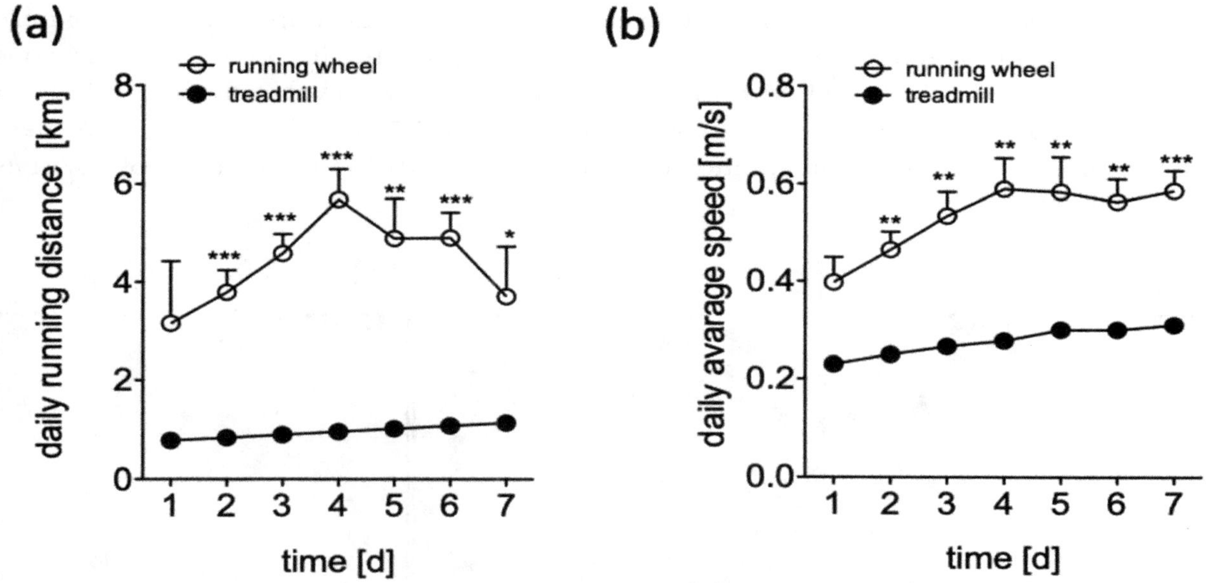

Figure 1. Daily running distance (**a**) and daily average speed (**b**) of C57BL/6 mice over time, during 7 days of adaptation in a treadmill receiving forced exercise (filled circles) or in a voluntary running wheel (open circles). Data are displayed as mean ± SEM. * $p < 0.05$; ** $p < 0.01$; *** $p < 0.005$.

2.2. Acceptance of Voluntary Training in ApoE$^{-/-}$ Mice after HFD and Post-Surgery

To further increase a similarity to patients presenting PAD we included ApoE$^{-/-}$ mice fed with a high fat diet (HFD; 21% butter fat, 1.5% cholesterol) to the exercise study. These mice showed numerous plaques throughout the whole arterial system including the femoral artery and the aortic root as well as fat deposition in the collateral arterioles (Figure 2a–c).

Given the health constraints of ApoE$^{-/-}$ mice following 12 weeks of HFD, we intended to evaluate whether they were able to cover the same distance as healthy C57BL/6 mice pre- and post-FAL. During the adaptation the mean distance covered was 3.93 ± 0.28 km/d which was not significantly different to C57BL/6 mice ($p = 0.36$). Post-FAL the re-adjustment period was similar to C57BL/6 mice, with no significant difference, as visualized in the equal progression of running performance (Figure 2d). Both strains, before and after surgery, recovered quickly to their initial distance when they had access to a voluntary running wheel.

2.3. Reperfusion Recovery after FAL in C57BL/6 and ApoE$^{-/-}$ Mice with and without Training

In order to evaluate training effects on reperfusion recovery, 18-week-old ApoE$^{-/-}$ mice that had been fed with an HFD for 12 weeks and 12-week-old healthy C57BL/6 mice were subjected to the experimental protocols shown in Figure 3a,b. Both mouse strains were randomly subdivided into training or control groups. The control group was housed in motion-restricting cages. The training group was held in single cages containing a free-to-access running wheel starting 7 days prior surgery. FAL was performed on day 0 and perfusion of the hind-limb was measured by LDPI pre- and postoperatively and on postoperative days, d3, d7, and d14. Adductor muscle tissue was harvested from ApoE$^{-/-}$ mice at different time points following FAL. The ratio of hind-limb perfusion in the operated leg to that in the non-operated leg dropped to 10% on average in C57BL/6 mice (training: 11 ± 4%, $n = 12$, control: mean 8 ± 1%, $n = 16$; $p > 0.05$), whereas perfusion recovery increased similarly within 14 days in the control (69 ± 10%) and training group (69 ± 4%) (Figure 3c).

In contrast, exercising ApoE$^{-/-}$ mice showed a significantly faster approximation of perfusion with training ($n = 19$). A maximum of 78 ± 8% perfusion of the hind limbs could be reached within 7 days postoperatively, compared with the control group ($n = 21$) averaging 53 ± 3% ($p = 0.012$) (Figure 3d,e). Interestingly, immediately postoperatively ApoE$^{-/-}$ mice showed a baseline perfusion of 25% independent of a training adaptation that was significantly higher than that of C57BL/6 mice ($p = 0.001$) (Figure 3f).

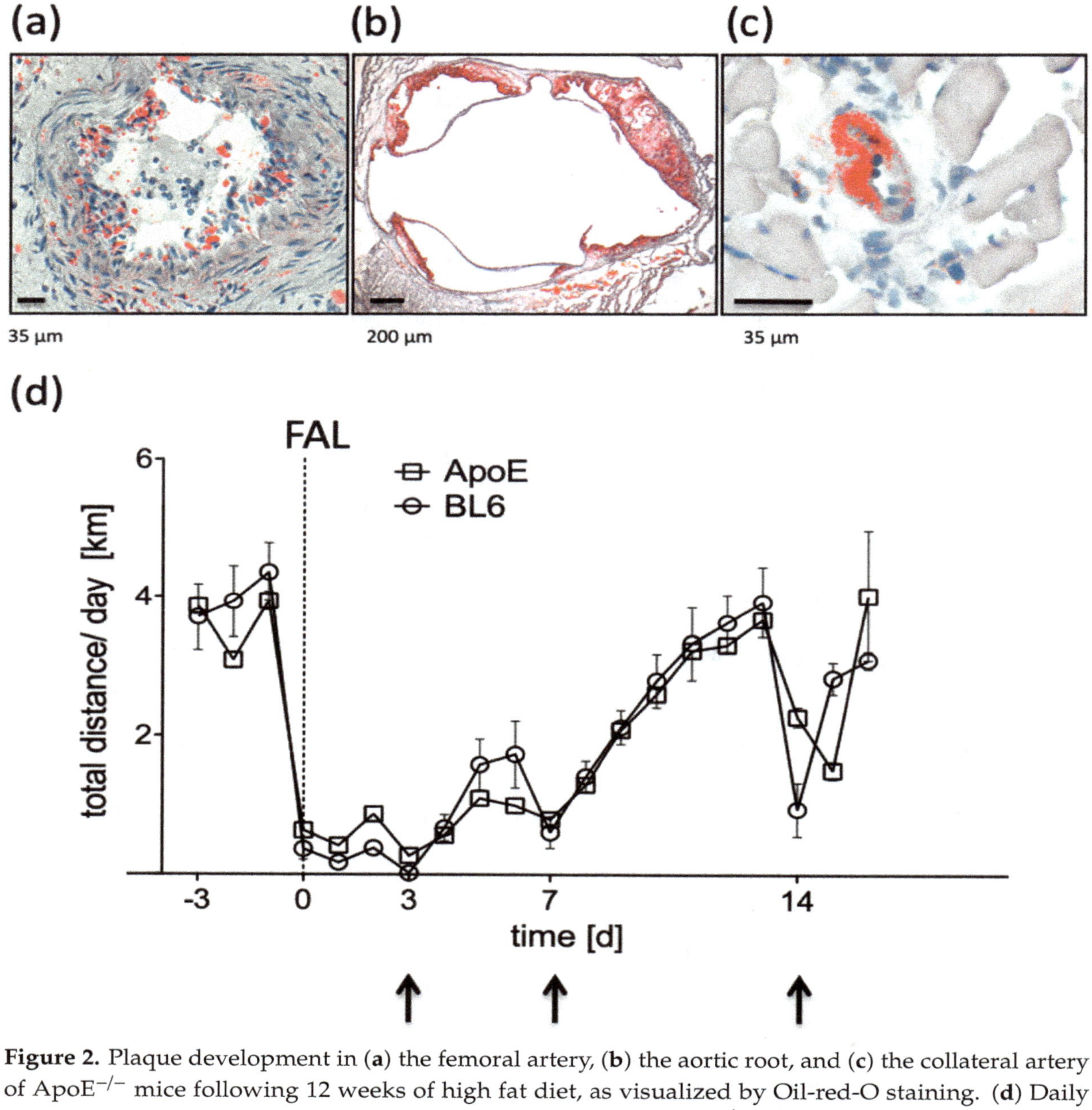

Figure 2. Plaque development in (**a**) the femoral artery, (**b**) the aortic root, and (**c**) the collateral artery of ApoE$^{-/-}$ mice following 12 weeks of high fat diet, as visualized by Oil-red-O staining. (**d**) Daily running distances of C57BL/6 mice (BL6, circles) compared to ApoE$^{-/-}$ mice (ApoE, squares) over time, pre- and post-ligation of the femoral artery (FAL). Arrows indicate short term running breaks due to anesthesia during perfusion measurements.

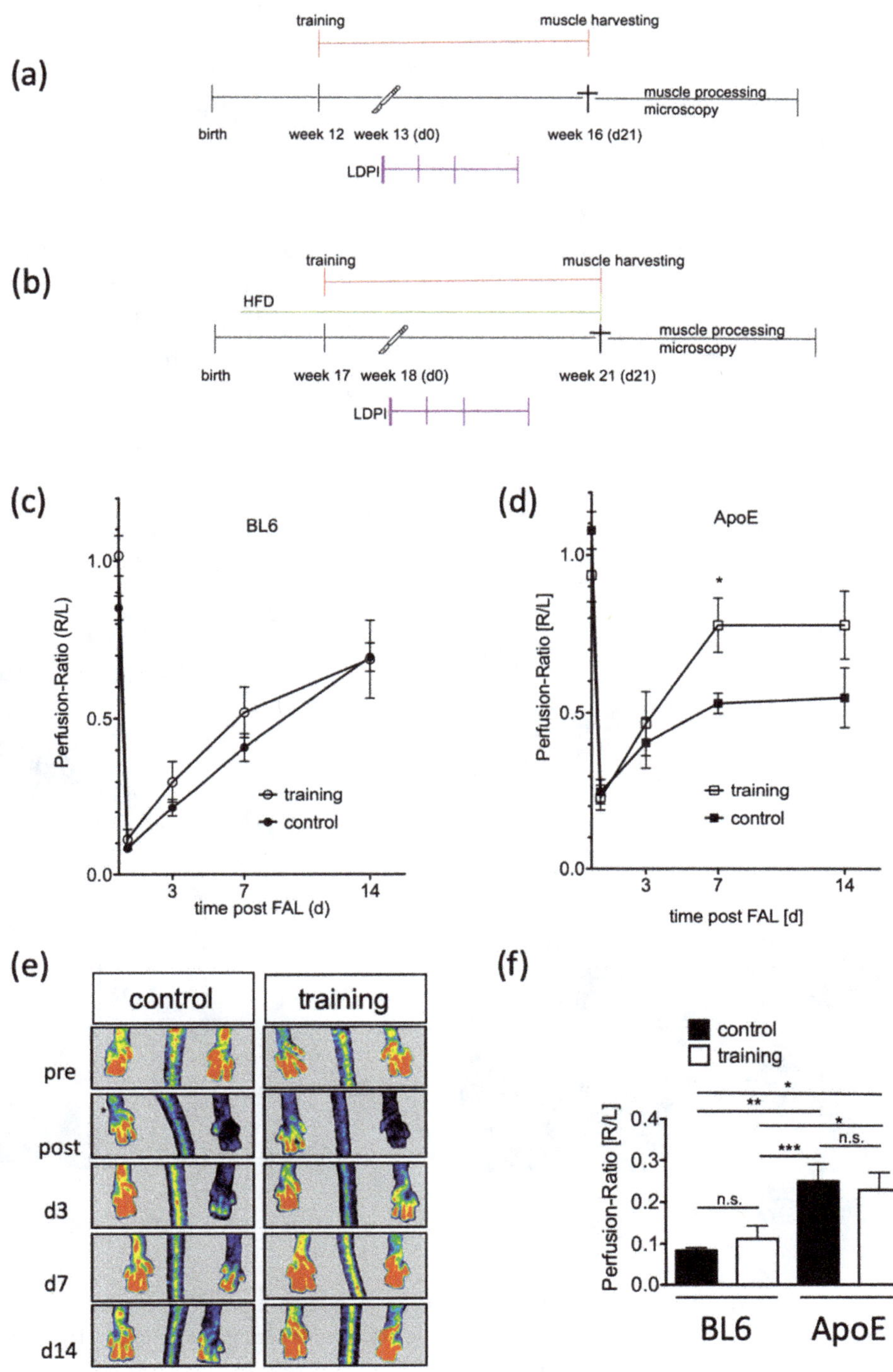

Figure 3. Functional effects on hind limb perfusion in response to training. (**a**) Schematic of experimental setup in C57BL/6, (**b**) schematic of experimental setup in ApoE$^{-/-}$, and (**c**,**d**) laser Doppler perfusion imaging in C57BL/6 and ApoE$^{-/-}$ as indicated. Data are expressed as ratio of the operated leg to the non-operated leg and represent mean ± SEM. Open symbols show the data of the training group whereas filled symbols represent the control group. As a statistical test, the unpaired t-test was used; * $p < 0.05$. (**e**) Representative laser Doppler perfusion images indicate the effect of training in the operated hind limb when compared to the control group. (**f**) Postoperative perfusion ratio (R/L). Open symbols show the data of the training group whereas filled symbols represent the control group. As a statistical test, the one-way ANOVA was used; * $p < 0.05$; ** $p < 0.01$; *** $p < 0.005$; n.s. not significant.

2.4. Increased Accumulation of Macrophages after Training in ApoE$^{-/-}$ Mice

In order to investigate the beneficial influence of exercise training on the vascular remodeling process in ApoE$^{-/-}$ mice, adductor muscle tissue was harvested from these mice 21 days following FAL. Early perfusion benefits were not reflected by morphometric examination at the end of the experimental period. There was no difference of the size of the wall area between training and control groups on day 21 post-surgery (2.15 ± 0.53 mm^2 and 2.46 ± 0.53 mm^2, respectively; $p > 0.05$; Figure 4a,b).

In the initial phase, collateral growth is critically driven by pericollateral macrophage assembly. Therefore, adductor muscle tissue was harvested from ApoE$^{-/-}$ mice 3 or 7 days following FAL and the macrophage number was quantified in the vascular nerve sheath of the collateral vessels. Seven days after FAL the number of macrophages in close proximity of growing collaterals was significantly higher in the training group with an average of 3.9 ± 0.8 compared to the control group with an average of 2.3 ± 0.4 ($p = 0.042$; Figure 4c,d).

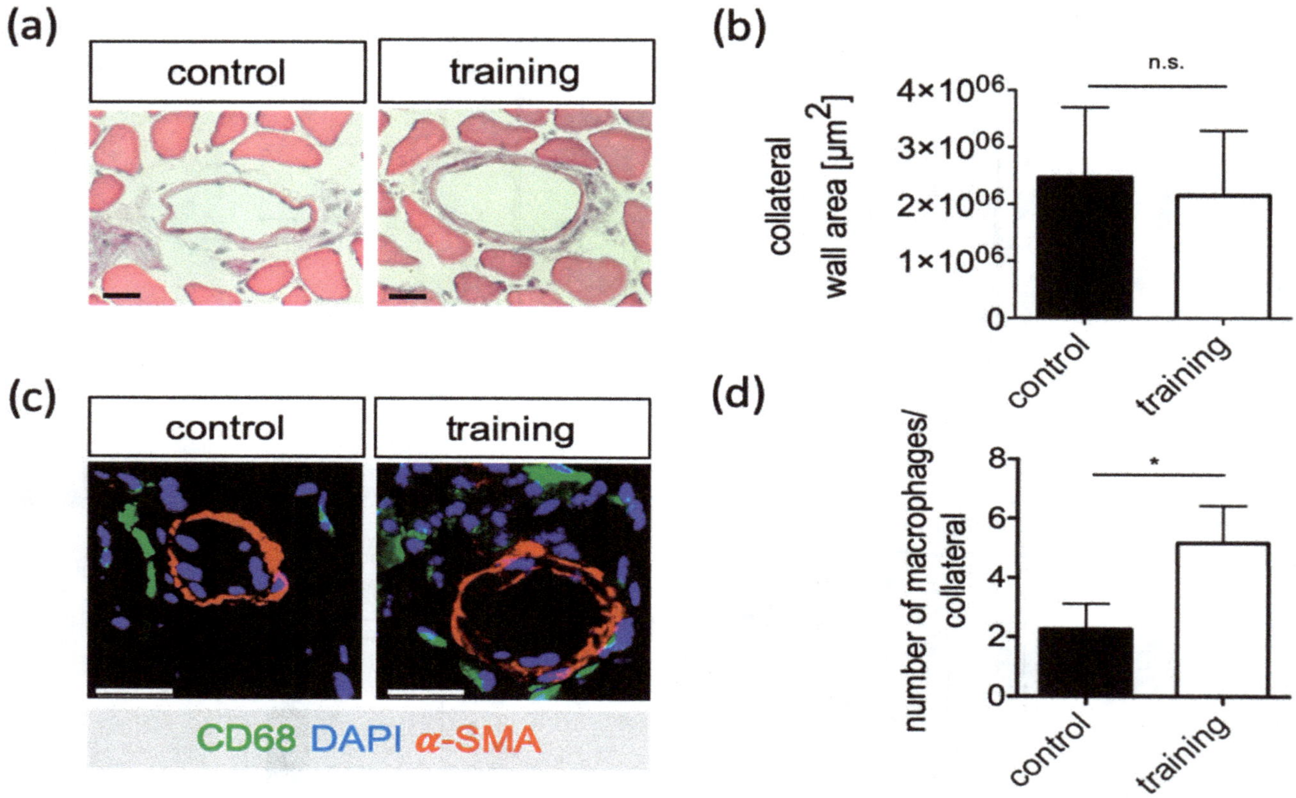

Figure 4. Histological evaluation of collateral growth in cross sections of the adductor muscles of ApoE$^{-/-}$ mice in response to training. (**a**) Representative micrographs of collateral arteries for morphometry. Scale bar: 200µm. (**b**) Quantification of wall area 21 days after FAL of the training and control group. (**c**) Immunostaining to determine macrophage accumulation around collaterals 7 d after FAL of the training and control groups. Representative images of CD68 (green) and αSMA (red) immunostaining. Blue staining indicates nuclei and scale bars are 25 µm. (**d**) Quantification of macrophage number. Data are expressed as mean ± SEM of three collateral cross-sections per mouse of at least three mice per group ($n \geq 3$). As a statistical test, the unpaired *t*-test was used; * $p < 0.05$.

3. Discussion

Arteriogenesis is the natural compensation mechanism through which collateral circulation develops. This formation is stimulated by an increase of shear stress on the endothelium [20]. An increase of blood flow can be achieved by a high demand and walking exercise is the best possibility to maximize the flow physiologically [6]. Therefore, the aim of the study was to establish a training protocol in a murine model of PAD that increases arteriogenesis through exercise. Our results suggest that a FAL surgery in ApoE$^{-/-}$ mice having free access to a voluntary running wheel serves best for future studies of exercise-induced arteriogenesis.

To increase physiologic shear stress on the arterioles it is preferable to develop an exercise program that maximizes intensity.

Initially we compared activity of healthy young C57BL/6 mice trained either with forced exercise by treadmill twice daily or with a 24 h accessible running wheel. Forced exercise is controlled and reproducible, but usually depends on a negative impulse. In models with forced exercise regimens, increased distress values, depressive behavior, inflammation reactions, and elevated corticosterone levels have been shown [26,28–30]. Distress, for example, may limit physiological remodeling normally associated with exercise training in humans [31,32]. The transferability of forced exercise models into humans may thus be limited. In contrast, similar structural and functional cardiac changes occurred in forced and voluntary exercise regimens [33]. The pros and cons of a forced versus a voluntary exercise model are thus not finally delineated.

We further showed that voluntary training leads to a much greater distance covered than forced exercise. Furthermore, voluntary running resulted in a higher running speed. Resulting from this higher exercise dose, a higher training effect response of voluntary running than of forced treadmill walking would be expected. Free-to-access running wheels are an easy way to record and store activity data without disturbing the habitual behavior. Likewise, voluntary access to running wheels permits reasonable adaptation to exercise after surgery and provides an excellent tool to monitor the behavior of mice. We could show that mice do tolerate this voluntary training much better with an increase of the distance travelled compared to forced exercise. For the reasons given above we continued our studies with voluntary training knowing well that this cannot be directly translated to the human situation. There is a discrepancy in intrinsic exercise capacity and response to exercise training between mice and humans. Mice do have a natural drive for running. Humans with sedentary behavior do not push their maximum limit. The focus of our study was to establish a protocol in mice which was adapted to their natural behavior and allowed for future investigations on collateral growth.

Since in PAD a stenosis is progressing over time and involves the whole arterial system, there is an uncertainty if healthy animals can be used to simulate the human patient's illness [3,23,34,35]. An acute occlusion in healthy participants by e.g., arterial emboli or trauma demands an instant intervention. The sudden tissue hypoxia can lead to an acute inflammatory–angiogenic–myogenic response which could result in massive loss of tissue. Patients suffering from PAD usually better tolerate an acute occlusion [36].

In order to increase the similarity to patients presenting PAD we used ApoE$^{-/-}$ mice fed with a HFD, that show numerous plaques throughout the whole arterial system [21,23,24,37] including fat deposition in collaterals.

It was expected that different mouse strains don't have similar responses to voluntary training [27,38]. Our findings showed that C57BL/6 and ApoE$^{-/-}$ animals accepted the voluntary training without a notable difference between the two strains. In this study we showed that there was just a short postoperative readjustment period of 10 days needed to get mice back to the initial distance. Whether this delay was due to the surgical intervention alone (opening and closing of the skin) cannot be fully excluded, because a sham treatment group without FAL was not investigated.

Next, the voluntary training protocol (running wheel) was tested in both strains to evaluate the reperfusion recovery after FAL.

The LDPI data acquired showed a significant higher perfusion immediately after the occlusion in ApoE$^{-/-}$ mice. This could be explained due to an increased collateral growth as a result of arteriosclerotic plaques in the major arteries [21]. C57BL/6 as well as ApoE$^{-/-}$ mice presented a maximum re-perfusion up to 69% and 77% with no significant difference in between the two strains.

It could be shown that having training possibility allowed ApoE$^{-/-}$ mice to reach the maximum reperfusion alignment one week post-FAL.

In order to correlate the increased perfusion to arteriogenesis we performed histological analyses of collateral tissue of $ApoE^{-/-}$ mice with and without exercise training. It is well accepted that mechanical, cellular, and molecular factors influence collateral growth [39]. Macrophages accumulate around the growing collaterals and cytokine secretion improves that process [40,41]. After training, $ApoE^{-/-}$ mice show a higher accumulation of $CD68^{+}$ macrophages in the vascular nerve sheath of the collateral vessels than without training.

The presented experimental setup involves atherosclerotic $ApoE^{-/-}$ mice subjected to an acute FAL. Functional as well as histological findings implicate an improvement of arteriogenesis after exercise training in the proposed model.

4. Materials and Methods

4.1. Ethics Statement

Animal handling and all experimental procedures carried out were in full compliance with the Directive 2010/63/EU of the European Parliament on protection of animals used for scientific purposes. Approval was given by the responsible local authority, the Darmstadt governmental council for animal protection and handling (permit reference numbers V54-19c20/15-B2/360, permit date: 30 October 2013). Throughout this study all mice had access to water and food ad libitum.

4.2. Femoral Artery Ligation (FAL)

Twenty-eight male C57BL/6 mice (Charles River, Sulzfeld, Germany) and 40 male $ApoE^{-/-}$ mice were subjected to FAL as described [22]. The contralateral leg served as the reference. During the surgical procedure mice were kept on a heating plate with a temperature of 38 °C. Anesthesia was applied using ketamine (120 mg/kg BW) and xylazine (16 mg/kg BW) i.p.. For postoperative analgesia carprofen (5 mg/kg BW) was injected s.c.. After termination of experiments the mice were euthanized by an anesthetic overdose.

4.3. Forced Exercise on Treadmill

Mice were first accustomed by using a treadmill (Exer 3/6, Columbus Instruments, Columbus, OH, USA) with a motivation grid for 15 min/day. This applied small amounts of electric shock for conditioning when the mice stopped running.

After being conditioned, the mice started training at a light intensity with a preset speed of 0.2 m/s leading up to a maximum of 0.3 m/s with no further resistance. Training frequency was 2 times per day. Training was terminated at exhaustions. Exhaustion was defined as pause of more than 5 s at a time, or three times for two or more seconds on the shock pad without trying to get back on the treadmill.

4.4. Voluntary Running Wheels

To evaluate voluntary training each animal was individually housed in a cage equipped with a free-to-access running wheel. The running wheels were connected to a computer equipped with TSE PhenoMaster V5.1.6 (2014-4115) (TSE Systems GmbH, Bad Homburg, Germany). This setup gave accurate data on each animal, recording time and traveled distances and it allowed evaluation of activity patterns during an adaptation period as well as identifing post-surgery effects.

4.5. Restraining Cages

For simulating inactivity, mice were kept as a reference (control) group in smaller cages without the possibility to climb in order to minimize movement.

4.6. *Laser Doppler Perfusion Imaging (LDPI)*

Perfusion of the paws was recorded using the laser Doppler imaging device PIM3 (Perimed Instruments, Järfälla, Sweden; Software: LDPIwin for PIM3 3.1.3), on a heating plate at 38 °C, before FAL (d0 pre), immediately after FAL (d0 post), as well as at d3, d7, and d14 after FAL.

The mean perfusion was shown as the ratio of the ligated hind limb to the contralateral, non-ischemic hind limb.

4.7. *Histology*

Mice were perfused with 10 mL vasodilation buffer (100 μg adenosine, 1 μg sodium nitroprusside, 0.05% BSA in PBS, pH7.4) followed by 10 mL 4% PFA post mortem. Adductor muscles from ligated or sham-operated mice were harvested and placed in 15% sucrose in PBS for 4 h and overnight at 4 °C in 30% sucrose in PBS. Tissue was cryopreserved in Tissue-Tek O.C.T. (Sakura, Alphen aan den Rijn, The Netherlands) and cut in 8 μm cryosections. Morphometric analyses were performed using a hematoxylin-eosin stain to evaluate the dimensions of collateral arteries.

4.8. *Immunohistochemistry*

Cryosections were stained with blue-fluorescent DNA stain DAPI (4′,6-Diaminidino-2-phenyllindole-dilactate; Thermo Fisher Scientific, Waltham, MA, USA) and counterstained for αSMA-Cy3 (C6198, Sigma-Aldrich GmbH, Taufkirchen, Germany) or αSMA-FITC (F3777, Sigma-Aldrich GmbH, Taufkirchen, Germany) and CD68 (MCA1957A448T, AbD Serotec, BioRad, Feldkirchen, Germany).

4.9. *Statistical Analysis*

All statistical analyses were supported by GraphPad software PRISM5 for Mac (GraphPad Software, La Jolla, CA, USA), JMP for Mac (Version 9.0.12010 SAS Institute Inc., Heidelberg, Germany), Image J (National Institutes of Health, Bethesda, Maryland, USA) and Microsoft Excel for Mac (Version16.15, Microsoft, Redmond, Washington, USA). Comparisons between groups were based on unpaired student's t-test. One-way or two-way ANOVA were used to determine differences between the means of three or more independent groups as indicated. Data were reported as standard error of mean (SEM). Data deviations were considered to be statistically significant differences at $p < 0.05$.

5. Conclusions

Femoral artery ligated ApoE$^{-/-}$ mice on HFD with running wheel training is a suitable model to simulate exercise induced collateral growth. This experimental set-up may provide a model for investigating molecular training effects on arteriogenesis.

Author Contributions: A.B., K.T., and T.S.-R. designed the experiments. A.B., J.V., D.N. and K.T. interpreted the findings. A.B. and K.T. wrote the first draft of the manuscript. A.B and K.T. analyzed and performed experiments, A.B. performed statistical analyses; D.G., J.V., D.N., and T.S.-R. discussed the results and revised the manuscript. All authors edited and approved the manuscript.

Acknowledgments: The authors thank Christina Reschke and Brigitte Matzke for excellent technical assistance and Amir Kauveh Panah for proofreading the manuscript.

Abbreviations

PAD	Peripheral artery disease
CVD	Cardiovascular disease
ApoE$^{-/-}$	Apolipoprotein E knockout
FAL	Femoral artery ligation
HFD	High fat diet

References

1. Naci, H.; Ioannidis, J.P. Comparative effectiveness of exercise and drug interventions on mortality outcomes: Metaepidemiological study. *Br. J. Sports Med.* **2015**, *49*, 1414–1422. [CrossRef] [PubMed]
2. Lyu, X.; Li, S.; Peng, S.; Cai, H.; Liu, G.; Ran, X. Intensive walking exercise for lower extremity peripheral arterial disease: A systematic review and meta-analysis. *J. Diabetes* **2016**, *8*, 363–377. [CrossRef] [PubMed]
3. Gardner, A.W.; Montgomery, P.S.; Parker, D.E. Physical activity is a predictor of all-cause mortality in patients with intermittent claudication. *J. Vasc. Surg.* **2008**, *47*, 117–122. [CrossRef] [PubMed]
4. Aherne, T.; McHugh, S.; Kheirelseid, E.A.; Lee, M.J.; McCaffrey, N.; Moneley, D.; Leahy, A.L.; Naughton, P. Comparing Supervised Exercise Therapy to Invasive Measures in the Management of Symptomatic Peripheral Arterial Disease. *Surg. Res. Pract.* **2015**, *2015*, 960402. [CrossRef] [PubMed]
5. Larsen, O.A.; Lassen, N.A. Effect of daily muscular exercise in patients with intermittent claudication. *Lancet* **1966**, *2*, 1093–1096. [CrossRef]
6. Haas, T.L.L.P.; Yang, H.-T.; Terjung, R.L. Exercise Training and Peripheral Arterial Disease. *Compr. Physiol.* **2012**, *2*, 2933–3017. [CrossRef] [PubMed]
7. Niessner, A.; Richter, B.; Penka, M.; Steiner, S.; Strasser, B.; Ziegler, S.; Heeb-Elze, E.; Zorn, G.; Leitner-Heinschink, A.; Niessner, C.; et al. Endurance training reduces circulating inflammatory markers in persons at risk of coronary events: Impact on plaque stabilization? *Atherosclerosis* **2006**, *186*, 160–165. [CrossRef] [PubMed]
8. Timmerman, K.L.; Flynn, M.G.; Coen, P.M.; Markofski, M.M.; Pence, B.D. Exercise training-induced lowering of inflammatory (CD14+CD16+) monocytes: A role in the anti-inflammatory influence of exercise? *J. Leukoc. Biol.* **2008**, *84*, 1271–1278. [CrossRef] [PubMed]
9. Michishita, R.; Shono, N.; Inoue, T.; Tsuruta, T.; Node, K. Effect of exercise therapy on monocyte and neutrophil counts in overweight women. *Am. J. Med. Sci.* **2010**, *339*, 152–156. [PubMed]
10. Higashi, Y.; Sasaki, S.; Kurisu, S.; Yoshimizu, A.; Sasaki, N.; Matsuura, H.; Kajiyama, G.; Oshima, T. Regular aerobic exercise augments endothelium-dependent vascular relaxation in normotensive as well as hypertensive subjects: Role of endothelium-derived nitric oxide. *Circulation* **1999**, *100*, 1194–1202. [CrossRef]
11. Guerreiro, L.F.; Rocha, A.M.; Martins, C.N.; Ribeiro, J.P.; Wally, C.; Strieder, D.L.; Carissimi, C.G.; Oliveira, M.G.; Pereira, A.A.; Biondi, H.S.; et al. Oxidative status of the myocardium in response to different intensities of physical training. *Physiol. Res.* **2016**, *65*, 737–749. [PubMed]
12. Huonker, M.; Halle, M.; Keul, J. Structural and functional adaptations of the cardiovascular system by training. *Int. J. Sports Med.* **1996**, *17* (Suppl. 3), S164–S172. [CrossRef]
13. Nash, M.S.; Montalvo, B.M.; Applegate, B. Lower extremity blood flow and responses to occlusion ischemia differ in exercise-trained and sedentary tetraplegic persons. *Arch. Phys. Med. Rehabil.* **1996**, *77*, 1260–1265. [CrossRef]
14. Dopheide, J.F.; Rubrech, J.; Trumpp, A.; Geissler, P.; Zeller, G.C.; Schnorbus, B.; Schmidt, F.; Gori, T.; Münzel, T.; Espinola-Klein, C. Supervised exercise training in peripheral arterial disease increases vascular shear stress and profunda femoral artery diameter. *Eur. J. Prev. Cardiol.* **2017**, *24*, 178–191. [CrossRef] [PubMed]
15. Sayed, A.; Schierling, W.; Troidl, K.; Ruding, I.; Nelson, K.; Apfelbeck, H.; Benli, I.; Schaper, W.; Schmitz-Rixen, T. Exercise linked to transient increase in expression and activity of cation channels in newly formed hind-limb collaterals. European journal of vascular and endovascular surgery. *Eur. J. Soc. Vasc. Endovasc. Surg.* **2010**, *40*, 81–87. [CrossRef] [PubMed]
16. Heil, M.; Eitenmüller, I.; Schmitz-Rixen, T.; Schaper, W. Arteriogenesis versus angiogenesis: Similarities and differences. *J. Cell. Mol. Med.* **2006**, *10*, 45–55. [CrossRef] [PubMed]
17. Ben Driss, A.; Benessiano, J.; Poitevin, P.; Levy, B.I.; Michel, J.B. Arterial expansive remodeling induced by high flow rates. *Am. J. Physiol.* **1997**, *272*, H851–H858. [CrossRef]
18. Vogel, J.; Niederer, D.; Engeroff, T.; Vogt, L.; Troidl, C.; Schmitz-Rixen, T.; Banzer, W.; Troidl, K. Effects on the Profile of Circulating miRNAs after Single Bouts of Resistance Training with and without Blood Flow Restriction-A Three-Arm, Randomized Crossover Trial. *Int. J. Mol. Sci.* **2019**, *20*, 3249. [CrossRef]
19. Hendrikx, G.; Voo, S.; Bauwens, M.; Post, M.J.; Mottaghy, F.M. SPECT and PET imaging of angiogenesis and arteriogenesis in pre-clinical models of myocardial ischemia and peripheral vascular disease. *Eur. J. Nucl. Med. Mol. Imaging* **2016**, *43*, 2433–2447. [CrossRef]

20. Eitenmuller, I.; Volger, O.; Kluge, A.; Troidl, K.; Barancik, M.; Cai, W.J.; Heil, M.; Pipp, F.; Fischer, S.; Horrevoets, A.J.; et al. The range of adaptation by collateral vessels after femoral artery occlusion. *Circ. Res.* **2006**, *99*, 656–662. [CrossRef]
21. Lee-Young, R.S.; Griffee, S.R.; Lynes, S.E.; Bracy, D.P.; Ayala, J.E.; McGuinness, O.P.; Wasserman, D.H. Skeletal muscle AMP-activated protein kinase is essential for the metabolic response to exercise in vivo. *J. Biol. Chem.* **2009**, *284*, 23925–23934. [CrossRef] [PubMed]
22. Limbourg, A.; Korff, T.; Napp, L.C.; Schaper, W.; Drexler, H.; Limbourg, F.P. Evaluation of postnatal arteriogenesis and angiogenesis in a mouse model of hind-limb ischemia. *Nat. Protoc.* **2009**, *4*, 1737–1746. [CrossRef] [PubMed]
23. Baltgalvis, K.A.; White, K.; Li, W.; Claypool, M.D.; Lang, W.; Alcantara, R.; Singh, B.K.; Friera, A.M.; McLaughlin, J.; Hansen, D.; et al. Exercise performance and peripheral vascular insufficiency improve with AMPK activation in high-fat diet-fed mice. *Am. J. Physiol. Heart Circ. Physiol.* **2014**, *306*, H1128–H1145. [CrossRef] [PubMed]
24. Lo Sasso, G.; Schlage, W.K.; Boue, S.; Veljkovic, E.; Peitsch, M.C.; Hoeng, J. The Apoe(-/-) mouse model: A suitable model to study cardiovascular and respiratory diseases in the context of cigarette smoke exposure and harm reduction. *J. Trans. Med.* **2016**, *14*, 146. [CrossRef] [PubMed]
25. Schirmer, S.H.; Millenaar, D.N.; Werner, C.; Schuh, L.; Degen, A.; Bettink, S.I.; Lipp, P.; van Rooijen, N.; Meyer, T.; Böhm, M.; et al. Exercise promotes collateral artery growth mediated by monocytic nitric oxide. *Arterioscler. Thromb. Vasc. Biol.* **2015**, *35*, 1862–1871. [CrossRef] [PubMed]
26. Morgan, J.A.; Corrigan, F.; Baune, B.T. Effects of physical exercise on central nervous system functions: A review of brain region specific adaptations. *J. Mol. Psychiatry* **2015**, *3*, 3. [CrossRef] [PubMed]
27. Manzanares, G.; Brito-da-Silva, G.; Gandra, P.G. Voluntary wheel running: Patterns and physiological effects in mice. *Braz. J. Med. Biol. Res.* **2019**, *52*, e7830. [CrossRef] [PubMed]
28. Slattery, D.A.; Cryan, J.F. Using the rat forced swim test to assess antidepressant-like activity in rodents. *Nat. Protoc.* **2012**, *7*, 1009. [CrossRef]
29. Cook, M.D.; Martin, S.A.; Williams, C.; Whitlock, K.; Wallig, M.A.; Pence, B.D.; Woods, J.A. Forced treadmill exercise training exacerbates inflammation and causes mortality while voluntary wheel training is protective in a mouse model of colitis. *Brain Behav. Immun.* **2013**, *33*, 46–56. [CrossRef]
30. Gong, S.; Miao, Y.L.; Jiao, G.Z.; Sun, M.J.; Li, H.; Lin, J.; Luo, M.J.; Tan, J.H. Dynamics and correlation of serum cortisol and corticosterone under different physiological or stressful conditions in mice. *PLoS ONE* **2015**, *10*, e0117503. [CrossRef]
31. Billman, G.E.; Cagnoli, K.L.; Csepe, T.; Li, N.; Wright, P.; Mohler, P.J.; Fedorov, V.V. Exercise training-induced bradycardia: Evidence for enhanced parasympathetic regulation without changes in intrinsic sinoatrial node function. *J. Appl. Physiol. (1985)* **2015**, *118*, 1344–1355. [CrossRef] [PubMed]
32. Bartolomucci, A.; Palanza, P.; Costoli, T.; Savani, E.; Laviola, G.; Parmigiani, S.; Sgoifo, A. Chronic psychosocial stress persistently alters autonomic function and physical activity in mice. *Physiol. Behav.* **2003**, *80*, 57–67. [CrossRef]
33. Lakin, R.; Guzman, C.; Izaddoustdar, F.; Polidovitch, N.; Goodman, J.M.; Backx, P.H. Changes in Heart Rate and Its Regulation by the Autonomic Nervous System Do Not Differ Between Forced and Voluntary Exercise in Mice. *Front. Physiol.* **2018**, *9*, 841. [CrossRef] [PubMed]
34. Ziegler, M.A.; Distasi, M.R.; Bills, R.G.; Miller, S.J.; Alloosh, M.; Murphy, M.P.; Akingba, A.G.; Sturek, M.; Dalsing, M.C.; Unthank, J.L. Marvels, mysteries, and misconceptions of vascular compensation to peripheral artery occlusion. *Microcirculation* **2010**, *17*, 3–20. [CrossRef] [PubMed]
35. Leeper, N.J.; Myers, J.; Zhou, M.; Nead, K.T.; Syed, A.; Kojima, Y.; Caceres, R.D.; Cooke, J.P. Exercise capacity is the strongest predictor of mortality in patients with peripheral arterial disease. *J. Vasc. Surg.* **2013**, *57*, 728–733. [CrossRef] [PubMed]
36. Dragneva, G.; Korpisalo, P.; Yla-Herttuala, S. Promoting blood vessel growth in ischemic diseases: Challenges in translating preclinical potential into clinical success. *Dis. Model. Mech.* **2013**, *6*, 312–322. [CrossRef] [PubMed]
37. Berger, J.S.; Hochman, J.; Lobach, I.; Adelman, M.A.; Riles, T.S.; Rockman, C.B. Modifiable risk factor burden and the prevalence of peripheral artery disease in different vascular territories. *J. Vasc. Surg.* **2013**, *58*, 673.e1–681.e1. [CrossRef] [PubMed]

38. Goh, J.; Ladiges, W. Voluntary Wheel Running in Mice. *Curr. Protoc. Mouse Biol.* **2015**, *5*, 283–290. [CrossRef] [PubMed]
39. Heil, M.; Schaper, W. Influence of mechanical, cellular, and molecular factors on collateral artery growth (arteriogenesis). *Circ. Res.* **2004**, *95*, 449–458. [CrossRef] [PubMed]
40. Troidl, C.; Jung, G.; Troidl, K.; Hoffmann, J.; Mollmann, H.; Nef, H.; Schaper, W.; Hamm, C.W.; Schmitz-Rixen, T. The temporal and spatial distribution of macrophage subpopulations during arteriogenesis. *Curr. Vasc. Pharmacol.* **2013**, *11*, 5–12. [CrossRef]
41. van Royen, N.; Piek, J.J.; Buschmann, I.; Hoefer, I.; Voskuil, M.; Schaper, W. Stimulation of arteriogenesis; a new concept for the treatment of arterial occlusive disease. *Cardiovasc. Res.* **2001**, *49*, 543–553. [CrossRef]

13

Local Mast Cell Activation Promotes Neovascularization

Ilze Bot [1], Daniël van der Velden [1], Merel Bouwman [1,2,3], Mara J. Kröner [1], Johan Kuiper [1], Paul H. A. Quax [2,3] and Margreet R. de Vries [2,3,*]

1 Division of BioTherapeutics, Leiden Academic Centre for Drug Research, Leiden University, 2333CC Leiden, The Netherlands; i.bot@lacdr.leidenuniv.nl (I.B.); daniel.vandervelden@hu.nl (D.v.d.V.); merel_bouwman@hotmail.com (M.B.); marakroner@hotmail.com (M.J.K.); j.kuiper@lacdr.leidenuniv.nl (J.K.)

2 Department of Surgery, Leiden University Medical Center, 2300RC Leiden, The Netherlands; p.h.a.quax@lumc.nl

3 Einthoven Laboratory for Experimental Vascular Medicine, Leiden University Medical Center, 2300RC Leiden, The Netherlands

* Correspondence: m.r.de_vries@lumc.nl

Abstract: Mast cells have been associated with arteriogenesis and collateral formation. In advanced human atherosclerotic plaques, mast cells have been shown to colocalize with plaque neovessels, and mast cells have also been associated with tumor vascularization. Based on these associations, we hypothesize that mast cells promote angiogenesis during ischemia. In human ischemic muscle tissue from patients with end-stage peripheral artery disease, we observed activated mast cells, predominantly located around capillaries. Also, in mouse ischemic muscles, mast cells were detected during the revascularization process and interestingly, mast cell activation status was enhanced up to 10 days after ischemia induction. To determine whether mast cells contribute to both arteriogenesis and angiogenesis, mast cells were locally activated immediately upon hind limb ischemia in C57Bl/6 mice. At day 9, we observed a 3-fold increase in activated mast cell numbers in the inguinal lymph nodes. This was accompanied by an increase in the amount of Ly6C^{high} inflammatory monocytes. Interestingly, local mast cell activation increased blood flow through the hind limb (46% at day 9) compared to that in non-activated control mice. Histological analysis of the muscle tissue revealed that mast cell activation did not affect the number of collaterals, but increased the collateral diameter, as well as the number of CD31^{+} capillaries. Together, these data illustrate that locally activated mast cell contribute to arteriogenesis and angiogenesis.

Keywords: arteriogenesis; angiogenesis; innate immunity; mast cell

---

1. Introduction

The mast cell, part of the innate immune system, generally resides in tissues such as the lung and the skin to protect against pathogens like bacteria and parasites. Mast cells have also been described to participate in diseases such as asthma, allergies, and rheumatoid arthritis. Over the last decades, the mast cell has been implicated in cardiovascular diseases as well, for example in atherosclerosis [1,2], the underlying pathology of acute cardiovascular diseases including peripheral artery disease (PAD) [3,4]. Interestingly, mast cell numbers in advanced human atherosclerotic plaques obtained after endarterectomy surgery were seen to be of predictive value for the incidence of a secondary cardiovascular event [5]. In those plaques, mast cell density associated with the number of CD31^{+} microvessels [5]. Mast cells have also been associated with arteriogenesis and collateral formation [6]. Mast cells can secrete growth factors and pro-inflammatory cytokines that can recruit immune cells such as neutrophils and monocytes to the site of inflammation, thus further enhancing a pro-inflammatory response [6–8]. Patients with systemic mastocytosis, a disease that is characterized by the excessive accumulation of mast cells in tissue or organs, experienced an increased prevalence of cardiovascular disease events, such as myocardial infarction, stroke, and importantly, peripheral artery disease, which is actually caused by the development of atherosclerosis in the arteries that supply oxygen to the extremities [9]. These associative data suggest that the mast cell may actively contribute to these underlying pathologies, and preclinical studies have been performed to elucidate underlying mast cell pathways that are causally related to vascular remodeling and the related disease outcome.

We speculate that mast cells may affect atherosclerotic plaque progression and PAD by increasing angiogenesis. Plaque angiogenesis has been shown to be related to atherosclerotic plaque progression and also, during tumor development, mast cells have been implicated in angiogenesis [10]. Mast cells have been shown to induce tumor endothelial proliferation by the release of Vascular Endothelial Growth Factor (VEGF) in response to the hypoxic environment in the tumor [10], which may be translatable to muscles in PAD patients, in which hypoxia occurs as well [11,12]. Although induction of neovascularization, in particular angiogenesis, maybe unfavorable for atherosclerosis progression, in PAD, the induction of neovascularization by mast cells, more precisely by inducing collateral formation and angiogenesis, may act as a repair pathway to resupply the ischemic limb tissue with oxygen. This neovascularization process requires a pro-inflammatory response, which is thus, on one hand, beneficial to resolve ischemia, but may on the other hand lead to enhanced progression of atherosclerosis. This two-faced process is also known as the Janus phenomenon [13]. Recently, the contribution of mast cells to arteriogenesis and collateral formation in a shear-stress induced mouse model of hind limb ischemia (HLI) has been described by Chillo and colleagues [6]. In that study, mast cells were systemically activated with the mast cell activator compound 48/80 upon ligation of the femoral artery, which resulted in increased hind limb perfusion. Treatment with the mast cell stabilizer cromolyn prevented the mast cell-induced effects on arteriogenesis and the investigators identified the neutrophil as a prominent effector cell involved in the mechanism behind mast cell-induced arteriogenesis. However, in that study, mast cell activation-dependent effects on angiogenesis in the ischemic muscles were not reported.

In this study, we aimed to investigate whether local induction of mast cell activation can stimulate blood flow recovery in a mouse hind limb ischemia model by inducing angiogenesis as well as arteriogenesis.

First, we analyzed the number and activation status of mast cells in human ischemic tissue, obtained after limb amputation. Next, we induced hind limb ischemia in mice by ligation of the femoral artery and at time of ligation, we activated mast cells in the hind limb by a skin sensitization/challenge protocol using a pluronic gel to apply the hapten DNP locally at the ligation site as described before [7,14], after which blood perfusion was measured using laser Doppler imaging. Mast cell activation increased reperfusion of the hind limb by not only increasing arteriogenesis, but also angiogenesis, which is at least partly induced by increasing the pro-inflammatory monocyte response.

2. Materials and Methods

2.1. Tissue Collection from Patients with End-Stage Peripheral Artery Disease

Sample collection of tissues from patients with end-stage peripheral artery disease undergoing limb amputation was approved by the Medical Ethics Committee of the Leiden University Medical Center (Protocol No. P12.265). Written informed consent was obtained from the participants. Inclusion criteria were a minimum age of 18 years and lower limb amputation, excluding ankle, foot, or toe amputations. Exclusion criteria were suspected or confirmed malignancy and inability to give informed consent. Gastrocnemius and soleus muscle samples obtained from 15 patients were formalin fixed, processed, paraffin embedded sectioned, and stained for mast cells. From these patients, $n = 1$ had type I diabetes and $n = 7$ suffered from type II diabetes.

2.2. *Hind Limb Ischemia Model*

This study was performed in accordance with the Directive 2010/63/EU of the European Parliament and Dutch government guidelines. All experiments were approved (reference number 14185) by the Leiden University and Leiden University Medical Center committee on animal welfare (Leiden, the Netherlands). Wild-type C57Bl/6J mice were bred in our in-house breeding facility. Male mice aged 8 to 12 weeks were housed in groups with free access to water and regular chow.

Before the unilateral hind limb ischemia, mice were anesthetized by i.p. injection of midazolam (8 mg/kg, Roche Diagnostics, Basel, Switzerland), medetomidine (0.4 mg/kg, Orion, Espoo, Finland), and fentanyl (0.08 mg/kg, Janssen Pharmaceuticals, Beerse, Belgium). Hind limb ischemia was induced by electrocoagulation on two locations of the left femoral artery; the first ligation proximal to the superficial epigastric artery and the second proximal to the bifurcation of the popliteal and saphenous artery [15,16]. After surgery, anesthesia was antagonized with with atipamezol (2.5 mg/kg, Orion, Espoo, Finland) and flumazenil (0.5 mg/kg, Fresenius Kabi, Bad Homburg vor der Höhe, Germany).and buprenorphine (0.1 mg/kg, MSD Animal Health, Keniworth, NJ, USA) was provided as a painkiller. For the time course, 5 mice per time point were used, whereas for both the long-term (t28) and short-term (t9) HLI experiments, 8–9 mice per group were used.

2.3. *Local Mast Cell Activation with DPN treatment*

Mice were skin-sensitized on the shaved abdomen and paws for 2 consecutive days with a dinitrofluorobenzene (DNFB (D1529) solution (0.5% *v*/*v* in acetone:olive oil (4:1), Sigma-Aldrich, St. Louis, MO, USA) as described previously to sensitize the mice for the hapten DNP [7,14]. In the control mice, a vehicle solution of acetone:olive oil (4:1) was applied. At the end of the hind limb ischemia procedure, which was scheduled one week after the skin-sensitization procedure, 50 μg dinitrophenyl hapten (DNP (D198501), Sigma-Aldrich, St. Louis, MO, USA) in a pluronic gel (25% *w*/*v*, Sigma-Aldrich, St. Louis, MO, USA) was applied around the ligated areas of the left hind limb to locally activate the mast cells. Empty pluronic gel was applied in the control mice. This model has been previously applied [7,14,17,18] and has been shown to specifically induce mast cells activation upon local hapten application.

2.4. *Laser Doppler Perfusion Measurements*

Before and directly after surgery and at 3, 7,10, 14, 21, and 28 days after surgery, blood flow recovery to the ligated hind limb and the unligated control paw were measured using Laser Doppler Perfusion Imaging (LDPI) (Moor Instruments, Axminster, UK). Before the LDPI measurements, mice were anesthetized by i.p. injection of midazolam (8 mg/kg) and medetomidine (0.4 mg/kg,). Next, mice were placed in a double glazed pot, perfused with water at 37 °C for 5 min [19]. After LDPI, anesthesia was antagonized by subcutaneous injection of flumazenil (0.7 mg/kg). LDPI measurements in the ligated paw were normalized to measurements of the unligated paw, as an internal control. At sacrifice, after the last LDPI measurement, analgesic fentanyl (0.08 mg/kg) was administered, blood was drawn, and mice were sacrificed via cervical dislocation. The adductor and soleus muscles were harvested and fixed in 4% formaldehyde. For a second short experiment, animals were sacrificed at day 9, where blood was collected by orbital bleeding and the inguinal lymph nodes were isolated for further analyses. Again, the adductor and soleus muscles were harvested and fixed in 4% formaldehyde for histology analysis.

2.5. *Immunohistochemistry*

Mast cells were visualized by staining using a naphthol AS-D chloroacetate esterase staining kit (#91C, Sigma-Aldrich, St. Louis, MO, USA) and counted manually. A mast cell was considered resting when all granula were maintained inside the cell, while mast cells were assessed as activated when granula were deposited in the tissue surrounding the mast cell (examples are shown in Figure 1A).

Tissue size was quantified by the Leica image analysis system (Leica Ltd., Cambridge, UK). Paraffin embedded adductor and soleus muscle were stained with alpha smooth muscle actin (aSMA) (1A4, DAKO, Glostrup, Denmark) to visualize smooth muscle cell positive collaterals. Soleus muscles were stained for capillaries using CD31 (Sc-1506, Santa Cruz, Dallas, TX, USA) and macrophages using MAC3 (550292, BD-Pharmingen, Franklin Lakes, NJ, USA) together with aSMA and DAPI (Sigma, Santa Clara, CA, USA) as nuclear staining. For each antibody, negative controls were included using specific isotype-matched antibodies. The Pannoramic MIDI digital slide scanner (3DHistech, Budapest, Hungary) was used to create high-resolution images of the muscles. Snapshots (9 representative images per muscle) were taken using the caseviewer software (3DHistech) with a 40× magnification. aSMA positive collaterals were analyzed by counting the number of collaterals and measuring the diameters of each collateral with a visible lumen to determine arteriogenesis. CD31 positive capillaries and the number of MAC3 positive macrophages were quantified. All quantifications were performed using FIJI Image J image analysis software (ImageJ, Bethesda, MD, USA).

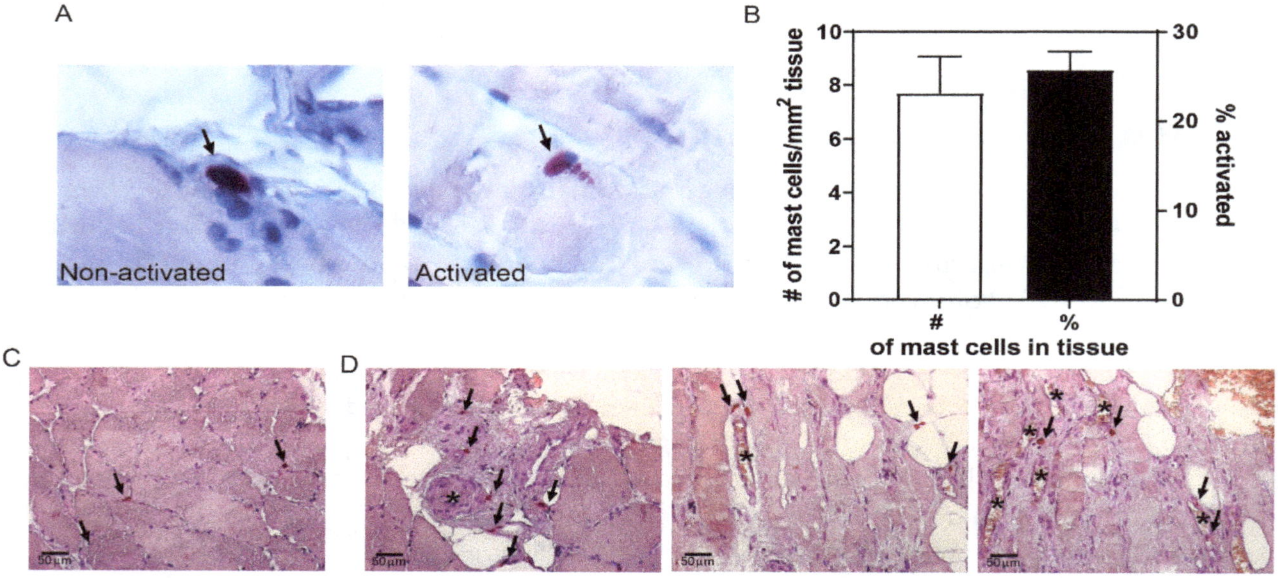

Figure 1. Mast cells in calf muscles of patients with peripheral artery disease. (**A**) Representative high-magnification image of a non-activated (left) and activated (right) mast cell, stained using a chloro-acetate esterase (CAE) staining and indicated by arrows. The non-activated mast cell shows the pink granula in the cytoplasm of the cell, whereas the pink granula are being released in the surroundings of the activated mast cell. (**B**) Quantification of the number of mast cells/mm^2 tissue, and the percentage of activated mast cells observed (n = 15). (**C**) Overview of a chloro-acetate esterase (CAE) staining of muscle tissue showing mast cells in pink (indicate by arrows) in between muscle fibers. (**D**) Representative overview images of mast cells surrounding microvessels (indicated by *) in human calf muscle tissue.

2.6. FACS Analysis

Blood was collected at sacrifice, after which red blood cells were lysed using an erythrocyte lysis buffer (0.1 mM EDTA, 10 mM $NaHCO_3$, 1 mM NH_4Cl, pH = 7.2). Subsequently, white blood cells were stained with the antibodies for flow cytometric analysis. Inguinal lymph nodes were harvested from all mice and processed through a 70 μm cell strainer to acquire single cell suspensions. Subsequently, the cell suspensions were stained for flow cytometry. In approximation, 200,000 cells per sample were stained with antibodies against extracellular proteins at a concentration of 0.1 μg/sample for 30 min as described previously [20,21]. All flow cytometry experiments were executed on a FACS Canto II (BDBiosciences, San Jose, CA, USA) and data were analyzed using FlowJo software (v10, BDBiosciences).

2.7. Statistical Analysis

Results are presented as mean ± standard error of the mean (SEM). A 2-tailed Student's t-test was used to compare individual groups. Non-Gaussian distributed data were analyzed using a 2-tailed Mann–Whitney U test. p-values < 0.05 were considered statistically significant and are indicated with *; p-values < 0.01 and < 0.001 are indicated by ** and ***, respectively.

3. Results

3.1. Mast Cells Localization in Calf Muscles of Peripheral Artery Disease Patients

To assess mast cell presence and its activation status in calf muscles of peripheral artery disease patients, we stained sections of ischemic muscle biopsies obtained after amputation surgery with a CAE staining and quantified the number of mast cells. On average, we detected 7.7 ± 1.4 mast cells/mm^2 tissue, of which 26 ± 2% was activated (Figure 1B). As shown in Figure 1C, mast cells, primarily non-activated, can be detected between the muscle fibers. Interestingly, mast cells, and in particular activated ones, generally appeared to colocalize with blood vessels in the muscle tissue (representative overview images in Figure 1D). The amount of mast cells in muscle tissue did not differ between patients that suffered from type I or II diabetes vs. patients that did not (7.5 ± 2.0 mast cells/mm^2 vs. 7.4 ± 2.1 mast cells/mm^2, respectively). Also, mast cell activation status in the muscle tissue was not affected by presence of diabetes (DM: 24.1 ± 2.3% vs. non-DM: 29.9 ± 3.1%).

3.2. Activation of Mast Cells upon Ischemia in a Murine Hindlimb Ischemia Model

To study whether mast cells accumulate in the murine muscle tissue upon hind limb ischemia, we quantified mast cell number and its activation status in adductor muscle tissue at 0, 7, 10, 21, and 28 days after the induction of hind limb ischemia. Similar to the human tissue, in murine muscles, mast cells were located in between muscle fibers and near blood vessels (Figure 2A). As the overall number of mast cells in this ischemic muscle tissue was relatively low, we included overview images of different locations in tissue to illustrate where mast cells reside (Figure 2A) Mast cell density, i.e., the number of mast cells per mm^2 tissue, did not change during the time-course of the experiment (Figure 2B), but mast cell activation status increased upon the induction of ischemia, in particular during the initial phase from day 0 up to day 10 (Figure 2C).

At day 7, a 33% increase in activated mast cells was observed compared to the percentage of activated mast cells at day 0, which further rose to a maximum of a 54% increase at 10 days after HLI. The number of activated mast cells then declined at 21 and 28 days to the level control (day 0; non-surgery) muscles (Figure 2B). Interestingly, most of these activated mast cells, as indicated by granules that reside outside the cell, were found in close proximity of capillaries in the muscle tissues (Figure 2A, lower panels) suggesting a direct relation between blood vessels and mast cells as we have shown previously in atherosclerosis [5].

3.3. Effect of Local Mast Cell Activation on Post Ischemic Blood Flow Recovery.

To study the effects of local mast cell activation on blood flow recovery, we applied the hapten DNP as part of our mast cell activation protocol on the gastrocnemius and adductor muscles directly after the hind limb ischemia procedure. We studied the subsequent blood flow recovery starting with eight mice per group, however between surgery and day 3, two mice in the DNP group and three mice in the control group had to be sacrificed because they reached humane end points. At day 10, a significant 44% increase in paw perfusion could be observed in the DNP treated group (left/right ratio of 0.70 ± 0.07) in comparison to the vehicle treated control group (left/right ratio of 0.49 ± 0.04). The enhanced increase in blood flow perfusion continued until the end of the experiment with significant differences between the groups at day 21 and day 28 (Figure 3A). We repeated the experiment, focusing on the early stage of blood flow recovery by sacrificing the mice at day 9 (short-term experiment). The experiment was started with nine mice per group; one mouse in the control and two mice in the DNP group reached the humane end point and were not included in the analysis. Similar to the t28 experiment, we observed an increase in paw perfusion in the DNP group at the day 9 time point of 46% (DNP: 0.66 ± 0.02 vs. control: 0.45 ± 0.05, Figure 3B).

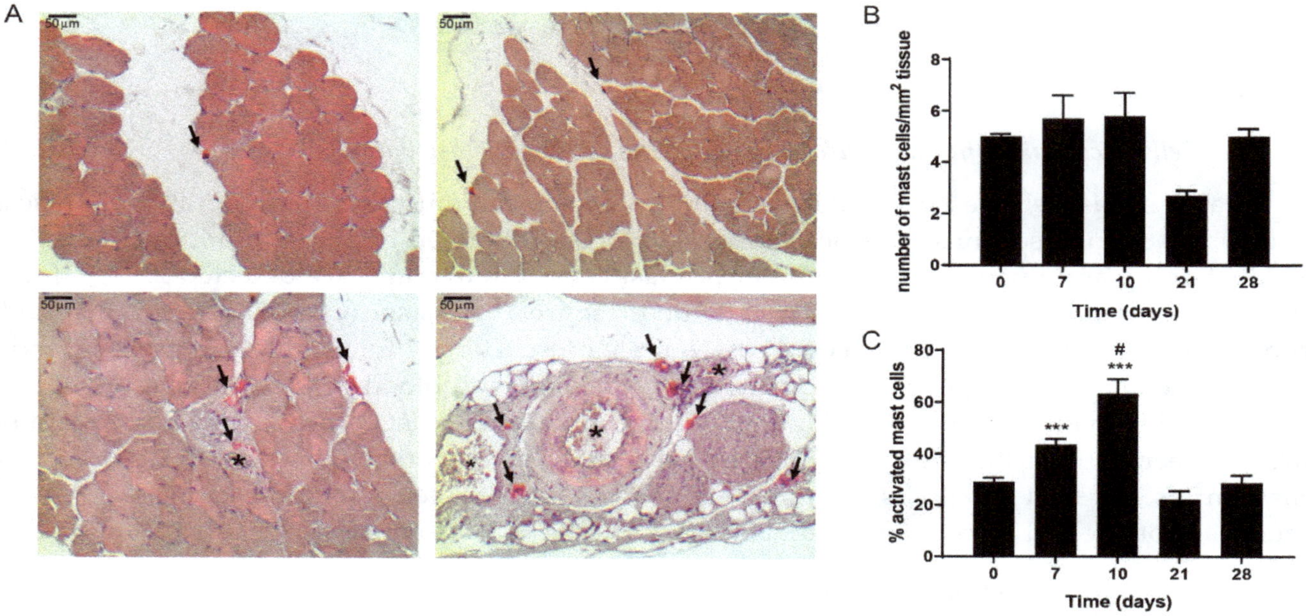

Figure 2. Mast cells in hind limb muscle tissue during ischemia in mice. (**A**) Representative images of mast cells in pink (CAE staining, indicated by arrows) in mouse ischemic muscle tissue (upper panels) and in close proximity to blood vessels (lower panels, indicated by *). (**B**) Mast cell density and (**C**) the percentage of activated mast cells in the hind limb muscle during recovery after ischemia. p-values of < 0.001 in comparison to t0 are indicated by *** p-value of < 0.05 in comparison to t7 is indicated by #.

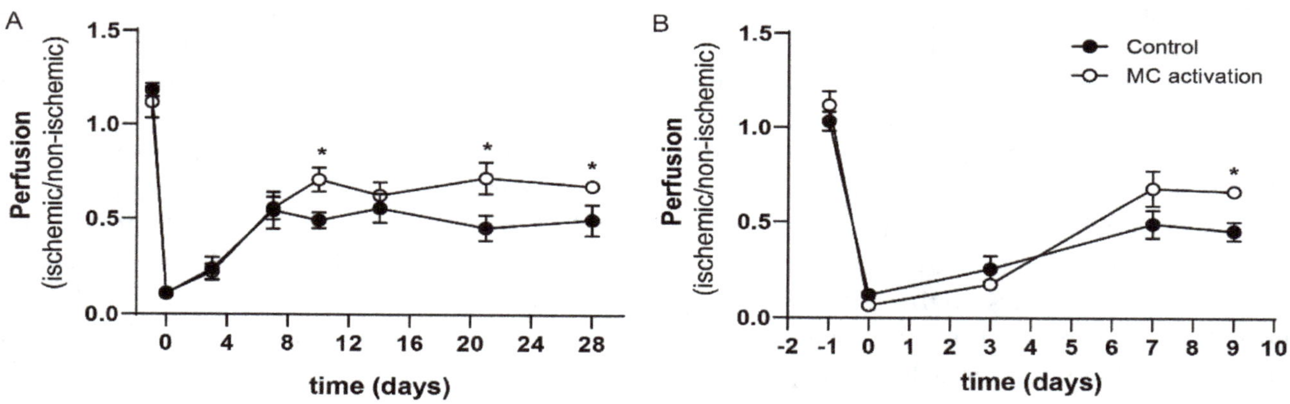

Figure 3. Perfusion of the ischemic hind limb in mast cell (MC) activated vs. control mice. Perfusion (ischemic/non-ischemic) as measured by Laser Doppler Perfusion Imaging (LDPI) from day 0 to day 28 in the long-term experiment (**A**) and in the short-term experiment from day 0 up to day 9 (**B**) after ligation of the femoral artery. * p-value of < 0.05 between the groups.

3.4. Local Mast Cell Activation Induced by DNP

We studied to what extent mast cell number and activation status were still affected after the single treatment with DNP of the ischemic hind limb. At nine days after ligation, the number of mast cell observed in the ligated and non-ligated adductor muscles were comparable (Figure 4A). In the ligated adductor muscles, the number of activated mast cells still tended to be increased at nine days after DNP treatment ($p = 0.11$), an effect that was lost at 28 days after ligation. In the soleus muscle of the DNP groups, both total mast cell numbers as well as the number of activated mast cells was still somewhat increased at nine days after ligation as compared to the controls (Figure 4B,C). Representative images of soleus muscle tissue are shown in Figure 4D.

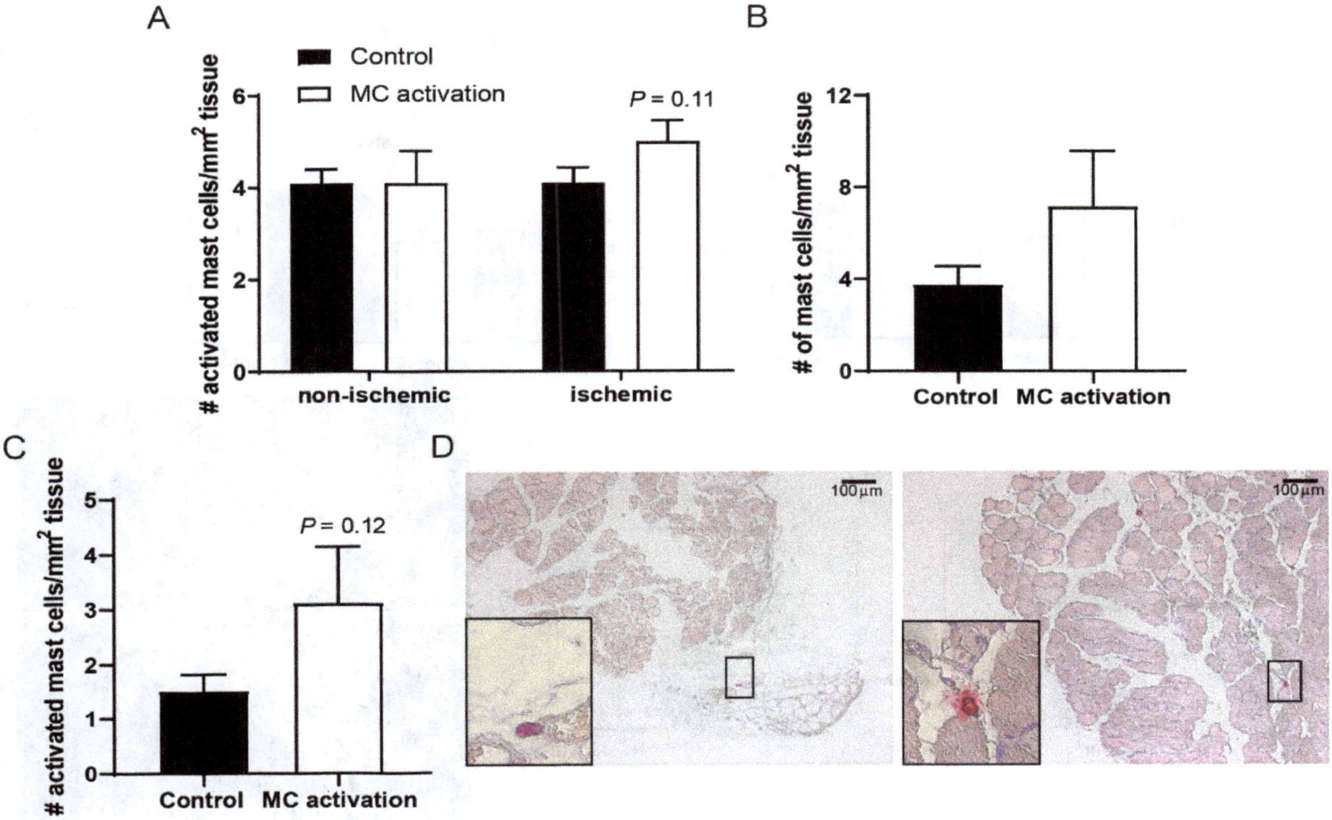

Figure 4. Activated mast cell numbers in muscle tissue of the ischemic hind limb. (**A**) The number of activated mast cells as measured by histology in the ischemic vs. non-ischemic adductor muscles of mice in which mast cells were activated compared to control mice at day 9 after the induction of ischemia. (**B**) Total mast cell numbers per mm^2 of ischemic soleus muscle tissue. (**C**) Number of activated mast cells per mm^2 of soleus muscle tissue at day 9 after ligation. (**D**) Representative overview images of the soleus muscles with a resting (control, left) and an activated mast cell (dinitrophenyl hapten, DNP, right) in high-magnification inserts.

Mast cell activation did not result in muscle hypertrophy, analyzed in both the ischemic and non-ischemic adductor muscles of the control and DNP-group at day 9 and day 28 after femoral artery ligation (data not shown).

3.5. Contribution of Arteriogenesis to the Increase in Blood Flow Recovery by Activated Mast Cells

Since restoration of blood flow recovery is a combination of shear stress induced arteriogenesis and ischemia induced angiogenesis [22], we studied these processes in the adductor muscle upstream of the ligation and in the soleus muscle, the ischemic region downstream of the ligation. Increased shear stress upstream of the ligation leads to arterialization of collaterals in the adductor muscle. At day 28, the number of collaterals did not differ between the ischemic and the non-ischemic adductor muscles in both the control and DNP treated group, nor did the number of collaterals differ between the control and DNP treated group (control: non-ischemic 32.7 ± 1.8, ischemic 28.7 ± 1.8, DNP: non-ischemic 34.6 ± 3.4, ischemic 32.2 ± 1.5). No differences in collateral numbers after ligation is frequently observed in hind limb ischemia studies since the pre-existing collaterals predominantly increase in size upon shear stress. Therefore, we also analyzed the surface area of the collaterals. The area of the collaterals in the ischemic muscles of the DNP treated mice was slightly increased compared to control mice (control: 318.4 ± 12.5 µm^2 vs. DNP: 381.2 ± 42.5 µm^2, $p = 0.205$) (Figure 5A). Also, the area of the collaterals in the non-ischemic vs. the ischemic hind limbs expressed as the ratio collateral area was somewhat increased between the control and DNP treated mice, but did not reach significance (control: 1.420±0.1 vs. DNP: 1.611 ± 0.2, $p = 0.509$).

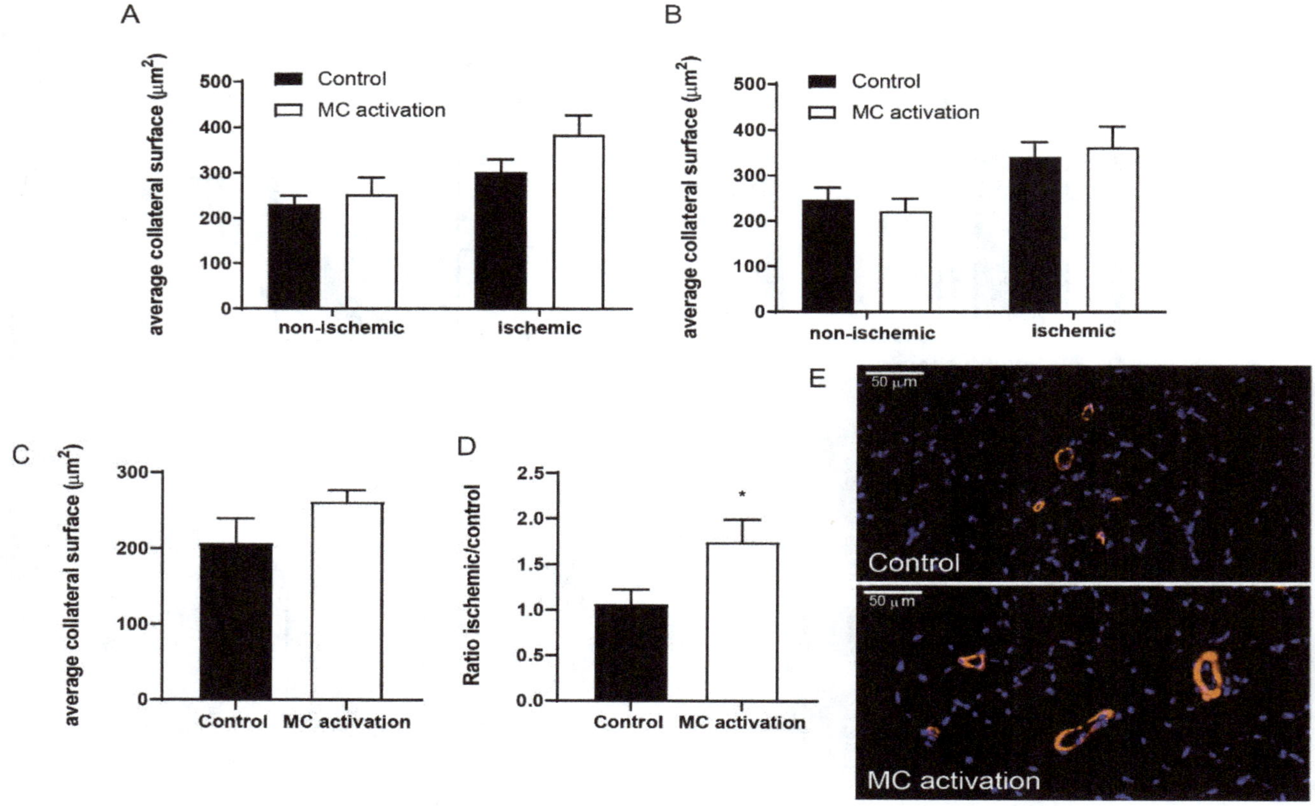

Figure 5. Arteriogenesis upon mast cell activation in the ischemic hind limb. The average collateral surface area in ischemic as compared to non-ischemic adductor muscles of mice in which mast cells were activated compared to controls at (**A**) 28 days after ligation and (**B**) 9 days after ligation. (**C**) The average collateral surface area in the soleus muscle of mice in which mast cells were activated compared to controls. (**D**) The collateral area ratio between ischemic and non-ischemic soleus muscles in mast cell activated compared to control mice at nine days after femoral artery ligation. (**E**). Representative pictures of smooth muscle cell actin positive collaterals in orange and nuclei in blue (DAPI) in both a control muscle and a muscle in which mast cells were activated. * $p < 0.05$.

In the short-term experiment with sacrifice at day 9, the number of collaterals also did not differ between the ischemic and the non-ischemic adductor muscles in both the control and DNP treated group, nor did the number of collaterals between the control and DNP treated group (control: Non-ischemic 27.3 ± 1.8, ischemic 30.7 ± 1.5, DNP: Non-ischemic 29.0 ± 1.8, ischemic 27.3 ± 1.8). Furthermore, no differences could be observed in collateral area in the ligated hind limbs between the control and DNP treated mice at day 9 (control 340.2 ± 29.2 μm^2 vs. DNP 362.1 ± 45.5 μm^2, $p = 0.680$) (Figure 5B) nor in the collateral area ratio (control 1.557 ± 0.3 vs. DNP 1.749 ± 0.3, $p = 0.633$).

In the downstream area of the ligation, the distal end of the collaterals in the soleus muscle are also exposed to increased shear stress. Comparable to the adductor muscle, the number of collaterals in the soleus muscle did not differ between the groups with or without ischemia at day 9 (control: Non-ischemic 23.8 ± 2.1, ischemic 26.3 ± 1.7, DNP: Non-ischemic 25.2 ± 2.0, ischemic 23.9 ± 1.9). A non-significant increase in soleus muscle collateral area could be observed in the ligated hind limbs of the DNP treated mice compared to the control mice (control 207.4 ± 31.7 μm^2 vs. DNP 261.7 ± 14.8 μm^2, $p = 0.163$) (Figure 5C). Interestingly, the collateral area ratio of the ischemic vs. the non-ischemic soleus of the individual mice was significantly increased in the DNP group vs. the control group (Control:

1.070 ± 0.2 vs. DNP: 1.751 ± 0.2, $p = 0.026$) (Figure 5D), suggesting that local mast cell activation does increase collateral diameter downstream of the ligation.

3.6. Effects of Mast Cell Activation on Angiogenesis

As a measure for the angiogenic response, CD31 positive capillaries were quantified in the right non-ischemic and the left ischemic soleus muscles. Local mast cell activation resulted in an increased number of angiogenic capillaries in the ischemic soleus muscles (Figure 6A). Quantification revealed a 66% significant increase in the number of capillaries (control: 211 ± 31 vs. DNP: 351 ± 55 μm^2, $p = 0.039$, Figure 6B), whereas in the control non-ischemic muscles, no significant difference in the number of capillaries were observed (control 176 ± 15 vs. DNP 196 ± 40 μm^2).

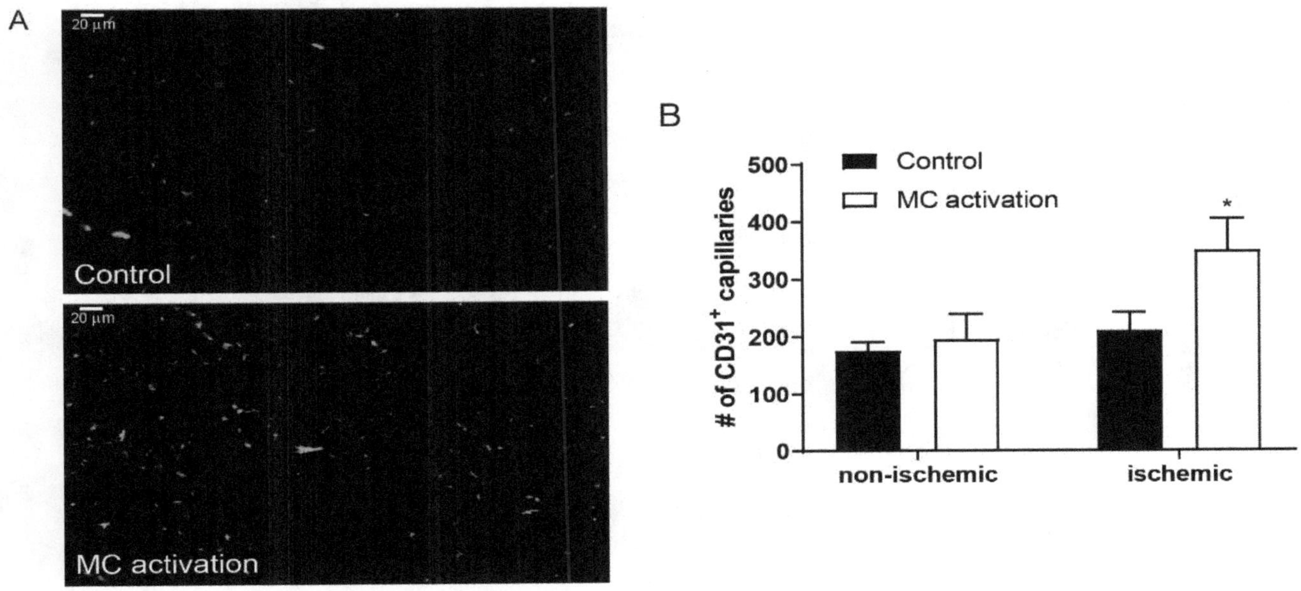

Figure 6. Activated mast cells induce angiogenesis in the ischemic hind limb. (**A**) CD31 staining of the ischemic soleus muscles shows the presence of $CD31^+$ capillaries in control mice and in mice in which mast cells were activated. (**B**) Quantification of the number of $CD31^+$ capillaries in non-ischemic and ischemic soleus muscle with (white bars) or without local (black bars) mast cell activation, measured at nine days after femoral artery ligation. $^*p < 0.05$.

3.7. Local Mast Cell Activation Induces a Pro-Inflammatory Monocyte Response

To determine whether local mast cell activation induced a pro-inflammatory response in the hind limb, we analyzed the inguinal lymph nodes draining from the hind limbs in which mast cells were activated at day 9 after ligation. To do so, we measured the number of $CD117^+Fc\varepsilon R^+$ cells and analyzed CD63 as a common mast cell activation marker. Interestingly, mast cells numbers were highly increased in the DNP group (Figure 7A), similarly to the number of activated mast cells (Figure 7B), which suggests that mast cells have drained from the muscle tissue to the lymph nodes. The number of $CD11b^+Ly6G^{high}$ neutrophils in the lymph nodes did not differ between the groups (Figure 7C), nor did the amount of T- and B-cells (data not shown). The number of $CD11b^+Ly6G^{low}$ monocytes in the draining lymph nodes was significantly increased upon mast cell activation (Figure 7D), which was due to an increase in both the $Ly6C^{low/mid}$ and the $Ly6C^{high}$ monocytes (Figure 7E,F). In the circulation, neutrophil and total monocyte numbers were not affected (Figure 7G,H), however within the monocyte population, the relative amount of inflammatory $Ly6C^{high}$ monocytes was significantly increased (Figure 7I). We also measured plasma IL-6 and CCL2 levels as markers of a systemic inflammatory response at 9 days after ligation but were unable to detect any differences between the control mice and those in which mast cells were locally activated (data not shown). To further investigate the local effect of mast cell activation on the pro-inflammatory response in the ischemic tissue, we used a MAC3 staining to quantify the number of macrophages present. Here, in contrast to the number of inflammatory monocytes in the draining lymph nodes, no effect on the macrophage numbers in the ischemic soleus muscles was observed at day 9 (control: 14.1 ± 3.2 vs. DNP 8.1 ± 1.8, $p = 0.141$, Figure 7J,K).

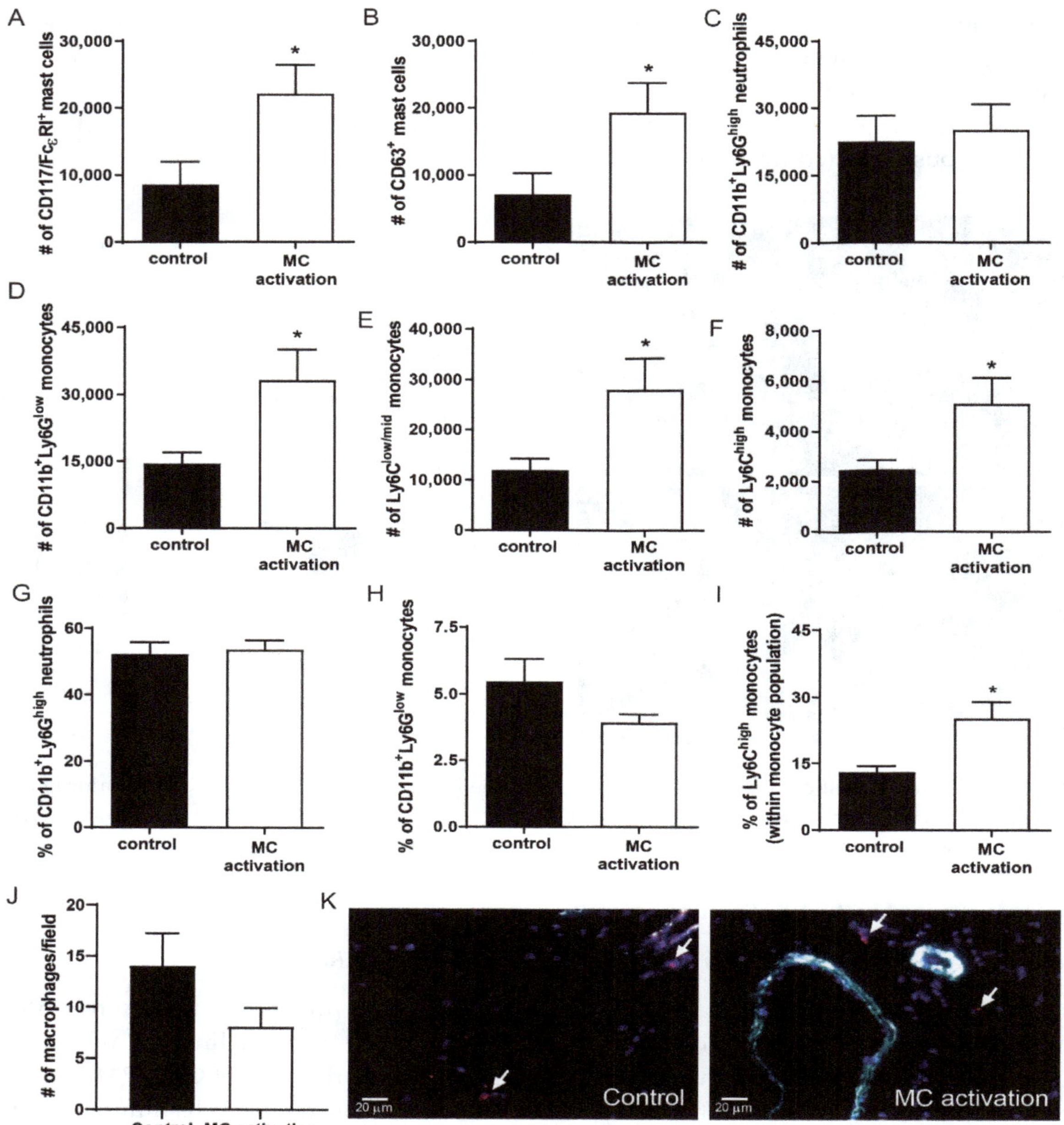

Figure 7. Inflammatory cell analysis in the ischemic hind limb at nine days after ischemia induction. (**A**) Total $CD117^+Fc\varepsilon RI^+$ mast cell numbers and (**B**) the number of $CD63^+$ activated mast cells were measured in the inguinal lymph node (iLN) draining from the ischemic hind limb of mice in the DNP-group and the controls using flow cytometry. (**C**) The number of $CD11b^+Ly6C^{high}$ neutrophils in the iLN. (**D**) The number of $CD11b^+Ly6G^{low}$ monocytes of which, (**E**) $Ly6C^{low/mid}$ and (**F**) $Ly6C^{high}$ monocytes. (**G**) Percentage of neutrophils, (**H**) percentage of total monocytes, and (**I**) percentage of inflammatory monocytes within the total monocyte population were measured in the circulation of control mice vs. mice in which mast cells were activated. (**J**) The number of macrophages per microscopic field in the ischemic soleus muscles of mice in which mast cells were activated vs. controls at nine days after ligation. (**K**) Representative micrographs of macrophages in red (indicated by arrows) and $aSMA^+$ collaterals in cyan and nuclei (DAPI) in blue. * $p < 0.05$.

4. Discussion

In this study, we aimed to determine the contribution of mast cell activation to angiogenesis in hind limb ischemia. First, we demonstrated the presence of mast cells in human ischemic limb tissue, and both non-activated and activated mast cells were observed. Interestingly, activated mast cells were predominantly present around the capillaries in the ischemic limb, similarly as that described previously in the atherosclerotic plaque, where mast cells were seen to colocalize with microvessels [5]. In addition, mast cells have previously been associated with microvessel density in the brain [23]. Although mast cells have been associated with obesity and diabetes in experimental models of disease [24], the presence of diabetes did not affect mast cell numbers in the human ischemic tissue, which is in line with previous human studies in which intraplaque mast cells numbers did not differ between cardiovascular patients with and without diabetes mellitus [5].

In ischemic mouse hind limbs, the mast cells that colocalized with capillaries were mostly activated early in the revascularization process. Apparently, the ischemic environment in the hind limb causes the mast cells to degranulate. However, the mechanisms via which mast cells are activated upon ischemia remain largely unknown. In ischemia/reperfusion studies, reactive oxygen species, but also alarmins/DAMPS, have been suggested to activate mast cells [24]. The composition of the mast cell secretome completely depends on the specific stimuli and receptors involved, which indicates that the ischemic microenvironment can influence how mast cells are activated and which mediators these cells secrete. In this study, we aimed to determine whether local mast cell activation using a sensitization and challenge protocol in the ischemic hind limb would improve limb perfusion by inducing neovascularization. Similarly as described previously [6], we have established that mast cell activation promotes limb perfusion as indicated by enhanced blood flow to the lower limbs. Previously, it was suggested that neutrophils were the culprit immune effector cells during the neovascularization process in the ischemic hind limb [6]. In our study, we actually show that mast cell activation induced a pro-inflammatory monocyte response, while not affecting neutrophil numbers, either systemically or locally in the draining lymph nodes. The difference in observed immune response between the studies may be explained by the fact that we analyzed these monocyte responses at nine days after the induction of ischemia, whereas neutrophils are usually early responders and act in the first few days after injury. Furthermore, the difference in mast cell activation methods used may have affected the composition of the releasate, resulting in a difference in immune responses in the two studies. The increased immune response in the draining lymph nodes from the ischemic hind limb was not reflected by a difference in macrophage count in the muscle tissue itself at nine days after ligation. Again, this may be due to the timeframe of the study or to local secretion of pro-inflammatory mediators.

To further elucidate the underlying mechanisms that have caused the increased limb perfusion, both angiogenesis and arteriogenesis processes in the ischemic hind limbs were analyzed. In the adductor muscle, we were unable to detect any significant differences in either the number or the surface area of the collaterals, both at 9 and 28 days after femoral artery ligation. In the soleus muscle downstream of the ischemia, however, at day 9 we did observe an increase in the collateral surface area ratio in the mice in which mast cells were activated, suggesting that mast cells increase limb perfusion by expansion of pre-existing collaterals, as arteriogenesis is defined. At the same time point, we observed that the number of CD31 positive capillaries in the soleus muscle was significantly increased upon mast cell activation, and as this did not occur in the non-ischemic muscles, we can conclude that this is a specific local effect of mast cell activation. Together, these effects early in the revascularization process can explain the increase in paw perfusion induced in our model and that both arteriogenesis and angiogenesis in the ischemic muscles are responsible for the increased perfusion. To further elucidate the underlying mechanisms, it would be of interest to study arteriogenesis and angiogenesis processes in mast cell deficient mouse models. However, in our hands, survival of mast cell deficient $Kit^{W\text{-}sh/W\text{-}sh}$ mice upon hind limb ischemia was too limited to study these processes (unpublished data), and we therefore decided to apply a more therapeutics mast cell activation protocol, which made use of a local delayed type hypersensitivity approach. Previously, we have established that this method induces a specific mast cell activation response [7], however it would also be of interest to study other local mast cell activation approaches to determine which method induces the best neovascularization response without side effects.

As our data imply that mast cell activation improves limb perfusion after an ischemic episode, it is of great interest to determine how we can use these data for therapeutic application. As mentioned earlier, excessive mast cell activation can have detrimental effects on atherosclerotic plaque stability, the lungs, and other tissues in which mast cells reside. Also, an enhanced systemic inflammatory response induced by activated mast cells may be beneficial upon ischemia, but may also negatively affect other sources of inflammation, the so-called Janus phenomenon [13]. Local mast cell activation in the ischemic area may be a more suitable option. Furthermore, the identification of ischemia-specific mast cell activation pathways may provide novel therapeutic strategies to specifically target mast cell activation in the ischemic area. Further research may shed more light on the therapeutic opportunities for intervention.

In conclusion, in this study, we show that mast cells colocalize with capillaries in human ischemic tissue and in ischemic mouse limbs, where mast cells are activated in the early phase after the induction of ischemia. Locally induced mast cell activation in the hind limb leads to an increase in recovery of paw perfusion, which was associated with increased arterio- and angiogenesis, and with an increased inflammatory response, suggesting that mast cells actively contribute to tissue neovascularization.

Author Contributions: Conceptualization, I.B. and M.R.d.V.; formal analysis, I.B., D.v.d.V., M.B. and M.R.d.V.; investigation, I.B., D.v.d.V., M.B., M.J.K. and M.R.d.V.; resources, I.B., J.K., P.H.A.Q. and M.R.d.V.; supervision, I.B and M.R.d.V.; visualization, I.B and M.R.d.V.; writing—original draft, I.B. and M.R.d.V.; writing—review and editing, I.B., J.K., P.H.A.Q. and M.R.d.V. All authors have read and agreed to the published version of the manuscript.

References

1. Kaartinen, M.; Penttila, A.; Kovanen, P.T. Accumulation of activated mast cells in the shoulder region of human coronary atheroma, the predilection site of atheromatous rupture. *Circulation* **1994**, *90*, 1669–1678. [CrossRef] [PubMed]
2. Kovanen, P.T.; Kaartinen, M.; Paavonen, T. Infiltrates of activated mast cells at the site of coronary atheromatous erosion or rupture in myocardial infarction. *Circulation* **1995**, *92*, 1084–1088. [CrossRef] [PubMed]
3. Bot, I.; Shi, G.P.; Kovanen, P.T. Mast cells as effectors in atherosclerosis. *Arter. Thromb. Vasc. Biol.* **2015**, *35*, 265–271. [CrossRef] [PubMed]
4. Shi, G.P.; Bot, I.; Kovanen, P.T. Mast cells in human and experimental cardiometabolic diseases. *Nat. Rev. Cardiol.* **2015**, *12*, 643–658. [CrossRef]
5. Willems, S.; Vink, A.; Bot, I.; Quax, P.H.; de Borst, G.J.; de Vries, J.P.; van de Weg, S.M.; Moll, F.L.; Kuiper, J.; Kovanen, P.T.; et al. Mast cells in human carotid atherosclerotic plaques are associated with intraplaque microvessel density and the occurrence of future cardiovascular events. *Eur. Heart J.* **2013**, *34*, 3699–3706. [CrossRef]
6. Chillo, O.; Kleinert, E.C.; Lautz, T.; Lasch, M.; Pagel, J.I.; Heun, Y.; Troidl, K.; Fischer, S.; Caballero-Martinez, A.; Mauer, A.; et al. Perivascular Mast Cells Govern Shear Stress-Induced Arteriogenesis by Orchestrating Leukocyte Function. *Cell Rep.* **2016**, *16*, 2197–2207. [CrossRef]
7. Bot, I.; de Jager, S.C.; Zernecke, A.; Lindstedt, K.A.; van Berkel, T.J.; Weber, C.; Biessen, E.A. Perivascular mast cells promote atherogenesis and induce plaque destabilization in apolipoprotein E-deficient mice. *Circulation* **2007**, *115*, 2516–2525. [CrossRef]
8. Sun, J.; Sukhova, G.K.; Wolters, P.J.; Yang, M.; Kitamoto, S.; Libby, P.; MacFarlane, L.A.; Mallen-St, C.J.; Shi, G.P. Mast cells promote atherosclerosis by releasing proinflammatory cytokines. *Nat. Med.* **2007**, *13*, 719–724. [CrossRef]

9. Indhirajanti, S.; van Daele, P.L.A.; Bos, S.; Mulder, M.T.; Bot, I.; Roeters van Lennep, J.E. Systemic mastocytosis associates with cardiovascular events despite lower plasma lipid levels. *Atherosclerosis* **2018**, *268*, 152–156. [CrossRef]
10. Albini, A.; Bruno, A.; Noonan, D.M.; Mortara, L. Contribution to Tumor Angiogenesis From Innate Immune Cells Within the Tumor Microenvironment: Implications for Immunotherapy. *Front. Immunol.* **2018**, *9*, 527. [CrossRef]
11. van Weel, V.; Seghers, L.; de Vries, M.R.; Kuiper, E.J.; Schlingemann, R.O.; Bajema, I.M.; Lindeman, J.H.; Delis-van Diemen, P.M.; van Hinsbergh, V.W.; van Bockel, J.H.; et al. Expression of vascular endothelial growth factor, stromal cell-derived factor-1, and CXCR4 in human limb muscle with acute and chronic ischemia. *Arter. Thromb. Vasc. Biol.* **2007**, *27*, 1426–1432. [CrossRef] [PubMed]
12. Campia, U.; Gerhard-Herman, M.; Piazza, G.; Goldhaber, S.Z. Peripheral Artery Disease: Past, Present, and Future. *Am. J. Med.* **2019**, *132*, 1133–1141. [CrossRef] [PubMed]
13. Epstein, S.E.; Stabile, E.; Kinnaird, T.; Lee, C.W.; Clavijo, L.; Burnett, M.S. Janus phenomenon: The interrelated tradeoffs inherent in therapies designed to enhance collateral formation and those designed to inhibit atherogenesis. *Circulation* **2004**, *109*, 2826–2831. [CrossRef] [PubMed]
14. de Vries, M.R.; Wezel, A.; Schepers, A.; van Santbrink, P.J.; Woodruff, T.M.; Niessen, H.W.; Hamming, J.F.; Kuiper, J.; Bot, I.; Quax, P.H. Complement factor C5a as mast cell activator mediates vascular remodelling in vein graft disease. *Cardiovasc. Res.* **2013**, *97*, 311–320. [CrossRef]
15. de Vries, M.R.; Seghers, L.; van, B.J.; Peters, H.A.; de Jong, R.C.; Hamming, J.F.; Toes, R.E.; van Hinsbergh, V.W.; Quax, P.H. C57BL/6 NK cell gene complex is crucially involved in vascular remodeling. *J. Mol. Cell Cardiol.* **2013**, *64*, 51–58. [CrossRef]
16. Simons, K.H.; Aref, Z.; Peters, H.A.B.; Welten, S.P.; Nossent, A.Y.; Jukema, J.W.; Hamming, J.F.; Arens, R.; de Vries, M.R.; Quax, P.H.A. The role of CD27-CD70-mediated T cell co-stimulation in vasculogenesis, arteriogenesis and angiogenesis. *Int. J. Cardiol.* **2018**, *260*, 184–190. [CrossRef]
17. Kraneveld, A.D.; Buckley, T.L.; van Heuven-Nolsen, D.; van, S.Y.; Koster, A.S.; Nijkamp, F.P. Delayed-type hypersensitivity-induced increase in vascular permeability in the mouse small intestine: Inhibition by depletion of sensory neuropeptides and NK1 receptor blockade. *Br. J. Pharm.* **1995**, *114*, 1483–1489. [CrossRef]
18. den Dekker, W.K.; Tempel, D.; Bot, I.; Biessen, E.A.; Joosten, L.A.; Netea, M.G.; van der Meer, J.W.; Cheng, C.; Duckers, H.J. Mast cells induce vascular smooth muscle cell apoptosis via a toll-like receptor 4 activation pathway. *Arterioscler. Thromb. Vasc. Biol.* **2012**, *32*, 1960–1969. [CrossRef]
19. Aref, Z.; de Vries, M.R.; Quax, P.H.A. Variations in Surgical Procedures for Inducing Hind Limb Ischemia in Mice and the Impact of These Variations on Neovascularization Assessment. *Int J. Mol. Sci* **2019**, *20*, 3704. [CrossRef]
20. Kritikou, E.; van der Heijden, T.; Swart, M.; van Duijn, J.; Slutter, B.; Wezel, A.; Smeets, H.J.; Maffia, P.; Kuiper, J.; Bot, I. Hypercholesterolemia Induces a Mast Cell-CD4(+) T Cell Interaction in Atherosclerosis. *J. Immunol.* **2019**, *202*, 1531–1539. [CrossRef]
21. Wezel, A.; Lagraauw, H.M.; van der Velden, D.; de Jager, S.C.; Quax, P.H.; Kuiper, J.; Bot, I. Mast cells mediate neutrophil recruitment during atherosclerotic plaque progression. *Atherosclerosis* **2015**, *241*, 289–296. [CrossRef] [PubMed]
22. Nowak-Sliwinska, P.; Alitalo, K.; Allen, E.; Anisimov, A.; Aplin, A.C.; Auerbach, R.; Augustin, H.G.; Bates, D.O.; van Beijnum, J.R.; Bender, R.H.F.; et al. Consensus guidelines for the use and interpretation of angiogenesis assays. *Angiogenesis* **2018**, *21*, 425–532. [CrossRef] [PubMed]
23. Ollikainen, E.; Tulamo, R.; Frosen, J.; Lehti, S.; Honkanen, P.; Hernesniemi, J.; Niemela, M.; Kovanen, P.T. Mast cells, neovascularization, and microhemorrhages are associated with saccular intracranial artery aneurysm wall remodeling. *J. Neuropathol Exp. Neurol.* **2014**, *73*, 855–864. [CrossRef] [PubMed]
24. He, Z.; Ma, C.; Yu, T.; Song, J.; Leng, J.; Gu, X.; Li, J. Activation mechanisms and multifaceted effects of mast cells in ischemia reperfusion injury. *Exp. Cell Res.* **2019**, *376*, 227–235. [CrossRef] [PubMed]

14

Control of Angiogenesis via a VHL/miR-212/132 Axis

Zhiyong Lei [1,†], Timothy D. Klasson [2,†], Maarten M. Brandt [3], Glenn van de Hoek [4], Ive Logister [2], Caroline Cheng [2,3], Pieter A. Doevendans [1,5,6], Joost P. G. Sluijter [1,7,*] and Rachel H. Giles [2,*]

1 Department of Cardiology, Division Heart and Lungs, University Medical Center Utrecht, Heidelberglaan 100, 3584 CX Utrecht, The Netherlands
2 Department of Nephrology & Hypertension, Division Internal Medicine, University Medical Center Utrecht, Heidelberglaan 100, 3584 CX Utrecht, The Netherlands
3 Experimental Cardiology, Department of Cardiology, Thoraxcenter, Erasmus MC, University Medical Center Rotterdam, 3015 GD Rotterdam, The Netherlands
4 Department of Medical Genetics, University Medical Center Utrecht, Heidelberglaan 100, 3584 CX Utrecht, The Netherlands
5 Netherlands Heart Institute, Catharijnesingel 52, 3511 GC Utrecht, The Netherlands
6 Central Military Hospital Utrecht, Lundlaan 1, 3584 EZ Utrecht, The Netherlands
7 UMC Utrecht Regenerative Medicine Center, University Medical Center, 3584 CT Utrecht, The Netherlands
* Correspondence: j.sluijter@umcutrecht.nl (J.P.G.S.); r.giles@umcutrecht.nl (R.H.G.)
† These authors contributed equally to this work.

Abstract: A common feature of tumorigenesis is the upregulation of angiogenesis pathways in order to supply nutrients via the blood for the growing tumor. Understanding how cells promote angiogenesis and how to control these processes pharmaceutically are of great clinical interest. Clear cell renal cell carcinoma (ccRCC) is the most common form of sporadic and inherited kidney cancer which is associated with excess neovascularization. ccRCC is highly associated with biallelic mutations in the von Hippel–Lindau (VHL) tumor suppressor gene. Although upregulation of the miR-212/132 family and disturbed VHL signaling have both been linked with angiogenesis, no evidence of a possible connection between the two has yet been made. We show that miRNA-212/132 levels are increased after loss of functional pVHL, the protein product of the VHL gene, in vivo and in vitro. Furthermore, we show that blocking miRNA-212/132 with anti-miRs can significantly alleviate the excessive vascular branching phenotype characteristic of vhl$^{-/-}$ mutant zebrafish. Moreover, using human umbilical vascular endothelial cells (HUVECs) and an endothelial cell/pericyte coculture system, we observed that VHL knockdown promotes endothelial cells neovascularization capacity in vitro, an effect which can be inhibited by anti-miR-212/132 treatment. Taken together, our results demonstrate an important role for miRNA-212/132 in angiogenesis induced by loss of VHL. Intriguingly, this also presents a possibility for the pharmaceutical manipulation of angiogenesis by modulating levels of MiR212/132.

Keywords: VHL loss of function; microRNA-212/132; angiogenesis

---

1. Introduction

Clear cell renal cell carcinoma (ccRCC), the most common form of sporadic and inherited kidney cancer, is highly associated with mutations in the von Hippel-Lindau (*VHL*) gene [1,2]. The protein product of the *VHL* gene (pVHL) is an E3 ubiquitin ligase involved in the degradation of hypoxia-inducible transcription factor subunits (HIF1α). Under normal oxygen tension, hydroxylated HIF1α can be recognized by the ubiquitin ligase complex containing pVHL and rapidly degraded. Upon hypoxia or loss of functional pVHL, HIF1α-subunits can no longer be hydroxylated and begin to accumulate. Stabilized HIF1α activates the expression of a large suite of downstream target genes (Erythropoietin (*EPO*), vascular endothelial growth factor (*VEGF*), etc), the actions of which are vital to promote angiogenesis. However, many of the changes initiated by the stabilization of HIF1α, such as increased angiogenesis, an upregulation of antiapoptotic signaling, and a shift to anaerobic glycolosis, can contribute to tumor growth and survival. People born with a mutation in one *VHL* allele may acquire somatic mutations in the second allele, resulting in consequent angiogenic symptoms and a variety of tumors, including ccRCC [3]. Another hallmark of ccRCC is the activated phosphatidylinositol-4,5-bisphosphate 3-kinase (PI3k)/AKT pathway signaling, higher levels of which is significantly correlated with a worse survival rate [2], although the mechanism by which this occurs is still not fully understood.

MicroRNAs (miRNAs) are small noncoding RNAs that posttranscriptionally regulate the expression of groups of target genes by inhibition of the translation of their targeting messenger RNAs (mRNAs) or marking these mRNAs for degradation. miRNAs are key regulators in many physiological and pathological processes [4], including the dynamic regulation of ccRCC during tumor progression [2]. By promoting the expression of vascular endothelial growth factor (*VEGF*), VHL/HIF1 signaling increases Cyclic adenosine monophosphate (cAMP) response element binding protein (CREB) levels, a transcription factor which upregulates the expression of pro-angiogenic miR-212/132 [5]. This implies that pVHL loss-of-function would stimulate miR-212/132 expression and therefore contribute to excessive angiogenesis. In this study, using a combination of cellular models, patient ccRCC material with biallelic loss of VHL and a previously described vhl$^{-/-}$ mutant zebrafish model, we show that miR-212/132 is upregulated after VHL knockdown or mutation and that this upregulation is at least partially responsible for pro-angiogenic effects. In order to grow, cancer tissues such as ccRCC have developed various strategies to provide sufficient blood supply by promoting angiogenesis [6]. Many of the common pharmaceutical treatments for ccRCC, such as sunitinib, use the strategy of reducing pathophysiological angiogenesis [7]. Conversely, many different strategies have been tested to improve perfusion of certain ischemic tissues or engineered tissue constructs by promoting neovascularization, which is essential for functional recovery of the organ after ischemic events or survival of transplanted engineered tissue constructs [8]. A scarcity of functional pVHL induces excessive vascular outgrowth, which further is enhanced by miR-212/132 expression, providing an exciting target for the modulation of angiogenesis.

2. Materials and Methods

2.1. MicroRNA In Situ Hybridization

microRNA in situ hybridization was performed with a modified microRNA in situ hybridization method as described [9]. Formalin-fixed paraffin-embedded tumor tissue from two ccRCCs and one healthy donor kidney dating from September 2006 were collected from the pathology archives of the University Medical Centre Utrecht (UMCU) after authorization of the UMCU institutional review board in accordance with Dutch medical ethical guidelines. Sequencing results of *VHL* identified no variants in the normal healthy kidney. However, in ccRCC #1, in addition to the already known germline deletion of *VHL* exons 1 and 2, an additional somatic mutation was found in the tumor (c.277delG/p.Gly93Ala_fs_x158). ccRCC #2 has a germline mutation c.266T> p.Leu89Pro and a somatic mutation of c.419-420delTC/p.Leu140Gln_fs_x142. Mutation analysis of these tumors has been previously published [10].

Paraffin samples were first deparaffinized with tissue clear (Cat# 1426, SAKURA) followed with 10 min of proteinase K treatment (5µg/ml, Cat# 03115828001, Roche). Hybridization was performed with 10 nM DIG-labeled miRCURY LNA miRNA detection probes in hybridization buffer (Urea (2 M), 2.5× SSC, 1× Denhardt's, 200 µg/ml yeast tRNA, 0.1% CHAPS, 0.1% Tween, and 50mg/ml heparin) for miR-132 (Cat# 38031-15, Exiqon). Sections were subsequently incubated with anti-DIG alkaline phosphatase antibody (1:1,500, Cat# 1093274, Roche). To block endogenous alkaline phosphatase activity, sections were incubated with levamisole solution (Cat. X3021, DAKO), followed by NBT/BCIP (Cat# K0598 DAKO) incubation for visualization. A light Eosin counter staining was performed to visualize histology of the tissue. Images were taken with an Olympus microscope (BX53) under bright field.

2.2. Cell Culture and Transfection

Human umbilical vascular endothelial cells (HUVECs) were cultured in EGM2 (Lonza, cat# cc-3156) according to manufacturer's instructions, and all experiments were performed before passage 7. HUVECS were either transfected with validated siVHL (ID: s14790), siPTEN (ID: s61222), silencer select negative control #1 (cat# 4390843), mirVana miRNA mimic negative control (cat# 4464085), hsa-miR-132-3p mimics (ID: MC10166), hsa-miR-212-3p mimics (ID: MC10340), mirVana miRNA inhibitor controll (cat# 4464077), hsa-miR-132-3p inhibitor (ID: AM10166), or hsa-miR-212-3p inhibitor (ID: AM10340) (all from Life Technologies) using Lipofectamine 2000 (Life Technologies). The transfection was performed with a final concentration of 20 nM in opti-MEM reduced-serum medium (Cat# 31985062, Life Technologies) and replaced with fresh EGM2 after 6 hours. Cells were harvested 72 hours after transfection for protein or RNA analysis.

2.3. RNA Isolation and RT-PCR

Total RNA was isolated with Tripure Isolation Reagent following manufactory's instructions (Roche Applied Science) and treated with Dnase to remove potential genome DNA contaminations. cDNA was synthesized using the iScript^{TM} cDNA Synthesis Kit (Bio-Rad). Quantitative real-time polymerase chain reaction (qRT-PCR) was performed with iQ SYBR Green Supermix (Bio-Rad). The following primers were used for detection of human genes: *GAPDH* forward 5′-GGCATGGACTGTGGTCAT GA-3′ and reverse 5′-TTCACCACCATGGAGAAGGC-3′; *PTEN* forward 5′-TGGATTCGACTTAGACT TGACCT-3′ and reverse 5′-GGTGGGTTATGGTCTTCAAAAGG-3′; *VHL* forward 5′-CAGCTACCGA GGTCACCTTT-3′ and reverse 5′-CCGTCAACATTGAGAGATGG-3′; the following primers are used for *zebrafish*: *ptena* forward 5′-CCAGCCAGCGCAGGTATGTGTA-3′ and reverse 5′-GCGGCTGAGGAAAC TCGAAGATC-3′; *ptenb* forward 5′-GCTACCTTCTGAGGAATAAGCTGG-3′ and reverse 5′-CTTGATG TCCCCACACACAGGC-3′; *rpl13α* forward 5′-TCTGGAGGACTGTAAGAGGTATGC-3′ and reverse 5′-AGACGCACAATCTTGAGAGCAG-3′ (All primers from Integrated DNA Technologies, Coralville, IA, USA).

2.4. In Vitro Angiogenesis Assay

HUVECs (Lonza) and human brain vascular pericytes (Cat#1200, Sciencell) were cultured on gelatin-coated plates in EGM2 medium (Lonza cat# cc-3156) and DMEM (10% FCS; Lonza), respectively, in 5% CO_2 at 37 °C. Lentiviral transduced HUVECs expressing green fluorescent protein (GFP) and pericytes expressing red fluorescent protein (RFP) were used between passage 6–8. HUVECs were transfected either with siRNA or anti-miRs as described above. In order to monitor the effects of miR-132 and miR-212 in angiogenesis, transfected HUVEC-GFP and Pericytes-dsRed were suspended in a 2.5 mg/ml collagen type I (BD Biosciences) as described by Stratman [11]. Cocultures were imaged after 48 h and 120 h incubation in 5% CO_2 at 37 °C by fluorescence microscopy, followed by automated thresholding and skeletonization of the images using a commercial analysis system (Angiosys, Buckingham, UK). These images were used for automated tubule length measurement, junction measurement, and other analyses according to manufacturer's instructions.

2.5. Zebrafish

Experiments were conducted in accordance with Dutch guidelines for the care and use of laboratory animals, with the approval of the Animal Experimentation Committee (DEC) of the Royal Netherlands Academy of Arts and Sciences (KNAW). Mutant *zebrafish* possessed the previously described vhl^{hu2117} mutation [12]. For RNA collection, *zebrafish* embryos were collected at 5 dpf based on these phenotypes and RNA was collected using Trizol reagent (Ambion) as per manufacturer's instructions.

2.6. Injections and Visualizations

Wild-type and mutant *Zebrafish* embryos were injected at the 1–2-cell stage with 1 nL of 5 uM of the same miRNA mimics and antagonists used for the cell culture experiments described above. Mimics and antagonists were diluted in pure water with 0.1% phenol red for visualization and injected using a nanoject2000 microinjector (World Precision Instruments). *Zebrafish* were selected without bias at 5dpf and then imaged using an LSM700 microscope (Zeiss). DNA was then collected from theses embryos using lysis buffer, and then embryos were genotyped using a KASP™ genotyping system (LGC Genomics, Teddington, Middlesex, England) kit designed against the vhl^{hu2117} mutation or by sanger sequencing using the following primers: Fw: 5′-TAA GGG CTT AGC GCA TGT TC-3′ and Rv: 5′-CGA GTT AAA CGC GTA GAT AG-3′.

2.7. Statistical Analysis

Data was analyzed with Graphpad Prism 6 and comparisons were performed with student t-test or paired *t*-test between two groups and with ANOVA for more than two groups. Data are presented as mean ± SEM. *p*-values are indicated as follows: * $p < 0.05$; ** $p < 0.01$; *** $p < 0.001$; $p < 0.05$ is considered significant.

3. Results

miRNA-212/132 are transcribed as a single RNA transcript and subsequently processed into two different mature microRNA miR-132 and miR-212. Due to the different efficiency in pre-miR processing, miR-132 is the dominant family member, as shown in Figure 1F. In most of the tissues, the expression of miR-212 are hardly detectable with the only exception being the brain. For this reason, mir-132 was used as the primary target in this study. We first examined the expression of miR-132 in relation to VHL loss-of-function and (pseudo)-hypoxic signaling. We found that endothelial cells grown in hypoxic conditions display significantly elevated levels of miR-132 expression (Figure 1A). We observe similar effects in HUVECs transfected with siRNA targeting *VHL* mRNA relative to those treated with non-targeting siRNA (Figure 1B). miR-212/132 are well conserved in most species, including zebrafish (Supplementary Figure S1A). To confirm this effect in vivo, we used a previously established zebrafish model of *VHL* deficiency [12–14]. Like our cell models, $vhl^{-/-}$ zebrafish also show an increased level of expression of miR-132 (Figure 1C). In isogenic cell lines taken from human ccRCC $VHL^{-/-}$ tumors, the expression of miR-132 is reduced upon *VHL* reconstitution with ectopic *VHL* (Figure 1E). The reduction of miR-132 expression is present in all cell lines upon VHL introduction but less pronounced in the RCC10, which might be related to a cell-line-specific genetic alteration on top of the VHL disruption that affects the miR-132 pathway. To assess the functional consequences of miR-212/132 loss in these cells, we examined the expression of a known target mRNA of this miRNA family. PTEN, phosphatidylinositol-3,4,5-trisphosphate 3-phosphatase, antagonizes the activity of phosphatidylinositol-4,5-bisphosphate 3-kinase (PI3K), suppressing cellular proliferation, cell survival, and angiogenesis by inactivating the PI3K-driven AKT signaling pathway [15]. *PTEN* has been predicted to be a potential target of miR-212/132 in humans by targetscan (Supplemental Figure S1B), and the rat homologue of *PTEN* has been shown to be targeted by miR-212/132 in rat vascular smooth muscle cells [16]. Moreover, downregulation of PTEN has been significantly correlated with lower survival rate in ccRCC patients [2]. We reasoned that upregulated miR-212/132 upon mutation or silencing of *VHL* could result in the subsequent reduction of PTEN. We therefore examined PTEN expression in HUVEC cells transfected with miR-212/132 mimics and found that the expression of PTEN was significantly reduced in these cells (Figure 1D). In order to assess the relative effects of miR-212 versus miR-132, we examined the differential expression of these miRNA in different mouse tissues. miR-212 is found at extremely low levels in the tissues tested, except brain tissue (Figure 1F). Based on this information, we examined miR-132 expression in histology slides taken from ccRCC tumors using microRNA in situ hybridization. In agreement with our previous qPCR results, we observed widespread overexpression of miR-132 in tumor material from ccRCC samples with biallelic *VHL* mutations proven by sequencing (Figure 1E). These results demonstrate that miR-132 is increased in response to the pseudo-hypoxia induced by the lack of functional pVHL, which eventually leads to overexpression of miR-132.

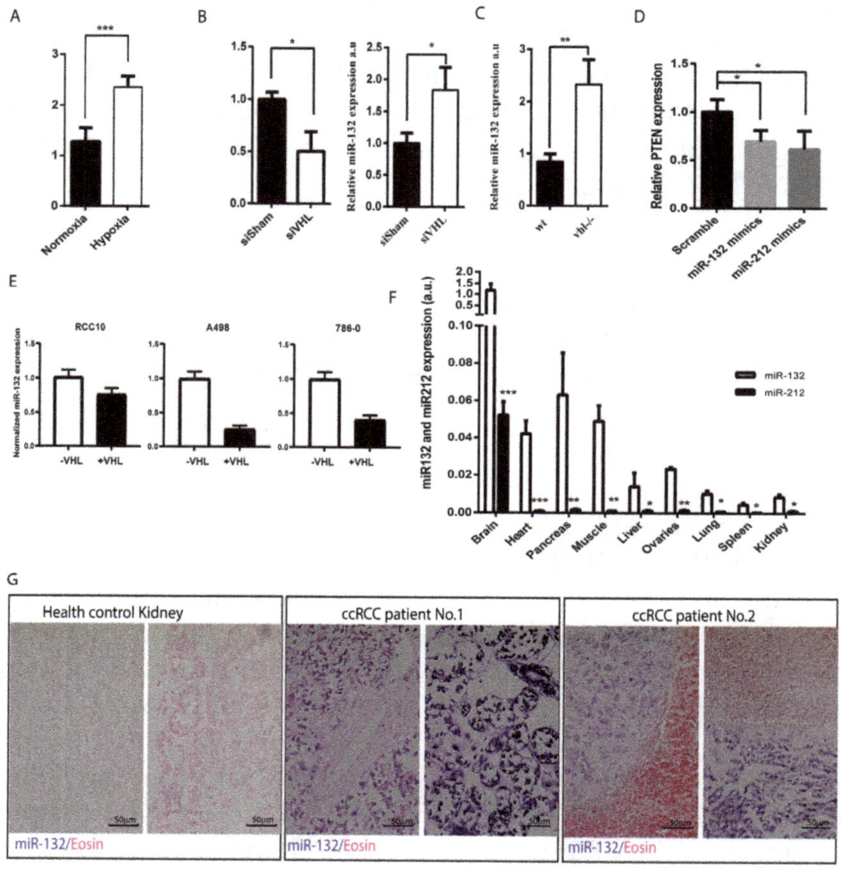

Figure 1. Characterization of miR-132 expression under hypoxic and pseudo-hypoxic conditions: (**A**) The expression of miR-132 in human umbilical vascular endothelial cells (HUVECs) under normoxia and hypoxia as compared by qPCR. (**B**) The expression of von Hippel–Lindau (VHL) in HUVECs after transfection with siRNA against VHL and the expression of miR-132 in siSham and siVHL transfected HUVECs as compared by qPCR. (**C**) The expression of miR-132 in wildtype (WT) and vhl$^{-/-}$ mutant zebrafish as compared by qPCR. (**D**) The expression of known miR-132 target PTEN (phosphatidylinositol-3,4,5-trisphosphate 3-phosphatase) in HUVECs treated with miR-132/212 mimics versus control as compared by qPCR. (**E**) The expression of miR-132 in established VHL$^{-/-}$ lines RCC10, A498, and 786-0 as well as the same lines reconstituted with ectopic VHL. The presented data is a mean of 3 in-depended PCR experiments with counting error. (**F**) Relative expression of miR-132 and 212 in different tissues in mouse. Note miR-132 expression is considerably higher than miR-212. $n = 3$. (**G**) The expression of miR-132 in healthy kidney tissue and ccRCC from two patients with known bilateral VHL mutations in their tumor as shown by miR-132 in situ hybridization. miR-132 in situ is in purple blue. Light eosin counterstaining appears pink. * $p < 0.05$; ** $p < 0.01$; *** $p < 0.001$

To assess the functional consequences of miR-212/132 expression in a *VHL*-null environment, we used an in vitro coculture assay designed to gauge angiogenesis. In agreement with the important role of VHL in HIF1 degradation, knockdown of VHL in HUVEC/pericyte coculture shows significantly more vascular junctions, tubule number, and total tubular length as compared to siSham control treatment (Figure 2A–C). To evaluate whether the pro-angiogenic effects of *VHL* silencing are mediated by a downstream increase in miR-212/132, GFP-labelled HUVECs were treated with anti-miRs against miR-212/132 in combination with siRNA targeting *VHL*. Inhibiting the action of miR-212/132 reduced the excessive angiogenetic response induced by the silencing of *VHL* significantly (Figure 2D), suggesting that VHL-regulated angiogenesis is at least partially mediated by the upregulation of miR-212/132.

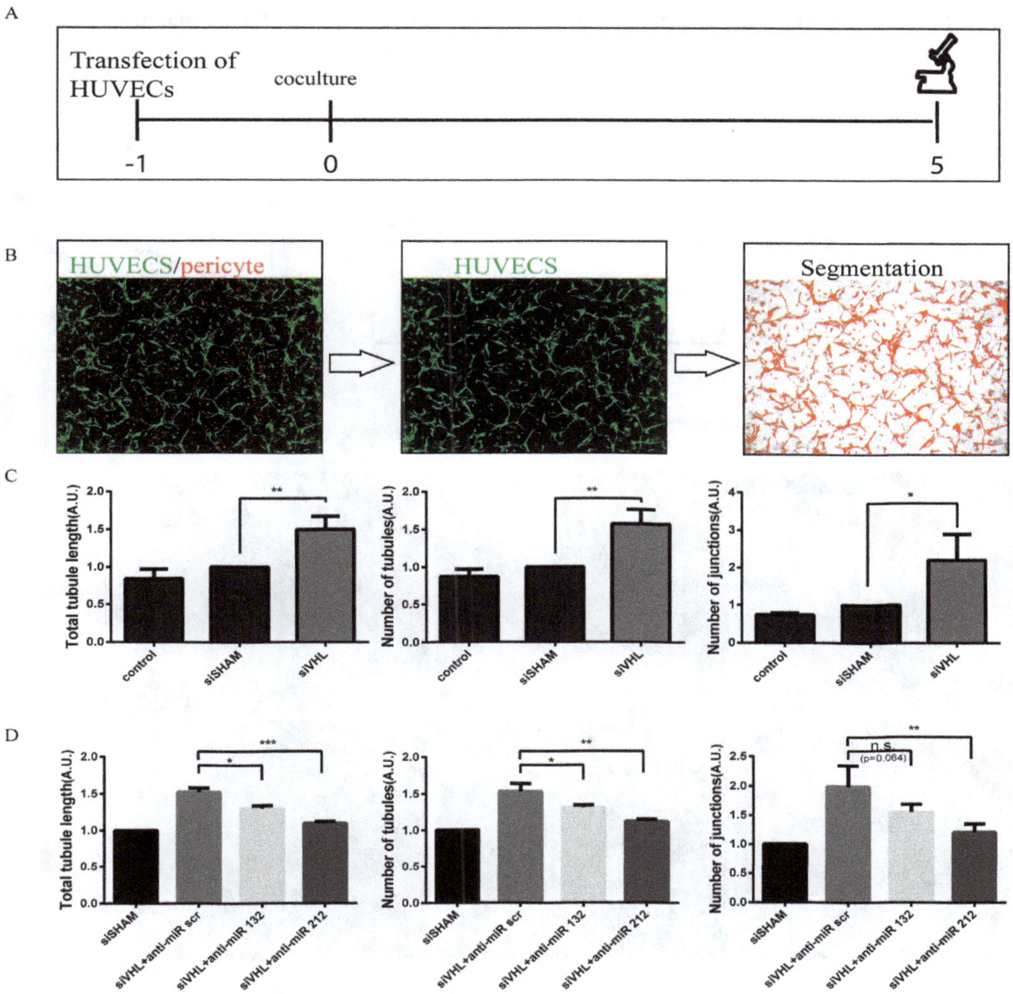

Figure 2. Reduced levels of VHL enhances endothelial cell neovascularization capacity and can be inhibited by blocking miR-132 or miR-212. (**A**) Schematic outline of the coculture experiment with HUVECs and pericytes. (**B**) Representative images showing the analysis process of tubular structures in the endothelial cells and pericytes coculture assay. (**C**) VHL siRNA knockdown in HUVECs enhances endothelial cell neovascularization capacity. (**D**) Blocking miR-132/212 inhibits neovascularization enhancement induced by VHL knockdown. Cell images are used to produce skeletonized 2D images which can be analyzed automatically. * $p < 0.05$; ** $p < 0.01$; *** $p < 0.001$

vhl$^{-/-}$ zebrafish embryos display a phenotype of post-vascularization branching/sprouting around the intersomitic vessels in the tails. Counting these sprouts is known as a quantitative measure of angiogenesis in zebrafish [13]. *vhl*$^{-/-}$ zebrafish were injected at a one-cell stage with anti-miRs directed against miR-132 or miR-212, and four days later, tails of the living fish were imaged with a confocal microscope (Figure 3A). The cloaca of the zebrafish is placed in the center of the image, and the branches sprouting from the inter-somitic vessels were counted for the four vessels anterior and the four vessels posterior to the cloaca (Figure 3B). Anti-miR injections against miR-212/132 significantly reduced the extent of intersomitic vessel sprouting in *vhl*$^{-/-}$ fish (Figure 3C,D). In addition, injecting wild-type zebrafish with miR-212/132 mimics partially recapitulated the *vhl* mutant vessel sprouting phenotype (Supplemental Figure S1C,D). In light of the fact that miR-212/132 expression is therefore linked to vessel sprouting in *vhl*$^{-/-}$ zebrafish, we proceeded to look at the expression of PTEN in our VHL-null models, as we had previously done in HUVECs. Zebrafish, as opposed to mammals, have two copies of the *pten* gene: *ptena* and *ptenb*. Zebrafish with loss of both *ptena* and *ptenb* [17] also display a vessel sprouting phenotype that phenocopies the one found in zebrafish injected with miR-212/132 mimics. *ptenb* is a predicted target of miR-212/132 in targetscan but not *ptena* (Supplemental Figure S1E). Accordingly, we found significantly reduced *ptenb* expression in $vhl^{-/-}$ zebrafish with no significant changes observed in *ptena* (Figure 4E).

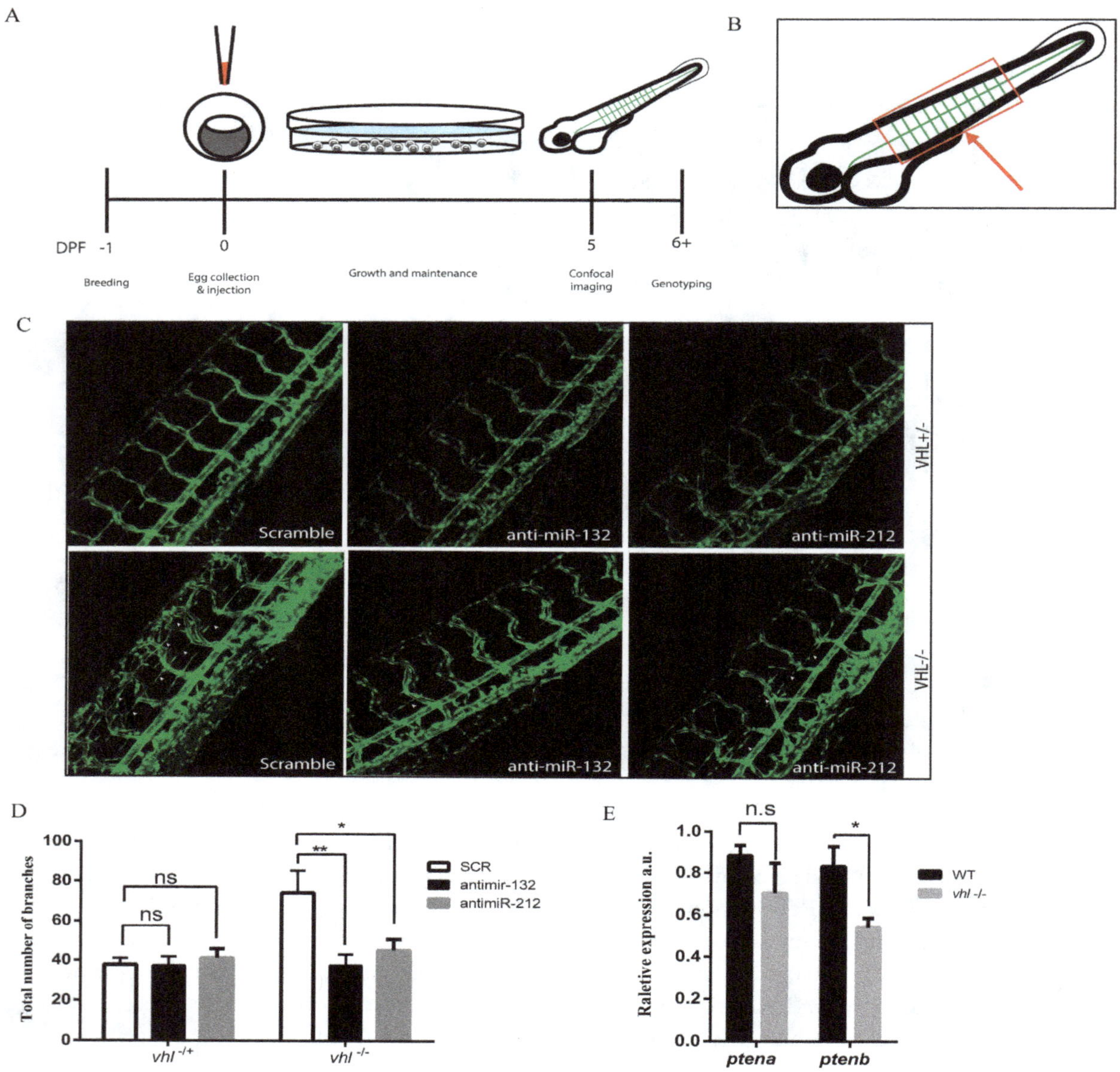

Figure 3. Inhibition of miR-132 or miR-212 suppresses VHL loss of function-induced vasculature outgrowth in zebrafish. (**A**) Schematic outline of the zebrafish embryo microinjection experiment. microRNA mimics and anti-miRs are injected into the yolk of the eggs on day 0 and imaged with a confocal microscope on day 5. (**B**) Schematic cartoon showing the area of the zebrafish embryo that is imaged after microinjection. The cloaca is marked with a red arrow. The imaging area is shown with a red box. The vessels of the tail are shown in green. (**C**) Representative images of zebrafish tail vascular structures in $vhl^{+/-}$ and $vhl^{-/-}$ zebrafish after injection with scrambled or miR-132 and miR-212 inhibitors. White arrows designate examples of structures which have been scored as branches. (**D**) Quantification of vascular branching in zebrafish tail structures after injection with scrambled control inhibitors, miR-132 inhibitors, or miR-212 inhibitors. (**E**) The expression levels of ptena and ptenb in WT and $vhl^{-/-}$ zebrafish determined by qPCR. * $p < 0.05$; ** $p < 0.01$.

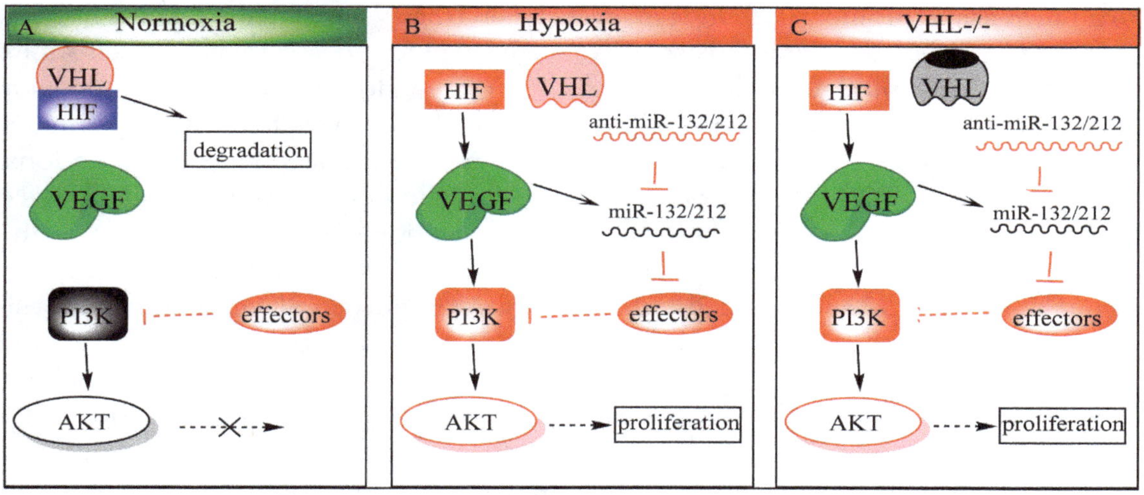

Figure 4. Proposed mechanism of miR-132/212 in modulation of the VHL/phosphatidylinositol-4, 5-bisphosphate 3-kinase (PI3K)/Protein kinase B(AKT)pathways. (**A**) During normoxia, hypoxia-inducible transcription factor 1 (HIF1) is ubiquitinated by the VHL-ubiquinition complex, targeting it for degradation. Some effectors, such as *PTEN*, antagonizes PI3k to prevent AKT from being activated. (**B**) Upon hypoxia, HIF1 can no longer be hydroxylated, which prohibits VHL-regulated degradation, and allows stabilized HIF1 to translocate to the nucleus, upregulating its downstream targets such as *vascular endothelial growth factor* (*VEGF*). VEGF in turn activates the PI3k-AKT pathway and upregulates miR-132/212 expression as well. Upregulated miR-132/212 inhibits effector (e.g., *PTEN)* expression, which in turn prolongs AKT activity. (**C**) *VHL* loss-of-function phenocopies hypoxic conditions even in the presence of oxygen (pseudo-hypoxia).

4. Discussion

In this study, we used patient material, human cells, and zebrafish to examine the role of the miRNA-212/132 family in ccRCC tumor neovascularization caused by the loss-of-functional pVHL. We observed that miR-212/132 is upregulated in response to *VHL* mutation both in zebrafish model systems and in human patient ccRCC tumor material carrying biallelic inactivating *VHL* mutations. We demonstrated that the excessive angiogenesis attributable to *VHL* mutation is strongly affected by miR-212/132. Indeed, targeting these miRNAs with anti-miRs can significantly reduce angiogenesis in both in vitro and in vivo models of *VHL* deficiency. We identified the tumor suppressor PTEN as one of the targets affected by miRNA-212/132 in *VHL*-null models. Taken together, our results implicate miRNA-212/132 as an important intermediate in angiogenesis after loss-of-functional pVHL or tissue hypoxia.

The miR-212/132 family is clustered in the genome and is highly conserved in vertebrates. miR-212/132 is initially expressed as one primary miRNA and then processed into two mature miRNA with the same target-defining "seed" sequence [18]. This miRNA family plays a number of roles in the promotion of angiogenesis. Mice without functional miR-212/132 show impaired arteriogenesis response after hindlimb ischemia [19]. The pro-angiogenic potential of miR-132 has been used to increase angiogenesis in endothelial cell grafts and after ischemic injury [20]. miR-212/132 frequently act as a promoter of cell proliferation, and increases in their expression levels have also been suggested as contributors to tumorigenesis in addition to their angiogenic role. miR-132 has previously been shown to induce neovascularization in the endothelium by targeting p120 Ras GTPase-activating protein [5]. In addition, anti-miR-132 has also been shown to reduce tumor burden in a mouse xenograft model of human breast carcinoma [5].

This study supports the previously reported role of miR-212/132 in angiogenesis and expands upon its role in the context of VHL-regulated hypoxia signaling. When VHL is mutated or downregulated, miR-212/132 is consequently upregulated. miR-212/132 targeting of mRNA such as *PTEN* ensures that downstream effectors are upregulated. For example, in the case of *PTEN*, PI3K may activate AKT, leading to an increase in proliferation. Indeed, cysts taken from VHL patients display hyperactivation of PI3K signaling [21]. Due to technical reasons, we were not able to detect this increased AKT signaling directly in our zebrafish model. In addition, *Pten* $^{-/-}$ *Vhl* $^{-/-}$ double mutant mice develop benign squamous metaplasia and cystadenoma [21] and display kidney cysts that are very similar to those taken from the kidneys of human VHL patients, while mouse models with *Vhl* mutations only do not develop renal tumors [22]. Uncontrolled proliferation and angiogenesis are hallmarks of cancer, and many tumors contain mutations leading to hyperactivation of signaling networks which act to promote these processes [23–25]. Differential expression of miRNA has been previously reported in tumors including ccRCC [26] and is widely believed to be an important player in tumorigenesis [27–29]. A group of miRs, termed hypoxamiRs, has been shown to be upregulated in hypoxia and play a role in the modulation of cellular responses to a lack of oxygen. The hypoxamiRs include miR-21; 23; 24; 26; 103/107; 373; and, most well studied, miR-210. Hypoxia is also considered a hallmark of the microenvironment of solid tumors, and a number of hypoxamiRs have been implicated in tumorigenesis [30,31]. Thus, the action of miRNA may play an important role in tumorigenesis and therefore presents an interesting potential target for the treatment of cancer.

One of the hallmarks of ccRCC is resistance to cytotoxic treatment. Antiapoptotic signaling is upregulated after HIF1α hyper-stabilization in ccRCC tumors. Many experimental treatments focus on inhibiting the action of downstream antiapoptosis proteins such as mammalian target of rapamycin (mTOR), an important pro-survival protein induced by activated AKT signaling [32]. Our results and the results of other studies suggest that miR-212/132 may act as a promoter of tumorigenesis by targeting inhibitors of proliferation, survival, and angiogenesis, presenting an interesting opportunity for pharmaceutical intervention. Currently, medications which target miRNA are largely unexplored as an avenue by which to target cancer. Here, we have shown that antagonizing the activity of this miRNA family can reduce angiogenesis in relevant models of *VHL* deficiency. *PTEN*, which we have confirmed to be a target of the miR-212/132 family in these models, is frequently mutated in cancer. Another miRNA, miRNA-21, has previously been shown to target PTEN in multiple cancer types and has been implicated in tumorigenesis [33]. Loss of PTEN leads to upregulation of mTOR signaling, and mTOR inhibitors have been used to treat multiple cancer types. Therefore, we envision that treatments designed to antagonize the effect of miRNA-212/132 or other miRNA might be able to reduce the angiogenic burden of tumors in patients, to reduce tumor resistance to other chemotherapeutic agents, or to slow or halt tumor growth.

Conversely, treatments with miR-212/132 might also be a useful method to promote angiogenesis and to increase neovascularization in the cases where neovascularization would be helpful, such as certain ischemic tissues or newly transplanted engineered tissue constructs. In fact, ex vivo transfection of mir-132 into endothelial cells has been shown to be beneficial for transplantation and vascularization of transplanted endothelial cells [34]. Based on our results and the results of other studies, further work is warranted in this area.

Author Contributions: Z.L., T.D.K., J.P.G.S., and R.H.G. conceived and designed the experiments. T.D.K., Z.L., M.M.B., G.v.d.H. and I.L. performed the experiments. C.C., P.A.D., J.P.G.S. and R.H.G supervise the study. T.D.K., Z.L., and M.M.B. analysed the data. T.D.K., Z.L., P.A.D., C.C., J.P.G.S., and R.H.G. wrote the paper. All authors have read and agreed to the published version of the manuscript.

References

1. Baldewijns, M.M.; van Vlodrop, I.J.; Vermeulen, P.B.; Soetekouw, P.M.; van Engeland, M.; de Bruine, A.P. VHL and HIF signalling in renal cell carcinogenesis. *J. Pathol.* **2010**, *221*, 125–138. [CrossRef]
2. Cancer Genome Atlas Network. Comprehensive molecular characterization of human colon and rectal cancer. *Nature* **2012**, *487*, 330–337. [CrossRef]
3. Frantzen, C.; Kruizinga, R.C.; van Asselt, S.J.; Zonnenberg, B.A.; Lenders, J.W.; de Herder, W.W.; Walenkamp, A.M.; Giles, R.H.; Hes, F.J.; Sluiter, W.J.; et al. Pregnancy-related hemangioblastoma progression and complications in von Hippel-Lindau disease. *Neurology* **2012**, *79*, 793–796. [CrossRef] [PubMed]

4. Shen, J.; Hung, M.C. Signaling-mediated regulation of MicroRNA processing. *Cancer Res.* **2015**. [CrossRef] [PubMed]
5. Anand, S.; Majeti, B.K.; Acevedo, L.M.; Murphy, E.A.; Mukthavaram, R.; Scheppke, L.; Huang, M.; Shields, D.J.; Lindquist, J.N.; Lapinski, P.E.; et al. MicroRNA-132-mediated loss of p120RasGAP activates the endothelium to facilitate pathological angiogenesis. *Nat. Med.* **2010**, *16*, 909–914. [CrossRef] [PubMed]
6. Qian, C.N. Hijacking the vasculature in ccRCC—Co-option, remodelling and angiogenesis. *Nat. Rev. Urol.* **2013**, *10*, 300–304. [CrossRef] [PubMed]
7. Schmid, T.A.; Gore, M.E. Sunitinib in the treatment of metastatic renal cell carcinoma. *Adv. Urol.* **2016**, *8*, 348–371. [CrossRef] [PubMed]
8. Rouwkema, J.; Rivron, N.C.; van Blitterswijk, C.A. Vascularization in tissue engineering. *Trends Biotechnol.* **2008**, *26*, 434–441. [CrossRef]
9. Lei, Z.; van Mil, A.; Xiao, J.; Metz, C.H.G.; van Eeuwijk, E.C.M.; Doevendans, P.A.; Sluijter, J.P.G. MMISH: Multicolor microRNA in situ hybridization for paraffin embedded samples. *Biotechnol. Rep. (Amst)* **2018**, *18*, e00255. [CrossRef]
10. Nordstrom-O'Brien, M.; van der Luijt, R.B.; van Rooijen, E.; van den Ouweland, A.M.; Majoor-Krakauer, D.F.; Lolkema, M.P.; van Brussel, A.; Voest, E.E.; Giles, R.H. Genetic analysis of von Hippel-Lindau disease. *Hum. Mutat.* **2010**, *31*, 521–537. [CrossRef]
11. Stratman, A.N.; Malotte, K.M.; Mahan, R.D.; Davis, M.J.; Davis, G.E. Pericyte recruitment during vasculogenic tube assembly stimulates endothelial basement membrane matrix formation. *Blood* **2009**, *114*, 5091–5101. [CrossRef] [PubMed]
12. Van Rooijen, E.; Voest, E.E.; Logister, I.; Korving, J.; Schwerte, T.; Schulte-Merker, S.; Giles, R.H.; van Eeden, F.J. Zebrafish mutants in the von Hippel-Lindau tumor suppressor display a hypoxic response and recapitulate key aspects of Chuvash polycythemia. *Blood* **2009**, *113*, 6449–6460. [CrossRef] [PubMed]
13. Van Rooijen, E.; Voest, E.E.; Logister, I.; Bussmann, J.; Korving, J.; van Eeden, F.J.; Giles, R.H.; Schulte-Merker, S. von Hippel-Lindau tumor suppressor mutants faithfully model pathological hypoxia-driven angiogenesis and vascular retinopathies in zebrafish. *Dis. Models Mech.* **2010**, *3*, 343–353. [CrossRef]
14. Van Rooijen, E.; Santhakumar, K.; Logister, I.; Voest, E.; Schulte-Merker, S.; Giles, R.; van Eeden, F. A zebrafish model for VHL and hypoxia signaling. *Methods Cell Biol.* **2011**, *105*, 163–190. [CrossRef] [PubMed]
15. Jiang, B.H.; Liu, L.Z. PI3K/PTEN signaling in angiogenesis and tumorigenesis. *Adv. Cancer Res.* **2009**, *102*, 19–65. [CrossRef]
16. Jin, W.; Reddy, M.A.; Chen, Z.; Putta, S.; Lanting, L.; Kato, M.; Park, J.T.; Chandra, M.; Wang, C.; Tangirala, R.K.; et al. Small RNA sequencing reveals microRNAs that modulate angiotensin II effects in vascular smooth muscle cells. *J. Biol. Chem.* **2012**, *287*, 15672–15683. [CrossRef]
17. Choorapoikayil, S.; Weijts, B.; Kers, R.; de Bruin, A.; den Hertog, J. Loss of Pten promotes angiogenesis and enhanced vegfaa expression in zebrafish. *Dis. Models Mech.* **2013**, *6*, 1159–1166. [CrossRef]
18. Remenyi, J.; Hunter, C.J.; Cole, C.; Ando, H.; Impey, S.; Monk, C.E.; Martin, K.J.; Barton, G.J.; Hutvagner, G.; Arthur, J.S. Regulation of the miR-212/132 locus by MSK1 and CREB in response to neurotrophins. *Biochem. J.* **2010**, *428*, 281–291. [CrossRef]
19. Lei, Z.; van Mil, A.; Brandt, M.M.; Grundmann, S.; Hoefer, I.; Smits, M.; El Azzouzi, H.; Fukao, T.; Cheng, C.; Doevendans, P.A.; et al. MicroRNA-132/212 family enhances arteriogenesis after hindlimb ischaemia through modulation of the Ras-MAPK pathway. *J. Cell. Mol. Med.* **2015**. [CrossRef]
20. Gomes, R.S.; das Neves, R.P.; Cochlin, L.; Lima, A.; Carvalho, R.; Korpisalo, P.; Dragneva, G.; Turunen, M.; Liimatainen, T.; Clarke, K.; et al. Efficient pro-survival/angiogenic miRNA delivery by an MRI-detectable nanomaterial. *ACS Nano* **2013**, *7*, 3362–3372. [CrossRef]
21. Frew, I.J.; Minola, A.; Georgiev, S.; Hitz, M.; Moch, H.; Richard, S.; Vortmeyer, A.O.; Krek, W. Combined VHLH and PTEN mutation causes genital tract cystadenoma and squamous metaplasia. *Mol. Cell. Biol.* **2008**, *28*, 4536–4548. [CrossRef] [PubMed]
22. Ma, W.; Tessarollo, L.; Hong, S.-B.; Baba, M.; Southon, E.; Back, T.C.; Spence, S.; Lobe, C.G.; Sharma, N.; Maher, G.W. Hepatic vascular tumors, angiectasis in multiple organs, and impaired spermatogenesis in mice with conditional inactivation of the VHL gene. *Cancer Res.* **2003**, *63*, 5320–5328. [PubMed]
23. Kumar, A.; Rajendran, V.; Sethumadhavan, R.; Purohit, R. AKT kinase pathway: A leading target in cancer research. *Sci. World J.* **2013**, *2013*, 756134. [CrossRef] [PubMed]

24. Hubbard, P.A.; Moody, C.L.; Murali, R. Allosteric modulation of Ras and the PI3K/AKT/mTOR pathway: Emerging therapeutic opportunities. *Front. Physiol.* **2014**, *5*, 478. [CrossRef] [PubMed]
25. Samatar, A.A.; Poulikakos, P.I. Targeting RAS-ERK signalling in cancer: Promises and challenges. *Nat. Rev. Drug Discov.* **2014**, *13*, 928–942. [CrossRef]
26. Ge, Y.Z.; Wu, R.; Xin, H.; Zhu, M.; Lu, T.Z.; Liu, H.; Xu, Z.; Yu, P.; Zhao, Y.C.; Li, M.H.; et al. A tumor-specific microRNA signature predicts survival in clear cell renal cell carcinoma. *J. Cancer Res. Clin. Oncol.* **2015**. [CrossRef]
27. Acunzo, M.; Romano, G.; Wernicke, D.; Croce, C.M. MicroRNA and cancer—A brief overview. *Adv. Biol. Regul.* **2015**, *57*, 1–9. [CrossRef]
28. Braicu, C.; Cojocneanu-Petric, R.; Chira, S.; Truta, A.; Floares, A.; Petrut, B.; Achimas-Cadariu, P.; Berindan-Neagoe, I. Clinical and pathological implications of miRNA in bladder cancer. *Int. J. Nanomed.* **2015**, *10*, 791–800. [CrossRef]
29. Qin, X.; Xu, H.; Gong, W.; Deng, W. The Tumor Cytosol miRNAs, Fluid miRNAs, and Exosome miRNAs in lung cancer. *Front. Oncol.* **2014**, *4*, 357. [CrossRef]
30. Greco, S.; Martelli, F. MicroRNAs in hypoxia response. *Antioxid. Redox Signal.* **2014**, *21*, 1164–1166. [CrossRef]
31. Gee, H.E.; Ivan, C.; Calin, G.A.; Ivan, M. HypoxamiRs and cancer: From biology to targeted therapy. *Antioxid. Redox Signal.* **2014**, *21*, 1220–1238. [CrossRef] [PubMed]
32. Lin, Y.C.; Lu, L.T.; Chen, H.Y.; Duan, X.; Lin, X.; Feng, X.H.; Tang, M.J.; Chen, R.H. SCP phosphatases suppress renal cell carcinoma by stabilizing PML and inhibiting mTOR/HIF signaling. *Cancer Res.* **2014**, *74*, 6935–6946. [CrossRef]
33. Leslie, N.R.; Foti, M. Non-genomic loss of PTEN function in cancer: Not in my genes. *Trends Pharm. Sci.* **2011**, *32*, 131–140. [CrossRef] [PubMed]
34. Devalliere, J.; Chang, W.G.; Andrejecsk, J.W.; Abrahimi, P.; Cheng, C.J.; Jane-wit, D.; Saltzman, W.M.; Pober, J.S. Sustained delivery of proangiogenic microRNA-132 by nanoparticle transfection improves endothelial cell transplantation. *FASEB J.* **2014**, *28*, 908–922. [CrossRef] [PubMed]

Permissions

All chapters in this book were first published by MDPI; hereby published with permission under the Creative Commons Attribution License or equivalent. Every chapter published in this book has been scrutinized by our experts. Their significance has been extensively debated. The topics covered herein carry significant findings which will fuel the growth of the discipline. They may even be implemented as practical applications or may be referred to as a beginning point for another development.

The contributors of this book come from diverse backgrounds, making this book a truly international effort. This book will bring forth new frontiers with its revolutionizing research information and detailed analysis of the nascent developments around the world.

We would like to thank all the contributing authors for lending their expertise to make the book truly unique. They have played a crucial role in the development of this book. Without their invaluable contributions this book wouldn't have been possible. They have made vital efforts to compile up to date information on the varied aspects of this subject to make this book a valuable addition to the collection of many professionals and students.

This book was conceptualized with the vision of imparting up-to-date information and advanced data in this field. To ensure the same, a matchless editorial board was set up. Every individual on the board went through rigorous rounds of assessment to prove their worth. After which they invested a large part of their time researching and compiling the most relevant data for our readers.

The editorial board has been involved in producing this book since its inception. They have spent rigorous hours researching and exploring the diverse topics which have resulted in the successful publishing of this book. They have passed on their knowledge of decades through this book. To expedite this challenging task, the publisher supported the team at every step. A small team of assistant editors was also appointed to further simplify the editing procedure and attain best results for the readers.

Apart from the editorial board, the designing team has also invested a significant amount of their time in understanding the subject and creating the most relevant covers. They scrutinized every image to scout for the most suitable representation of the subject and create an appropriate cover for the book.

The publishing team has been an ardent support to the editorial, designing and production team. Their endless efforts to recruit the best for this project, has resulted in the accomplishment of this book. They are a veteran in the field of academics and their pool of knowledge is as vast as their experience in printing. Their expertise and guidance has proved useful at every step. Their uncompromising quality standards have made this book an exceptional effort. Their encouragement from time to time has been an inspiration for everyone.

The publisher and the editorial board hope that this book will prove to be a valuable piece of knowledge for researchers, students, practitioners and scholars across the globe.

List of Contributors

Bin Ren
Department of Surgery, University of Alabama at Birmingham, Birmingham, AL 35294, USA
O'Neal Comprehensive Cancer Center, University of Alabama at Birmingham, Birmingham, AL 35294, USA
Nutrition & Obesity Research Center, University of Alabama at Birmingham, Birmingham, AL 35294, USA
Diabetes Research Center, University of Alabama at Birmingham, Birmingham, AL 35294, USA
Department of Biomedical Engineering, University of Alabama at Birmingham, Birmingham, AL 35294, USA
Graduate Biomedical Science Program of the Graduate School, University of Alabama at Birmingham, Birmingham, AL 35294, USA

J. Bart Rose and Carlo Contreras
Department of Surgery, University of Alabama at Birmingham, Birmingham, AL 35294, USA
O'Neal Comprehensive Cancer Center, University of Alabama at Birmingham, Birmingham, AL 35294, USA

Adam Beck
Department of Surgery, University of Alabama at Birmingham, Birmingham, AL 35294, USA

Renata Jaskular-Sztul
Department of Surgery, University of Alabama at Birmingham, Birmingham, AL 35294, USA
O'Neal Comprehensive Cancer Center, University of Alabama at Birmingham, Birmingham, AL 35294, USA
Department of Biomedical Engineering, University of Alabama at Birmingham, Birmingham, AL 35294, USA

Herbert Chen
Department of Surgery, University of Alabama at Birmingham, Birmingham, AL 35294, USA
O'Neal Comprehensive Cancer Center, University of Alabama at Birmingham, Birmingham, AL 35294, USA
Department of Biomedical Engineering, University of Alabama at Birmingham, Birmingham, AL 35294, USA
Graduate Biomedical Science Program of the Graduate School, University of Alabama at Birmingham, Birmingham, AL 35294, USA

Yehe Liu
Department of Biomedical Engineering, Case Western Reserve University, Cleveland, OH 44106, USA

Nicolas Ricard, Jiasheng Zhang and Zhen W. Zhuang
Yale Cardiovascular Research Center, Department of Internal Medicine, Yale University School of Medicine, New Haven, CT 06511, USA

Srinivasan Vedantham
MedGenome Labs Ltd., Bangalore, Karnataka 560099, India
School of Chemical Biotechnology, SASTRA University, Thanjavur 613401, India

Anna-Kristina Kluever and Elisabeth Deindl
Walter-Brendel-Centre of Experimental Medicine, University Hospital, LMU Munich, 80336 Munich, Germany

Ilze Bot, Daniël van der Velden, Mara J. Kröner, Johan Kuiper and Merel Bouwman
Division of BioTherapeutics, Leiden Academic Centre for Drug Research, Leiden University, 2333CC Leiden, The Netherlands
Department of Surgery, Leiden University Medical Center, 2300RC Leiden, The Netherlands
Einthoven Laboratory for Experimental Vascular Medicine, Leiden University Medical Center, 2300RC Leiden, The Netherlands

Paul H. A. Quax and Margreet R. de Vries
Department of Surgery, Leiden University Medical Center, 2300RC Leiden, The Netherlands
Einthoven Laboratory for Experimental Vascular Medicine, Leiden University Medical Center, 2300RC Leiden, The Netherlands

Michael Simons
Yale Cardiovascular Research Center, Department of Internal Medicine, Yale University School of Medicine, New Haven, CT 06511, USA
Department of Cell Biology, Yale University School of Medicine, New Haven, CT 06511, USA

Özgür Uslu
Institute for Biochemistry, Justus-Liebig-University Giessen, 35392 Giessen, Germany

Joerg Herold
Department of Angiology, Clinic for Vascular Medicine, Klinikum Darmstadt, 64283 Darmstadt, Germany

Sandip M. Kanse
Institute for Basic Medical Sciences, University of Oslo, Sognvannsveien 9, 0372 Oslo, Norway

Farah Abdel Rahman and Victoria Jurisch
Klinik & Poliklinik für Innere Medizin I, Klinikum rechts der Isar, Technical University of Munich, 81675 Munich, Germany

A. Yaël Nossent
Department of Surgery and Einthoven Laboratory for Experimental Vascular Medicine, Leiden University Medical Center, 2333 ZA Leiden, The Netherlands
Department of Laboratory Medicine and Department of Internal Medicine II, Medical University of Vienna, 1090 Vienna, Austria

Reginald V.C.T. van der Kwast
Department of Surgery and Einthoven Laboratory for Experimental Vascular Medicine, Leiden University Medical Center, 2333 ZA Leiden, The Netherlands

Tilman Ziegler and Christian Kupatt
Klinik & Poliklinik für Innere Medizin I, Klinikum rechts der Isar, Technical University of Munich, 81675 Munich, Germany
DZHK (German Center for Cardiovascular Research), Partner Site Munich Heart Alliance, 80802 Munich, Germany

Laura Parma and Hendrika A. B. Peters
Department of surgery; Leiden University Medical Center, 2300 RC Leiden, The Netherlands Einthoven laboratory for experimental vascular medicine, Leiden University Medical Center, 2300 RC Leiden, The Netherlands

Georg Jung
Department of Vascular and Endovascular Surgery, University Hospital Frankfurt, Theodor-Stern-Kai 7, 60590 Frankfurt, Germany

Hellen Ishikawa-Ankerhold
Walter-Brendel-Centre of Experimental Medicine, University Hospital, LMU Munich, 80539 Munich, Germany
Department of Internal Medicine I, Faculty of Medicine, University Hospital, LMU Munich, 80539 Munich, Germany

Fabiana Baganha and Margreet R. de Vries
Department of Surgery, Leiden University Medical Center, 2333 ZA Leiden, The Netherlands
Einthoven Laboratory for Experimental Vascular Medicine, Leiden University Medical Center, 2333 ZA Leiden, The Netherlands
Department of surgery; Leiden University Medical Center, 2300 RC Leiden, The Netherlands
Einthoven laboratory for experimental vascular medicine, Leiden University Medical Center, 2300 RC Leiden, The Netherlands

Laila Ritsma
Department of Cell and Chemical Biology, Leiden University Medical Center, 2333 ZC Leiden, The Netherlands

Johanna Vogel and Daniel Niederer
Department of Sports Medicine and Exercise Physiology, Goethe University Frankfurt/Main, Ginnheimer Landstr. 39, 60487 Frankfurt, Germany

Kerstin Troidl
Department of Vascular and Endovascular Surgery, University Hospital Frankfurt, Theodor-Stern-Kai 7, 60590 Frankfurt, Germany
Department of Pharmacology, Max-Planck-Institute for Heart and Lung Research, Ludwigstrasse 43, 61231 Bad Nauheim, Germany

Zhiyong Lei
Department of Cardiology, Division Heart and Lungs, University Medical Center Utrecht, Heidelberglaan 100, 3584 CX Utrecht, The Netherlands

Timothy D. Klasson, Ive Logister and Rachel H. Giles
Department of Nephrology & Hypertension, Division Internal Medicine, University Medical Center Utrecht, Heidelberglaan 100, 3584 CX Utrecht, The Netherlands

Caroline Cheng
Department of Nephrology & Hypertension, Division Internal Medicine, University Medical Center Utrecht, Heidelberglaan 100, 3584 CX Utrecht, The Netherlands
Experimental Cardiology, Department of Cardiology, Thoraxcenter, Erasmus MC, University Medical Center Rotterdam, 3015 GD Rotterdam, The Netherlands

Sarah Meister
Department of Obstetrics and Gynaecology, University Hospital, LMU Munich, 80539 Munich, Germany

Paul H. A. Quax
Department of Surgery and Einthoven Laboratory for Experimental Vascular Medicine, Leiden University Medical Center, 2333 ZA Leiden, The Netherlands
Department of surgery; Leiden University Medical Center, 2300 RC Leiden, The Netherlands
Einthoven laboratory for experimental vascular medicine, Leiden University Medical Center, 2300 RC Leiden, The Netherlands

Manuel Lasch
Walter-Brendel-Centre of Experimental Medicine, University Hospital, LMU Munich, 80539 Munich, Germany
Department of Otorhinolaryngology, Head and Neck Surgery, University Hospital, LMU Munich, 80539 Munich, Germany

Maarten M. Brandt
Experimental Cardiology, Department of Cardiology, Thoraxcenter, Erasmus MC, University Medical Center Rotterdam, 3015 GD Rotterdam, The Netherlands

Glenn van de Hoek
Department of Medical Genetics, University Medical Center Utrecht, Heidelberglaan 100, 3584 CX Utrecht, The Netherlands

Elisabeth Deindl
Walter-Brendel-Centre of Experimental Medicine, University Hospital, LMU Munich, 80539 Munich, Germany

Pieter A. Doevendans
Department of Cardiology, Division Heart and Lungs, University Medical Center Utrecht, Heidelberglaan 100, 3584 CX Utrecht, The Netherlands
Netherlands Heart Institute, Catharijnesingel 52, 3511 GC Utrecht, The Netherlands
Central Military Hospital Utrecht, Lundlaan 1, 3584 EZ Utrecht, The Netherlands

Joost P. G. Sluijter
Department of Cardiology, Division Heart and Lungs, University Medical Center Utrecht, Heidelberglaan 100, 3584 CX Utrecht, The Netherlands
UMC Utrecht Regenerative Medicine Center, University Medical Center, 3584 CT Utrecht, The Netherlands

Index